The Khecarīvidyā of Ādinātha

A critical edition and annotated translation of an early text of *haṭhayoga*

James Mallinson

Routledge
Taylor & Francis Group
LONDON AND NEW YORK

Transferred to digital printing 2010
First published 2007
by Routledge
2 Park Square, Milton Park, Abingdon, Oxon OX14 4RN

Simultaneously published in the USA and Canada
by Routledge
270 Madison Ave, New York, NY 10016

Routledge is an imprint of the Taylor & Francis Group, an informa business

Typeset in Adobe Garamond by
James Mallinson using LaTeX and Ledmac

British Library Cataloguing in Publication Data
A catalogue record for this book is available from the British Library

Library of Congress Cataloging in Publication Data
Ādinātha, 10th cent.
[Khecarīvidyā. English & Sanskrit]
The Khecarīvidyā of Ādinātha : a critical edition and annotated translation of an early text of haṭhayoga / James Mallinson.
p. cm. – (Routledge studies in tantric traditions series)
Includes bibliographical references and index.
ISBN-13: 978–0–415–39115–3 (hardback : alk. paper)
1. Hatha yoga–Early works to 1800. I. Mallinson, James, 1970- . II. Title.
BL1238.56.H38 A3513
294.5'436–dc22

2006033161

ISBN10: 0–415–39115–6
ISBN13: 978–0–415–39115–3

ISBN10: 0-415-58613-5 (pbk)
ISBN13: 978-0-415-58613-9 (pbk)

The Khecarīvidyā of Ādinātha

The Khecarīvidyā of Ādinātha, a Sanskrit text dated to pre-1400 CE, teaches *khecarīmudrā*, one of the most important exercises of *haṭhayoga*, in which the tongue is inserted above the palate in order to drink the *amṛta* or nectar of immortality dripping from the top of the skull. It is said to bestow immortality, the ability to remain in deep meditation for long periods and the power of flight upon its practitioners. The text has been edited for the first time and has never before been accessible to an English speaking readership. It is accompanied by an introduction and an extensively annotated translation. The author has drawn on twenty-seven Sanskrit manuscripts and original fieldwork amongst yogins in India to demonstrate how earlier tantric yogic techniques developed and mutated into the practices of *haṭhayoga*. The work sheds new light on the development of *haṭhayoga* and explains its practices.

James Mallinson has a BA and DPhil in Sanskrit from Oxford and an MA in South Asian ethnography from the School of Oriental and African Studies. He has spent several years living with sadhus and yogins in India and now translates Sanskrit poetry for the Clay Sanskrit Library and yoga texts for YogaVidya.com.

Routledge Studies in Tantric Traditions

Edited by Gavin Flood

Professor of Religious Studies, University of Stirling

The *Routledge Studies in Tantric Traditions* series is a major new monograph series which has been established to publish scholarship on South, East and Southeast Asian tantric traditions. The series aims to promote the serious study of both Hindu and Buddhist tantric traditions through the publication of anthropological and textual studies and will not be limited to any one method. Indeed, the series would hope to promote the view that anthropological studies can be informed by texts and textual studies informed by anthropology. The series will therefore publish contemporary ethnographies from different regions, philological studies, philosophical studies, and historical studies of different periods which contribute to the academic endeavour to understand the role of tantric texts and their meaning in particular cultural contexts. In this way, the series will hope to establish what the continuities and divergencies are between Buddhist and Hindu tantric traditions and between different regions. The series will be a major contribution to the fields of Indology, Sinology, History of Religions and Anthropology.

Identity, ritual and state in Tibetan Buddhism
Martin A. Mills

The Khecarīvidyā of Ādinātha
A critical edition and annotated translation of an early text of *haṭhayoga*
James Mallinson

Contents

Preface

The original impetus for the work contained in this book, which is a revision of the doctoral thesis I submitted for examination in Oxford in 2003, was my wish to use Sanskrit philology to investigate Hindu asceticism. It was clear to me that the practice of yoga, and in particular *haṭhayoga*, was one of the traits shared by most of the ascetic orders that flourish in India today, and the one most suited to philological research. I thus sought a Sanskrit text on *haṭhayoga* to edit critically. Christian Bouy's masterful survey of haṭhayogic literature, *Les Nātha-Yogin et les Upaniṣads*, threw up various possibilities, and I settled on the *Khecarīvidyā*. Not only was it important to the yogic textual tradition - it is cited by several commentators and verses from it are used in later texts - but its beautiful and unique teachings describe a practice still used by yogins in India today, so I could draw on their insights to elucidate the text.

Furthermore, the *Khecarīvidyā* appeared to suit my purposes for two practical reasons. Firstly, according to the catalogues I consulted, there were seven manuscripts of it to be collated, an easily manageable number for a text three hundred *śloka*s long. Secondly, unlike most other texts on *haṭhayoga*, it taught a single practice, so I thought it would be relatively easy to understand. How misguided I was! By discovering more names under which the text was known and more ways of searching for witnesses, I ended up unearthing twenty-seven manuscripts of the text, and I soon realised that to get to the bottom of its teachings would require an understanding of a wide range of subjects, in particular the vast and dauntingly complex world of tantric Śaivism.

I could not have been in a better place for help in overcoming these problems. The presence in Oxford of my thesis supervisor, Professor Alexis Sanderson, had attracted a group of doctoral and post-doctoral students whose energy and enthusiasm for philological research into tantric Śaivism were a constant inspiration to me, and they helped to reassure me of the importance for understanding Indian religion of the often tedious business of collating and editing manuscripts. Many helped directly with this book but a few were particularly generous with their time and learning. I must first thank Professor Sanderson who was always ready to help me with his encyclopedic knowledge and expert guidance. Dr. Somdev Vasudeva is responsible for any elegance in the book's presentation and provided me with a great deal of useful textual material as well as encouragement and advice. Dr. Dominic Goodall spurred me into going to India in search of manuscripts and helped me with the south Indian witnesses. Csaba Kiss was very generous with the fruits of his work on the *Matsyendrasaṃhitā*. Other Oxford contemporaries whom I wish to thank by name for their comments and help are Dr. Harunaga Isaacson, Dr. Alex Watson, Dr. Isabelle Onians, Dr. Jim Benson, Professor Richard Gombrich and Dr. Csaba Dezső. From outside of Oxford I thank Christian Bouy, whose work inspired me to start the thesis and who has helped me in my search for sources, Sebastian Pole, who with his practical expertise in yoga and his knowledge of *āyurveda* both encouraged and aided me in my work, Professor Arlo Griffiths, who made several improvements and corrections to the original thesis, Dr. Matthew Clark, who provided me with a copy of his doctoral thesis on Indian asceticism and answered my many questions, and the late Dr. Manmath Gharote who obtained several manuscripts for me and gave me copies of his editions of Sanskrit works on *haṭhayoga*.

Thanks are due to the many people who have helped me obtain copies of manuscripts, in particular Simon Stocken, Dr. David White, Cassia Smith-Bingham, His Highness Gaj Singh, Maharaja of Jodhpur, M. Ram, Dr. Dominik Wujastyk and the staff at the following institutions: the Maharaja Man Singh Library, Jodhpur (especially Kr. Mahendra Singh Tanwar), the Indian Institute Library, Oxford, the Wellcome Institute for the History of Medicine, London, the Government Oriental Manuscripts Library, Madras, the Scindia Oriental Research Institute, Ujjain, the Sarvajanik Library, Nasik, the Prajñāpāṭhaśālā, Wai, the National Archives, Kathmaṇdu, the Nepal-German Manuscript Preservation Project, the Oriental Institute, Baroda, the Institut français de Pondichéry, the Bhandarkar Oriental Research Institute, Pune, the Bombay University Library, the Rajasthan Oriental Research Institute, Jodhpur, and the Oriental Research Institute, Bikaner.

For funding my studies and field trips I thank the British Academy for Humanities Research, the Boden Fund, Eton College and the Spalding Trust.

Finally, this book could not have been completed without the help of my wife Claudia, my family and all the yogins in India who shared their knowledge and insights with me, in particular Śrī Rām Bālak Dās.

Introduction

The *Khecarīvidyā*

The *Khecarīvidyā* is a dialogue between Śiva and his consort, Devī. It calls itself a tantra[1] and consists of 284 verses divided into four *paṭala*s. In the colophons of its manuscripts its authorship is ascribed to Ādinātha, the first of the gurus of the Nātha order, who is usually identified with Śiva.[2] The first *paṭala* (77 verses) starts with praise of the text itself, followed by a coded description of the *khecarīmantra* and detailed instructions for the key physical practice of the text. This practice is called *khecarīmudrā*,[3] and involves the freeing and lengthening of the tongue of the yogin in order that it might be turned back and inserted above the soft palate to break through the *brahmadvāra*, the door of Brahmā, so that the yogin can drink the *amṛta*, the nectar of immortality, which is stored behind it. The second *paṭala* (124 verses) describes the different *kalā*s in the body where *amṛta* is stored, the rewards to be gained from accessing the *amṛta* in these *kalā*s, and how to cure the problems that may arise in the course of the practice. The third *paṭala* (69 verses) describes practices involving the insertion of the tongue into the abode of Brahmā and the raising of Kuṇḍalinī in order to flood the body with *amṛta* and defeat death by temporarily or permanently leaving the body. The short fourth *paṭala* (14 verses) describes herbal preparations which can effect various magical results (*siddhi*s) for the yogin.

The *Khecarīvidyā* is the source of four verses in the vulgate of the *Haṭhapradīpikā*, eleven verses in its ten-chapter recension and at least sixty-four verses in its long recension.[4] It is also the source of all 49 *śloka*s of the second *adhyāya* of the *Yogakuṇḍalyupaniṣad* and of two verses in the *Haṭharatnāvalī*. It is cited by Nārāyaṇa in his commentaries on 52 atharvan *upaniṣad*s and is quoted in the *Gorakṣasiddhāntasaṃgraha*, an anthology of passages connected with Gorakṣanātha, who is said to be the original teacher of *haṭhayoga*. The *Matsyendrasaṃhitā*, a collection of haṭhayogic and tantric lore associated with Matsyendranātha, who is claimed by the Nātha school to have been Gorakṣanāṭha's guru, has among its 55 *paṭala*s all four *paṭala*s of the *Khecarīvidyā*. The *Khecarīvidyā* was the subject of a lengthy commentary by Ballāla called the *Bṛhatkhecarīprakāśa*. Jayatarāma used it extensively when composing his Hindī manual of *haṭhayoga*, the *Jogpradīpakā*.[5] The *Khecarīvidyā* was thus regarded as an authority on *haṭhayoga* and associated with the Nātha order of yogins.[6]

The text has received little attention from modern scholars. R.G. Harshe, in

Summaries of Papers submitted to the 17th Session of the All-India Oriental Conference, Ahmedabad, 1953, under the heading "*Mahākālayogaśāstra*: *Khecarīvidyā* by Ādinātha", wrote: "It is not published so far as it is known and a critical edition is being presented for the first time". It has not been possible to ascertain whether this edition was in fact ever presented or published. Bouy (1994) noticed the borrowings from the *Khecarīvidyā* in the *Haṭhapradīpikā* and *Yogakuṇḍalyupaniṣad*; it was his pioneering work that first drew my attention to the text. White (1996:169–170) gives a synopsis of the text and Roşu (1997:429 n.40) mentions it in passing.[7]

The date and place of composition of the text

The *terminus a quo* of the *Khecarīvidyā* is the date of composition of the *Vivekamārtaṇḍa*, a work mentioned at *Khecarīvidyā* 1.14cd.[8] *Vivekamārtaṇḍa* (or °*mārtāṇḍa*) is one of the many names by which the work now usually known as the *Gorakṣaśataka* has been called.[9] No internal references allow us to establish a *terminus a quo* for the *Vivekamārtaṇḍa*, so its mention in the text is not especially helpful in dating the *Khecarīvidyā*. As noted by Bouy (ibid.:15 n.30), two verses of the *Vivekamārtaṇḍa* are cited without attribution in the *Śārṅgadharapaddhati*, a lengthy anthology of verses on a wide range of subjects.[10] This establishes a *terminus ad quem* for the *Vivekamārtaṇḍa* of 1363 CE (Sternbach 1974:17).

The *terminus ad quem* of the *Khecarīvidyā* is the date of composition of the *Haṭhapradīpikā* which, as mentioned above, borrows four *śloka*s from the *Khecarīvidyā*. The *Haṭhapradīpikā* is an anthology of passages from various texts.[11] The four borrowed verses are not found in any work other than the *Khecarīvidyā*, so one can be confident that the *Haṭhapradīpikā* has borrowed from the *Khecarīvidyā* and was therefore composed after it. Bouy (1994:81–85) summarises earlier attempts at dating the *Haṭhapradīpikā* and, adding further evidence, concludes "Dans l'état actuel des connaissances, il y a tout lieu de penser que la *Haṭhapradīpikā* est une anthologie qui a été composée dans le courant du xve siècle".[12] Thus the most that can be said about the date of the composition of the *Khecarīvidyā* is that it was almost certainly prior to 1400 CE.

About the place of composition of the text nothing definite can be said. Its witnesses are found all across the subcontinent, from Jodhpur in the west to Calcutta in the east, and from Kathmandu in the north to Pondicherry in the south. An origin in southern India is hinted at by the superiority of the readings found in the manuscripts of the *Matsyendrasaṃhitā*, parts of which show evidence of origins in the Tamil region of south India, and by the good readings found in a Grantha manuscript from Pondicherry (witness G) which is unique in showing no signs of contamination with the other manuscript traditions.[13]

The witnesses of the text

The manuscript witnesses of the *Khecarīvidyā* fall into five groups:[14]

- The *Khecarīvidyā* manuscripts (S$\alpha\beta\gamma$)

- The *Matsyendrasaṃhitā* manuscripts (μ)
- Manuscript G
- Manuscript R_2
- The *Yogakuṇḍalyupaniṣad (U)* and manuscript T.

The five manuscript groups are now examined in detail.

The *KhV* manuscripts

Twenty-two manuscripts form a discrete group on account of their similarity. Their sigla are: S, NW_1 MK_1K_3 (=subgroup α), $J_2J_4VK_4K_2PJ_3FK_5K_6C$ (=subgroup β) and $J_1J_5W_2R_1B$ (=subgroup γ). In the following pages these witnesses are referred to collectively as "the *KhV* manuscripts". The edited text as presented corresponds most closely to the text as found in these witnesses.

The twenty-two *KhV* manuscripts present similar versions of the text but can be divided into three distinct subgroups which I have called α, β and γ. See for example the list of *siddhi*s given at 1.75cd (this verse is omitted in G):[15]

pādukākhaḍgavetālasiddhidravyamanaḥśilāḥ //75//
75d °manaḥśilāḥ] μ; °m abhīpsitaṃ Sα, °manaḥśilā β, °m anekaśaḥ γ

Of these three subgroups, α is perhaps the best, sharing the most readings with μ and G (which as will be shown below often preserve the best readings). β is the largest and least homogeneous subgroup while γ is the most idiosyncratic. The subgroups themselves can be further divided. Thus K_1 and K_3 make up α_3. The rest of α, i.e. N, W_1 and M, make up α_1, which is in turn further divided because of the close similarity of N and W_1 (=α_2). J_2, J_4, V and K_4 make up β_1 on account of their similarity while in γ B is distinct on account of its corrected readings, leaving γ_1 (=J_1, J_5, W_2 and R) which contains γ_2 (=J_1 and J_5). Because of extensive contamination between and within the subgroups it has not been possible to use stemmatic analysis to decide which readings are to be adopted.[16] The *KhV* manuscripts are divided into subgroups in order to make the apparatus less cluttered.

The text as presented in the *Bṛhatkhecarīprakāśa* (witness S) is derived from witnesses in the tradition of groups α and β. Several times in his extensive commentary Ballāla gives alternative readings and these can all be found among the witnesses of α and β.[17]

The *Matsyendrasaṃhitā* manuscripts

Three manuscripts of a text entitled *Matsyendrasaṃhitā* have been collated. Their sigla are AJ_6J_7 and they are referred to collectively as "the *MaSaṃ* manuscripts", or as the group μ.[18] Verses 14.1–17.1 of the *Matsyendrasaṃhitā* correspond to the first three *paṭalas* of the *Khecarīvidyā* and *Matsyendrasaṃhitā paṭala* 28 corresponds to *Khecarīvidyā paṭala* 4.

The *Matsyendrasaṃhitā* is a long treatise in 55 *paṭalas* on Śaiva tantric ritual and *haṭhayoga*.[19] It is ascribed to Matsyendranātha, the second in the traditional list of gurus of the Nātha order[20] with which the *Khecarīvidyā* is usually affiliated.[21] As far as I am aware, the *Matsyendrasaṃhitā* is neither mentioned nor cited in any other works.[22] Evidence helpful in dating the text is scant, but there are clues as to where some parts of it were composed. The mention of cannabis *(siddhimūlikā)* in *paṭalas* 29 and 39 suggests an origin in eastern India after the advent of Islam in that region.[23] There is strong evidence for other parts of the text having been composed in the Tamil region of south India. At 55.3 the frame story mentions a king from the south whose city is called Allūra. The city has not been identified, but the suffix *-ūra* suggests the Tamil region.[24] References to the predominantly south Indian *paścimāmnāya* stream of Śaivism are found throughout the text. Southern origins can also be inferred from the injunction at 8.31 to worship the god Śāstṛ, a village deity found only in the Tamil region.[25] Furthermore the yoga taught in the text is often described as *śāmbhava*, a name commonly used in south India to describe Śaiva yoga.[26]

The layers of narrative in the text are complex—it is a dialogue between Śiva and Pārvatī which was overheard by Matsyendranātha while in the belly of a fish and which he then told to an unnamed Cola king who had it written down. The *Khecarīvidyā* as a dialogue between Śiva and the goddess fits neatly into the didactic section of the text but appears to have been added to an earlier layer. At the beginning of the *Matsyendrasaṃhitā* when Pārvatī asks Śiva for instruction in *śāmbhava* yoga she lists the subjects about which she wants to know. These subjects correspond closely to the subject matter of *paṭalas* 2–7 and 22–38, and she does not mention *Khecarīvidyā*.[27] The inclusion of the *Khecarīvidyā* causes some internal contradictions in the text: for example, a hand-gesture *khecarīmudrā* unlike those described at *Khecarīvidyā* 2.81–82 or 3.54 is mentioned in the eleventh *paṭala*,[28] and the praise of cannabis as the ultimate drug at 29.1–2 contrasts sharply with its not being mentioned in *paṭala* 28 (=*Khecarīvidyā paṭala* 4).[29] This evidence suggests that the *Khecarīvidyā* is a later addition to an earlier version of the *Matsyendrasaṃhitā*. However the *Khecarīvidyā* does tie in well with the subject matter of the *Matsyendrasaṃhitā*, which for the most part is a blend of Kaula ritual and *haṭhayoga*. In style and language too the texts are very similar. *Matsyendrasaṃhitā* 17.2–18.63 (particularly 17.20c–37b) echoes parts of the *Khecarīvidyā* and appears to be derived from it. For example, 17.24c–31, about the use, protection and worship of the book in which the text is written, is very similar to 14.18–28 (= *Khecarīvidyā* 1.18–28). The *Matsyendrasaṃhitā* is not entirely derivative when it covers subjects found in the *Khecarīvidyā*. Parts of its earliest layer are helpful for understanding the *Khecarīvidyā*. Thus *Matsyendrasaṃhitā paṭala* 27 covers in greater detail the practices described at *Khecarīvidyā* 2.72–79.[30]

Many of the readings found in μ are different from, and often superior to, those of the other *Khecarīvidyā* witnesses. Their superiority can be seen at 3.24a where we find *prapibet pavanaṃ yogī*, "the yogin should breathe in air". Only μ

and G have the reading *pavanaṃ*; the other witnesses read *paṃcamaṃ*. Similarly at 2.64ab, in the description of the location of the vessel of nectar in the head, only J6 and J7 read *parāmṛtaghaṭādhārakapāṭaṃ*, "the doorway at the base of the vessel of the supreme *amṛta*". For °*ghaṭā*°, A reads °*caṭā*°, G has °*ghaḍā*° and R2 and the *KhV* manuscripts have °*ṣaḍā*°. At 1.22cd, in the instructions for the worship of the written text, only μ has *granthiṃ (em.; granthi codd.) nodgranthayed asya vinā kaulikatarpaṇāt*, "one should not untie its knot without [carrying out] a Kaula libation"; for the first *pāda* G and α have variants on the unlikely *granthaṃ samarpayed asya*, R2, S and β retain the negative with *granthaṃ tu nārcayed asya* while γ has *granthaṃ tu cārcayed devi*.[31] Again, at 3.13a–14b, in a description of Kuṇḍalinī, the edition reads:

> *siñcantī yogino deham āpādatalamastakam* |
> *sudhayā śiśirasnigdhaśītayā parameśvari* ||13||
> *punas tenaiva mārgeṇa prayāti svapadaṃ priye* |
>
> "...sprinkling the body of the yogin from the soles of his feet to his head with dewy, unctuous, cool nectar, o supreme goddess, she then returns by that same pathway to her own abode, my dear."

For 13cd all the witnesses other than μ have variants on *atha sā śaśiraśmisthā śītalā parameśvari*, "then she, cool [and] sitting on a moonbeam, o supreme goddess". The particle *atha* and the omission of *sudhayā śiśirasnigdhaśītayā* leave the participle *siñcantī* with neither a main verb nor anything with which to sprinkle the yogin's body.

As hinted at in the example of °*ghaṭā*° above, μ and G (and sometimes R2) often share readings not found elsewhere and generally these readings are superior to those of the other witnesses. A very clear example of this is found at 1.69. This verse is found only in μ, G and R2 and is necessary to make sense of the passage in which it occurs. Similarly, at 2.37a, μ, G and R2 read *tatrastham amṛtaṃ* while the *KhV* manuscripts have the inferior *tatra sthāne 'mṛtaṃ* and *tatra saṃsthāmṛtaṃ*.

So far, the superior variants found in μ (and occasionally G and R2) that have been pointed out are simple and obvious improvements to the syntax or meaning of the readings found elsewhere. If we turn to 3.55a–69b, however, the differences become more interesting.[32]

The passage as found in μ is a Kaula eulogy of *madirā*, alcohol. In G, R2 and the *KhV* manuscripts, it has been redacted to make it more palatable to orthodox practitioners of *haṭhayoga*.[33] Thus μ's *madirā* becomes *khecarī* (see 3.56a, 57a and 65c) and the necessity of alcohol for success becomes the necessity of *śivabhakti*: *madirārādhanaṃ* at 3.59b becomes *madīyārādhanaṃ*; where μ has *tatprasādavihīnānāṃ tannindāparacetasām* at 3.59cd the *Khecarīvidyā* manuscripts substitute *mat*° and *man*° for *tat*° and *tan*°; *pūjāṃ saṃtyajya mādirīm* at 3.60d becomes *pūjāṃ saṃtyajya māmakīm*; *vāruṇyā tarpayet* at 3.62a becomes *bhaktyā saṃtarpayet* and so on.[34] Other passages in μ were so alcoholic that they had to be omitted altogether (see the entries in the last register of the critical edition apparatus at 3.62b, 3.64b and 3.67c). G, R2 and the *Khecarīvidyā* manuscripts probably derive from a single archetype, in which the text as it is found in μ was first redacted to remove the

Kaula references. There are several differences between them, however, and it is likely that their traditions diverged early on in the transmission of the text. In G attempts have been made to alter some of the verses found in μ that are omitted in R_2 and the *Khecarīvidyā* manuscripts. Thus at 17.110cd μ has

asaṃpūjya pibed devi madirāṃ yaḥ sa pāpabhāk

which is found in G as

mām asaṃpūjya yogena pāpaṃ bhavati nānyathā

and where μ at 113c–114b has

saṃtarpya śivam īśānaṃ devīṃ devāṃś ca sarvaśaḥ
tatprasādena labhate samyagjñānam akhaṇḍitam

in G we find

saṃtarpya śivam īśānaṃ sarvadevotsavapradam
matprasādena mahatā sarvavijñānavān bhavet.

μ's 17.107ab, *asaktaḥ sumahāpūjāṃ yadi kartuṃ ca sādhakaḥ*, is found verbatim at G 273ab but is absent from the *Khecarīvidyā* manuscripts. μ follows this half-verse with *kuryād bindvekadānaṃ vā guruvākyāvalambakaḥ*, the *bindvekadānaṃ vā* of which is replaced with *ekaikayā devi* in G; the *Khecarīvidyā* manuscripts have this half-verse at 3.67ab but in a different context and replace the offending phrase with *ekaikam abhyāsaṃ*.

It might well be asked how one can be so certain of the direction of borrowing, especially since the *Matsyendrasaṃhitā* has borrowed the entire *Khecarīvidyā*. Several points indicate that μ's version of the passage is the oldest:

- As mentioned above, μ's primacy can be inferred elsewhere in the text from its preservation of good readings not found in the other witnesses, and from its containing a large number of *aiśa* forms that are found corrected in the other witnesses.[35]

- Contextually, μ's version seems to fit better. The first three lines of the passage suggest that the section on Khecarī is over.[36]

- At 3.61ab, the combination of *śivena* and *mādirīm* fits better than the *KhV* manuscripts' incongruous pairing of *śivena* with *māmakīm* (G has *mānavaḥ* for the latter).

- At 3.62a, μ's *vāruṇyā tarpayed* is more natural than the unlikely *bhaktyā saṃtarpayed* of G, R_2 and the *Khecarīvidyā* manuscripts.

- If one were altering a text, it is more likely that one would omit troublesome passages than insert extra ones. The passage in μ at 17.106c–107d, which is omitted in R_2 and the *Khecarīvidyā* manuscripts (apart from 17.107cd which is found slightly altered at *Khecarīvidyā* 3.67ab), fits well contextually as well as syntactically with the following half-verse while its omission in the *Khecarīvidyā* manuscripts gives the passage a disjointed feel.[37]

Analysis of the three witnesses of μ indicates that they all descend from a single hyparchetype and that the readings of A derive from those of J_7 which derive from those of J_6.[38]

Manuscript G

Witness G is a palm-leaf manuscript written in Grantha script in the collection of the Institut français de Pondichéry. Entitled *Khecarīvidyā*, it is missing its first two folios and starts at the edition's 1.20a. It has no *paṭala* divisions and does not include *paṭala* 4.

As stated above, G, R_2 and the *KhV* manuscripts probably derive from an earlier attempt to expunge the explicitly Kaula references found in μ. G often shares good readings with μ that are not found in the *Khecarīvidyā* manuscripts, and has unique readings that appear to be deliberate alterations. See for example G's *ca gurutarpaṇāt* at 1.22d, where μ, R_2 and the *KhV* manuscripts have *kaulikatarpaṇāt.*[39] G also regularly has good readings not found in any other witnesses and several of these have been adopted in the edition. See e.g. 1.70a, 2.3d, 2.22c, 2.40a, 2.88c and 2.92a. G shows no evidence of contamination with any of the other manuscript traditions.

Manuscript R_2

Witness R_2 is a paper manuscript of the *Khecarīvidyā* from the collection of the Asiatic Society of Bengal. Like G it does not include *paṭala* 4 of the *Khecarīvidyā*, but unlike G it breaks the text into three *paṭala*s in the same places as the *Khecarīvidyā* manuscripts.

R_2 shares several readings with μ or μ and G which are not found in the other witnesses. Twice it shares readings with G which are not found elsewhere. On the other hand, it often has readings which are not found in μ or G but are found in the *Khecarīvidyā* manuscripts. In the few verses for which witness *D* (Nārāyaṇa's *Dīpikā*) is a witness, R_2's readings are uniquely close to it.[40]

As stated above it seems likely that G, R_2 and the *Khecarīvidyā* manuscripts derive from a single archetype in which attempts were made to expunge references to the explicitly Kaula practices found in μ. R_2's preservation of readings found only in μ and/or G and its lack of a fourth *paṭala* indicate that it and the *Khecarīvidyā* manuscripts derive from another later archetype from which G does not descend. At this point, the manuscript tradition of R_2 branched off before the redaction of the archetype of the *Khecarīvidyā* manuscripts. Later, through contamination with the tradition of the *Khecarīvidyā* manuscripts, R_2 acquired some of their readings.

At two places (2.110ab, 3.49b), R_2 has good readings which are not found elsewhere but neither of these has been adopted in the edition.

The *Yogakuṇḍalyupaniṣad* (*U*) and manuscript T

The 49 *ślokas* of the second *adhyāya* of the *Yogakuṇḍalyupaniṣad* are all found in the first 64 *ślokas* of the first *paṭala* of the *Khecarīvidyā*. Witness T, like *U*, stops at what is 1.64b in my edition of the *Khecarīvidyā*, but it has the $14\frac{1}{2}$ *ślokas* that the *upaniṣad* omits.

Bouy (1994) has shown how in the eighteenth century a corpus of 108 *upaniṣads* was compiled in south India. In order to do this, some new *upaniṣads* had to be put together and the vogue at that time for the teachings of *haṭhayoga* led to haṭhayogic works being used for the task. The compilers were orthodox *vedāntins* and tried to keep their compositions within the limits of upaniṣadic and *advaita* convention. Thus *U* omits most of the *Khecarīvidyā*'s first *paṭala*'s explicit references to tantra and tantric practices. Fourteen of the *Khecarīvidyā*'s first sixty-three verses are omitted altogether in the *upaniṣad*. In these verses (13c–20b, 21a–25b, 26a–28b, 30ab, 61ab) Śiva calls the *Khecarīvidyā* a tantra and mentions other tantras in which the practice is taught. The verses omitted by the *upaniṣad* include (at 22–25) the directions for worship of the *grantha* in which the text is written down, a practice described in other tantric works but not possible in the case of a divinely-revealed *upaniṣad*. Verses in which the text is referred to abstractly as *śāstra* rather than the more tangible *grantha* are generally retained and in 11a only *U* and J3 have *śāstraṃ* as opposed to *granthaḥ*.[41] The first chapter of the *upaniṣad* is not presented as a dialogue.[42] Without introducing his interlocutors, the redactor presses on with the second chapter, keeping it as a dialogue but concealing the tantric leitmotif of the text as a conversation between Śiva and Pārvatī by substituting the vocative forms *brahman* and *mune* where the *Khecarīvidyā* has *devi* and *priye* respectively. For longer vocatives, he substitutes colourless verse-fillers. Thus at *Khecarīvidyā* 8b *parameśvari* becomes *guruvaktrataḥ* and at 1.50d *tiṣṭhaty amaravandite* becomes *tiṣṭhed eva na saṃśayaḥ*.

Witness T is curious in that like *U* it stops at the edition's 1.64b but it keeps the verses that *U* omits and the vocatives addressed to the goddess. This must be either the result of conflation between manuscripts of the *upaniṣad* and of the *Khecarīvidyā* or evidence that *Khecarīvidyā* 1.1–64b existed as a text in its own right before being redacted to make the *upaniṣad*'s first *adhyāya*.

On the next page is a stemmatic diagram of the relationships between the witnesses. In this diagram, only the positions of the witnesses themselves represent definite historical facts; the remaining nodes and the lines are conjectural, and no attempt has been made to indicate the widespread contamination between the witnesses and witness groups.

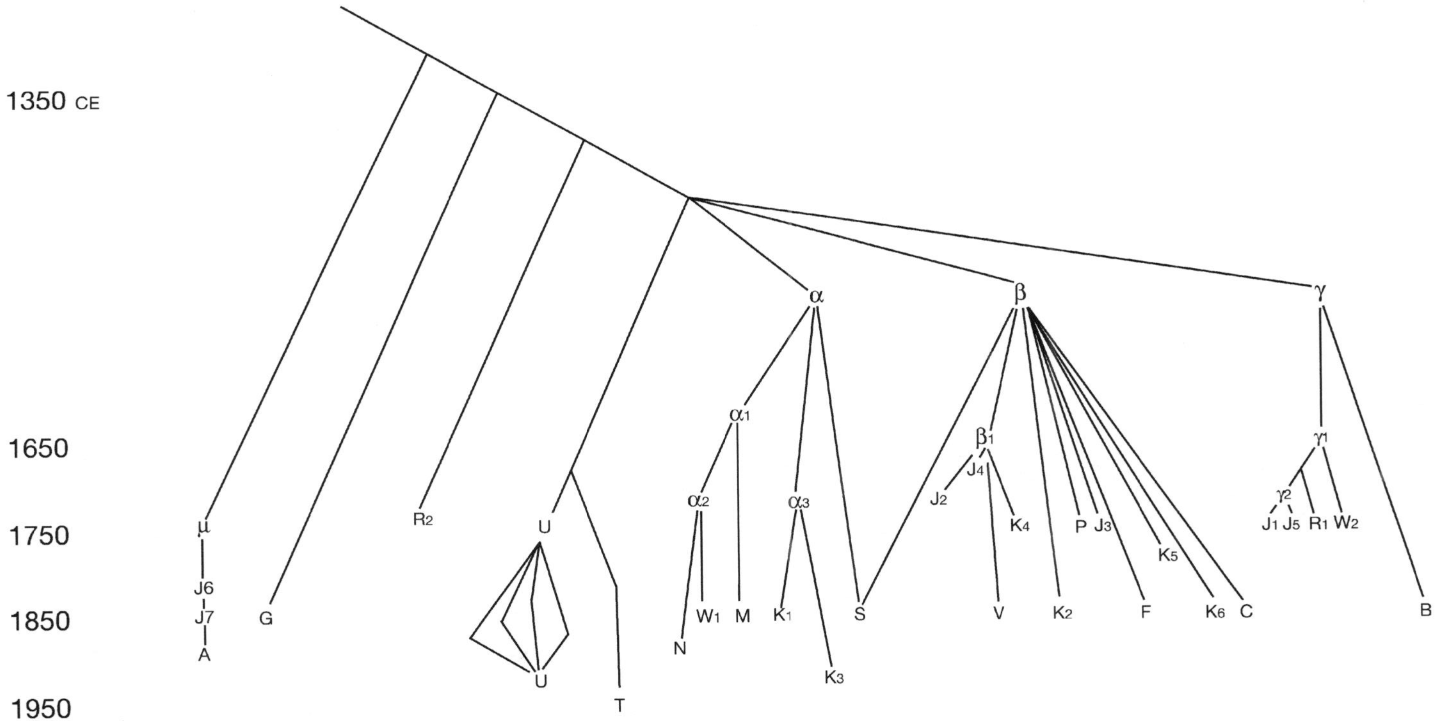

Figure 1: Stemmatic diagram of the relationship between the witnesses of the *Khecarīvidyā*

The *Khecarīvidyā*: part, whole or wholes?

The colophons of G, R_2 and the *Khecarīvidyā* manuscripts describe the *Khecarīvidyā* as being part of the *Mahākālayogaśāstra* of Ādinātha.[43] I have found no catalogue references to a manuscript by that name and the single textual reference to it that I have come across postdates the *Khecarīvidyā*'s composition by some centuries and may be derived from the *Khecarīvidyā*'s own attribution to the text.[44] This suggests that the *Mahākālayogaśāstra* never existed and that the *Khecarīvidyā* was connected with this fictitious text in order to anchor it within an appropriately weighty-sounding tradition.[45] Alternatively, the name *Mahākālayogaśāstra* may have been used to mean the teachings on yoga found in the *Mahākālasaṃhitā*, whose authorship is also ascribed to Ādinātha. As noted by Goudriaan (Goudriaan & Gupta 1981:78), the *Mahākālasaṃhitā* "functions as the locus of ascription for a number of *stotras* and other texts".[46] Its manuscript colophons say that the text originally consisted of 500,000 verses, but the manuscripts themselves provide only fragments of it (30 of at least 255 *paṭalas*).[47]

Whether or not the *Mahākālayogaśāstra* ever existed, examination of the *Khecarīvidyā* indicates that it was part of a larger work. The name of the text is very unusual—I know of no other tantric or haṭhayogic work called *vidyā*. In such texts *vidyā* may mean a mantra or a particular type of mantra and in all instances of the word in the text of the *Khecarīvidyā* this is what it means. Some tantras contain coded descriptions and instructions for the use of many different *vidyā*s.[48] It seems that the framework of the *Khecarīvidyā* was taken from a chapter of such a text in which the *vidyā* of Khecarī was described, and then filled out with instructions about the physical practice.[49]

The third *paṭala* ends with Śiva saying to the Goddess (3.68):

> "I have taught this yoga, which brings success in all yogas, out of fondness for you, o Goddess. What more would you like to hear?"

To which the Goddess replies (3.69):

> "O Śambhu, on whose head is the half-moon [and] who can be attained [only] by true devotion, may you be victorious. You have described well the secret *Khecarīvidyā*."

The second line is as it is found in the *KhV* manuscripts and fits with this being the end of the teaching of a text called *Khecarīvidyā*. In μ, however, we find the following:[50]

> ". . . you have taught the secret method of mastering the *vidyā* of Khecarī."

As we have seen above, μ often preserves older readings than those found in the *Khecarīvidyā* manuscripts and this reading suggests that we have come to the end of a section describing the form and practice of the Khecarī mantra rather than the end of the text itself.

The *Khecarīvidyā* manuscripts also have a fourth *paṭala* in just fourteen verses which makes no mention of Khecarī or the practice,[51] but describes drugs *(auṣadhāni)* for attaining magical powers. Besides its lack of continuity in subject matter, this *paṭala* is different in style from the preceding three, most noticeably in the variety and complexity of the metres that it uses. The first three *paṭala*s are entirely in *anuṣṭubh* metre with a few *vipulā*s. The fourth *paṭala* uses *vasantatilakā*, *upajāti*, and *sragdharā* metres as well as *anuṣṭubh*. Witnesses μ, G and R_2, which regularly have better readings than the *Khecarīvidyā* manuscripts, do not include this fourth *paṭala* with the other three.[52] The colophon to the Mysore *Khecarīvidyā* manuscript's fourth *paṭala* reads *iti siddhauṣadhāni* without ascribing it to the *Khecarīvidyā*, while in the colophons of the first three *paṭala*s it reads *iti śrīādināthaviracite mahākālayogaśāstre khecaryāṃ prathamaḥ/dvitīyaḥ/tṛtīyaḥ paṭalaḥ*. It seems likely that this fourth *paṭala* has been appended to the *Khecarīvidyā*, perhaps on the model of the *Yogasūtra*'s fourth *pāda*, which mentions drugs *(auṣadhi)* in its first *sūtra*. Similarly, DIGAMBARJĪ & JHĀ's edition of the *Haṭhapradīpikā* includes a short fifth *upadeśa*, found in only a small proportion of the witnesses, which details ways of curing physical imbalances through breath-control and diet.[53]

Analysis of the witnesses thus indicates that the text probably went through the following four stages in the course of its development:

1. It first existed as part of a longer text, in the form of a chapter describing the mantra *(vidyā)* of Khecarī. As such the text would probably have consisted of the edition's 1.1–44 and 3.55–69.[54]

2. This chapter was extracted from the larger text and the remaining verses found in the edition's first three *paṭala*s were added.[55] These verses contain instructions for the physical practice of *khecarīmudrā* and were probably gathered from a number of different sources.[56]

3. These three *paṭala*s were then redacted to remove the references to unorthodox Kaula practices found in the *Matsyendrasaṃhitā* manuscripts.

4. The fourth *paṭala*, on magical potions, was added to the text.

Editorial policy

The text has been presented in the form in which it is found in the *Khecarīvidyā* manuscripts. It is in this form that the text enjoyed its greatest popularity and it is this form for which there is the greatest amount of evidence. The composite nature of the text and the redaction it has undergone have resulted in internal contradictions that must have been present since at least the second stage outlined above. Rather than attempt the impossible task of creating a completely coherent text I am presenting it as an occasionally incoherent document whose incoherence tells the story of the development of both the text and *haṭhayoga*.

It has been impossible to adopt readings by means of the kind of stemmatic analysis advocated by WEST (1973) and others. There is considerable contamination between and within the witness groups to the extent that stemmatic analysis is impossible.[57] The following are among the most glaring indicators of this contamination:

- $\mu \leftarrow$ all other witnesses : 1.33c–35b is found after 1.53d in all witnesses. It is only found at 1.33c–35b in μ, which has the passage twice. It seems that it was originally at 1.33c–35b but was then mistakenly put after 1.53d and this mistake found its way into the μ manuscripts through conflation of sources.
- $\mu \leftarrow$ the *Khecarīvidyā* witnesses : these witnesses have *nābhi°* at 2.40a as opposed to G's correct *liṅga°*. Cf. 2.92a.
- $\alpha \leftrightarrow \beta$: as mentioned above, Ballāla mentions alternative readings in his commentary. These can all be found in α and β.
- $\mu \leftrightarrow \alpha_3$: e.g. 1.6a *abhyāsāl,* 1.9d *saṃsṛti,* 1.19d *vadet,* 1.74b *prajīvati,* 4.6d *labhet.*
- $R_2 \leftarrow$ everything else: R_2 is often the only other witness to share readings with μ, G or the *Khecarīvidyā* witnesses.
- $K_2PJ_3F \leftrightarrow \gamma$: these witnesses omit 2.90d–91a, 3.30 and 4.4ab.
- $K_4 \leftarrow \mu G\alpha$: K_4, uniquely among the witnesses of β and γ, has the reading *abhedyaḥ* found in $\mu G\alpha$ at 2.29a.
- $N \leftrightarrow J_1R_1$: these witnesses omit 2.107.
- $\alpha_1 \leftrightarrow K_2$: these witnesses omit 2.5b–6a.
- $\alpha_3 \leftrightarrow K_2 \leftrightarrow \gamma$: these witnesses omit 3.56cd.

As WEITZMANN (1977:229) has observed, in a contaminated tradition the true reading can easily survive in just one witness, so I have taken the merit of each individual variant to be the criterion for its selection.[58] As stated above, the text as found in the *Khecarīvidyā* manuscripts has been used as a blueprint, but where a variant reading from μ, G or *U* improves the text without conflicting with the ideological standpoint of the *Khecarīvidyā* manuscripts, it has been adopted.[59]

Where a plausible alternative can be found among the other witnesses, the readings of *U* have not been adopted. This is because *U* has undergone the most redaction so its variant readings are the least likely to be original. At 1.6cd, however, its reading has been adopted since it is the only one of which I can make any sense. There are two other places (1.38c, 1.51a) where the reading of *U* has been adopted over those of all the other witnesses.

Examples have been given above of how μ, G and R_2 often preserve better readings than the other witnesses. Where these are straightforward improvements to the text they have been adopted. Where their variants in the *Khecarīvidyā* manuscripts show signs of doctoring for ideological reasons they have not. Thus, in the example already given of μ and G's *pavanam* for the *Khecarīvidyā* manuscripts' *pañcamam* at 3.24a, *pavanam* has been adopted. Similarly, the verse found at 1.69 in μ, G and R2, which is missing from the *Khecarīvidyā* manuscripts, is adopted. On the other hand, the passage at 3.57–69 is presented as it is found in the *KhV* manuscripts despite μ's version being original and more coherent. Verses in which I have considered doctrine more important than originality include 2.39 (*°bhūtalayo bhavet* for *°bhūtajayaṃ labhet*), 2.50 (*yoginaḥ* for *yoginyaḥ*), 2.72 (*tālu°* for *bhāla°*), 3.11 (*sadāmṛtatanuḥ* for *parāmṛtatanuḥ*) and 3.31 (*nityadehamayam* for *tyaktvā deham imam*).

On matters such as how long a technique should be practised or how long it takes to produce results the readings of μ, G and R2 have usually been adopted if they differ from those of the *KhV* manuscripts. This approach could of course be flawed—the redactors of the *Khecarīvidyā* may have altered practical details as a result of first-hand observation.

My reliance on the quality of individual variants as the criterion for their adoption gives me considerable editorial licence. Where I feel that my reasons for adopting a particular variant may not be clear I have explained them in the notes to the translation.

Language

The *Khecarīvidyā* is written in simple Sanskrit, similar to that of other tantric and haṭhayogic works. *Aiśa* peculiarities are common, more so in μ than in the *Khecarīvidyā* manuscripts in which the *aiśa* forms found in μ have often been corrected. In the following list of *aiśa* forms I have for the most part only included those peculiarities which are found in the text as constituted or in μ.[60]

Aiśa peculiarities in the text

plural declined as singular 4.7a *pañcamāsena.*

neuters declined as masculines in dual and plural 2.59d *sthānāḥ*; 2.110b *phalān.*

masculine singular becoming neuter singular 1.4d *tadabhyāsaṃ ca durlabham* (μ only); 1.5a *abhyāsam*;[61] 1.54b, 1.55b *abhyāsam*; 2.89a, 2.124c *bhedam*; 2.107c *saṃgamam*; 3.14d *yogam*; 3.44a *kālam*; 3.59c *na sidhyati mahāyogam* (μ only); 3.68a *etad yogaṃ mayākhyātam* (μ only).

neuter singular becoming masculine singular 2.117a *divyadarśanaḥ.*

neuter singular becoming feminine singular 2.77b *adharā.*

dual *-ābhyām* for *-ayoḥ* 2.95c *karṇābhyām.*

***-in* stem declined as *-i* stem** *(metri causa)* 2.6c *parameṣṭhīnām.*

substantive for adjective 2.39c, 3.22d *śivasāmyaḥ*; 4.3c *mahāmārutasāmyavegaḥ*.

***-ya* for *-tvā* in the absolutive** 2.37a *tatrastham amṛtaṃ gṛhya* (μ only); after 3.62b *tāsām ekatamāṃ gṛhya* (μ only).

***-tvā* for *-ya* in the absolutive** 1.70a *saṃpītvā*.

active verb with causative sense 2.123d *viśet*; 3.2a *praviśya*; 3.3a *praviśet*.

incorrect verb-forms 1.46d, 1.47d *samucchinet*; 1.52a *kramati*; 1.57b *praviśyati*; 2.50c *samupāsante*; 2.96d *śṛṇutvā* (μ only); 2.110b *labhati*; 3.39b *grasatīm*.

consonant stem becomes vowel stem for purposes of sandhi 2.60b *śirordhve*; 3.8 *jyotirūpiṇī*.

incorrect sandhi 1.16c *asmin tantravare*;[62] 2.18d *vikhyātā 'maravandite*.[63]

awkward syntax 1.8cd *tadā tat siddhim āpnoti yad uktaṃ śāstrasaṃtatau*; 2.71cd *dambhakauṭilyaniratās teṣāṃ śāstraṃ na dāpayet*.[64]

Metre

The first three *paṭala*s of the text were composed in *anuṣṭubh* metre. In *paṭala* 4, verses 1, 5–9 and 11–14 are in *anuṣṭubh*, verse 2 is in *vasantatilakā*, verses 3 and 10 are in *upajāti* and verse 4 is in *sragdharā*. As I have presented it, the text contains the following *vipulā*s in its *anuṣṭubh* verses:

na-vipulā [17 in total]: 1.5c, 10c, 60c, 76c, 77a; 2.8a, 40c, 47c, 58a, 59a, 63a, 71c; 3.4a, 11a, 30a, 37a, 66a.

bha-vipulā [5]: 1.52a; 2.90a, 116a; 3.1c; 4.9a.

ma-vipulā [6]: 1.34c, 62c; 2.23a, 43c, 114c; 3.25a.

ra-vipulā [2]: 2.111a; 3.35c.

The haṭhayogic *khecarīmudrā*

This chapter starts with a survey of textual evidence for practices related to the haṭhayogic *khecarīmudrā* before the composition of the *Khecarīvidyā*.[65] This is followed by an examination of the practice as it is described in haṭhayogic texts. Next ethnographic data is drawn on to see how and why *khecarīmudrā* is practised today. The chapter finishes with a brief look at those who practised the technique in the past and those who practise it today.

Forerunners of the haṭhayogic *khecarīmudrā*

The Pali canon

A practice which has elements of the *Khecarīvidyā*'s *khecarīmudrā* is described in three passages in the Buddhist Pali canon. In two of the passages the technique is said to bring the mind under control and in the third it is said to suppress the appetite. The first passage is from the *Mahāsaccakasutta* (*Majjhima Nikāya* I, Book 9, pp. 242–246). The Buddha has been questioned by Saccaka, a Jaina who is also called Aggivessana, about *kāyabhāvanā*, "development of the body", and *cittabhāvanā*, "development of the mind". In his reply the Buddha describes his attempts to control his mind with physical practices including the pressing of the tongue against the palate, before describing further attempts involving *appānaka jhāna*, "non-breathing meditation", and fasting. The passage runs as follows:[66]

> "Then, Aggivessana, this occurred to me: 'Suppose now that I clench my teeth, press my palate with my tongue and restrain, suppress and torment my mind with my mind.' So, indeed, Aggivessana, I clenched my teeth, pressed my palate with my tongue and restrained, suppressed and tormented my mind with my mind. Aggivessana, as I clenched my teeth, pressed my palate with my tongue and restrained, suppressed and tormented my mind with my mind, sweat came from my armpits. Just as when, Aggivessana, a strong man, taking hold of a weaker man by the head or shoulders, restrains, suppresses and torments him, so when I clenched my teeth, pressed my palate with my tongue and restrained, suppressed and tormented my mind with my mind, sweat

> came from my armpits. But although, Aggivessana, unsluggish energy arose in me and unmuddled mindfulness came about, my body was impetuous, not calmed, while I was troubled by that painful exertion. And indeed, Aggivessana, this painful feeling arose in me and remained without taking over my mind. Then, Aggivessana, this occurred to me: 'Suppose I meditate the non-breathing meditation'..."

He goes on to hold his breath until he is afflicted by terrible headaches, strong winds in the stomach and a great heat that is like being roasted over burning coal. He then tries fasting until the skin of his belly touches his backbone, he falls over from fainting, his hair falls out and, finally, he loses his fair complexion. At this point he declares:[67]

> "Then, Aggivessana, this occurred to me: 'The ascetics or Brahmins of the past who experienced painful, sharp [and] severe sensations due to [self-inflicted] torture [experienced] this much at most, not more than this. And those ascetics or Brahmins who in the future will experience painful, sharp [and] severe sensations due to [self-inflicted] torture [will experience] this much at most, not more than this. And those ascetics or Brahmins who in the present experience painful, sharp [and] severe sensations due to [self-inflicted] torture [experience] this much at most, not more than this. But I indeed, by means of this severe and difficult practice, do not attain to greater excellence in noble knowledge and insight which transcends the human condition. Could there be another path to enlightenment?"

The Buddha is here clearly condemning the ascetic practices that he has undertaken, including the technique of pressing the tongue against the palate. However, in the following passage from the *Vitakkasanthānasutta* (*Majjhima Nikāya* I, Book 9, pp. 120–121), after being asked about *adhicitta*, "higher thought", he recommends the practice that we have just seen dismissed:[68]

> "Then if, monks, a monk concentrates on the thought function and the nature of those thoughts, but there still arise in him sinful and unwholesome thoughts associated with desire, aversion and confusion, then, monks, he should clench his teeth, press his palate with his tongue and restrain, suppress and torment his mind with his mind. Then, when he clenches his teeth, presses his palate with his tongue and restrains, suppresses and torments his mind with his mind, those sinful and unwholesome thoughts associated with desire, aversion and confusion are got rid of, they disappear. By getting rid of these the mind turns inward, becomes calm, one-pointed and focussed."

In the *Suttanipāta* (p. 138, vv. 716–718), when asked to explain *monam*, "sagehood", the Buddha says:[69]

> "[The sage] should be [as sharp] as a razor blade. Pressing his palate with his tongue he should be restrained with respect to his stomach.

> He should not have an inactive mind nor should he think too much. [He should be] without taint, independent and intent on the holy life. He should learn the practices of solitude and serving ascetics. Solitude is called sagehood. Solitary you will indeed be delighted and shine forth in the ten directions."

The *Paramatthajotikā* commentary on this passage describes the pressing of the palate with the tongue as a means of overcoming thirst and hunger. This is echoed both in medieval haṭhayogic texts,[70] and by contemporary Indian yogins who say that the haṭhayogic *khecarīmudrā* enables extended yogic practice by removing the need to eat or drink.

Here is not the place to attempt to ascertain the Buddha's true attitude towards this practice. For our purposes it is enough to conclude that these passages provide evidence that an ascetic technique involving the pressing of the tongue against the palate (but *not* its insertion above the palate) was current at the time of the composition of the Pali canon and that this practice had two aims: the control of the mind and the suppression of hunger and thirst.[71]

Early Sanskrit texts

The earliest Sanskrit reference that I have found to a practice similar to the *Khecarīvidyā*'s *khecarīmudrā* is in the *Viṣṇusmṛti*. Derrett (1973:32) describes this dharmaśāstric text as "a puzzle", standing "between the thought-world of Manu and that of the Vaiṣṇava Purāṇas". Kane (1968: vol. 1.2 p. 125) believes the text to consist of two layers, a prose nucleus composed between 300 and 100 BCE, and a later verse layer, added between 400 and 600 CE. The following passage (97.1) comes at the beginning of a prose section on *dhyāna*:[72]

> "With the feet placed on the thighs and facing upwards, with the right hand placed in the left, with the tongue unmoving and placed at the palate, not touching the teeth together, looking at the tip of his nose and not looking around, fearless and calm, he should think of that which is beyond the twenty-four elements...And for him who is devoted to meditation yoga manifests within a year."

Here the practice involving the tongue has no explicit purpose but is just one of various physical postures to be adopted by the meditator.

The next passage is from the *Maitrāyaṇīyopaniṣad*. This work is a later *upaniṣad* but its date is uncertain. In his edition of the text, van Buitenen makes no attempt at dating it. He does however distinguish between an early layer of the text and later interpolations, and includes the following passage among the interpolations (1962:85). The mention of Suṣumṇā *nāḍī* shows that the passage has been influenced by tantric physiology; it may be no older than the *Khecarīvidyā*.

At 6.18 yoga has been described as *ṣaḍaṅga*, consisting of *prāṇāyāma*, *pratyāhāra*, *dhyāna*, *dhāraṇā*, *tarka* and *samādhi*. The following passage (6.20–21) concerns *dhāraṇā*:[73]

"Elsewhere it has also been said: Next is the ultimate fixing of this [object of *dhyāna*]. By pressing the tip of the tongue and the palate [and there]by checking speech, mind and breath [the yogin] sees Brahman through consideration *(tarkeṇa)*. When, after the termination of mental activity [the yogin] sees the *ātman* by means of the *ātman*, more minute than an atom and shining, then having seen the *ātman* by means of the *ātman* he becomes without *ātman*. Because of his being without *ātman* he is to be conceived of as without thought, without origin; this is the definition of liberation. That is the ultimate mystery. For it is said thus:

'For by calmness of the mind
he destroys good and bad action.
Happy and abiding in the *ātman*
he attains eternal bliss.'

Elsewhere it has also been said: The upward-flowing channel called Suṣumṇā carries the breath and ends in the palate. By way of this [channel] which is joined with Om and the mind, the breath moves upward. Turning the tip [of the tongue] back over the palate and restraining the sense-organs greatness looks upon greatness. Then he becomes without *ātman*. Through being without *ātman* he does not partake of pleasure or pain and attains isolation."

Here the technique of turning the tongue back onto the palate seems to serve a similar purpose to that found in the first two Pali passages, namely that of controlling the activity of the mind. It is also connected with the raising of the breath by way of the Suṣumṇā *nāḍī*.

The Pali and Sanskrit passages cited above provide evidence (albeit rather scant) that a meditational practice involving pressing the tongue to the palate was known and used by Indian ascetics as early as the time of the composition of the Pali canon. The practice as described in these texts is however very different from the *khecarīmudrā* of the *Khecarīvidyā*, being merely its bare bones. We must turn to the texts of tantric Śaivism for the flesh.

Texts of tantric Śaivism[74]

A verse from the *yogapāda* of the *Kiraṇatantra* describes in brief a practice similar to that described in the *Maitrāyaṇīyopaniṣad* (which may well postdate the *Kiraṇatantra*):[75]

"Holding the breath and, while trembling (*sasphuram* ?), contracting the throat, by means of the conjunction of the tongue and palate there is instant rising [of the breath]."

Both this and the *Maitrāyaṇīyopaniṣad* passage describe a forerunner of the idea found in the *Khecarīvidyā* and other haṭhayogic texts that the insertion of the tongue into the cavity above the palate results in the raising of Kuṇḍalinī.[76] The later tantric and haṭhayogic emphasis on the raising of Kuṇḍalinī is not found in the *yogapādas* of early works of tantric Śaivism such as the *Kiraṇatantra*, where the emphasis is on the raising of the breath through the central channel.

We now turn to five passages from texts that are products of possession-based Yoginī cults or their Kaula derivatives. These passages describe methods of conquering death by drinking *a-mṛta*, "non-death". Similar techniques are described elsewhere in tantric Śaiva works but in these the yogin is instructed to visualise the body being flooded with the *amṛta* rather than to drink it.[77]

The first of these passages is from the *mudrāṣaṭka* of the *Jayadrathayāmala*. It is a description of a yogic *karaṇa* called *antarjala* and comes in the middle of a long passage describing several other such *karaṇas*.[78] These are all extremely obscure and the text is corrupt in several places. However the passage contains one of the earliest references to a yogic practice in which the tongue is definitely placed in *the hollow above* the palate and which links the practice with the drinking of *amṛta*. The previous twenty verses describe a technique of breath-retention by which the yogin can flood his body with *amṛta* and then increase the duration of the retention to attain various magical powers and worlds. I translate the passage thus:[79]

> "[The *sādhaka*] should drink that nectar of the stream which is milked as if from a cow's teats. Satiated by that *amṛta* he [becomes] free from wrinkles and grey hair. [...] When the tongue has reached the head of Viṣṇu, on union with the void it enters the aperture of the palate without even slightly touching [the side]. Then, o Brahmin, making the mouth like the hollow beak of a bird and then holding that sensation until [his] condition becomes steady, the yogin in the steady state floats comfortably. As a result of the relaxation of [the yogin] there and of the consideration of the two smells (?), the supreme nectar flows forth, struck by the tongue at the moon in the void. That which has the form of consciousness having tasted that *[amṛta]* assuredly moves upwards. This conjunction of Śiva and Śakti is the uprooting of the Key goddess.[80] †[The conjunction] in which the power of sight is above the pronunciation of an extended vowel is a garden created by the pervasiveness of Śiva.† Joining the tongue and the palate, [the yogin] joins the aperture of the palate above the throat with the energy of vibration up to the twelve levels."

Although there are many difficulties in this passage it is clearly the closest we have come so far to the *khecarīmudrā* of the *Khecarīvidyā*.[81]

In the *Maitrāyaṇīyopaniṣad* and *Kiraṇatantra* passages, the placing of the tongue at the palate is connected with the raising of the breath; in this passage, at 160a, *cidrūpam*, "that which has the form of consciousness", is said to rise. The breath is often associated with consciousness, but Kuṇḍalinī is also said to be *cidrūpā* (see e.g. *KMT* 6.4) so it may be that here we have the first instance of the placing of the tongue at the palate being associated with the raising of the goddess Kuṇḍalinī (or a forerunner of her), particularly in the light of the following half-verse, in which Śiva and Śakti are said to be united.

The next passage is from the *Mālinīvijayottaratantra*:[82]

> "And now the supreme secret, the acme of the *amṛta* of Śiva's gnosis is described for the destruction of disease and death in yogins. [The yogin] should visualise Parā in her own form pouring forth *amṛta* in the sixteen-spoked wheel in the void, whose hub is formed by the moon. Armed with the previously[-described] *nyāsa*, for an instant (?) the wise [yogin] should then lead his tongue to the uvula and insert it [there]. He should visualise the white heavenly *amṛta*, flowing from the orb of the moon. [If] his mouth fills with a slightly salty liquid that smells of iron then he should not drink it but spit it out. He should practise thus until [the liquid] becomes sweet-tasting. Drinking it, within six months he effortlessly becomes free of decrepitude and disease; after a year he becomes a conqueror of death. Once it has become sweet-tasting thenceforth his mouth fills up with whatever flowing substance he, with focussed mind, visualises in it, such as blood, alcohol or fat or milk or ghee and oil etc."[83]

Unlike in the other passages describing the defeat of death, in this passage the tongue is not explicitly said to enter the aperture above the uvula—*lambake viniyojayet* at 21.3d could mean either "[the yogin] is to place [his tongue] at the uvula" or "[the yogin] should place [his tongue] in [the cavity above] the uvula". However, in the light of the other passages, in which the insertion of the tongue above the palate is explicitly instructed, it seems likely that the same is intended here.[84]

The next passage is from the *Kaulajñānanirṇaya*:[85]

> "Next, a great secret which destroys all diseases. [The yogin] should point his tongue upwards and insert his mind in there. By regular practice he destroys death, my dear. In an instant he is freed from sickness, disease, death, decrepitude and the like. All diseases are destroyed, like deer by a lion. In an instant disease is destroyed, [there is] the destruction of severe leprosy. With a sweet taste, o great goddess, there is the removal of wrinkles and grey hair. With a milky taste, o wise one, a man becomes immortal. When [there is] a taste like ghee, o goddess, then autonomy arises."

The idea of a progression of tastes presented in the *Mālinīvijayottaratantra* and *Kaulajñānanirṇaya* passages is nowhere mentioned in the *Khecarīvidyā*, but is found at *Gorakṣaśataka*$_{\mathrm{N}}$ 149 (=*Haṭhapradīpikā* 3.49) and *Gheraṇḍasaṃhitā* 3.27–28.[86]

The next passage is another from the *Kaulajñānanirṇaya*, in a difficult section found at 6.15–28. The goddess asks Bhairava about *kālavañcana*, "cheating death". Bhairava answers:[87]

> "Stretching the uvula *(dantarāyam)* until he can reach the aperture of Brahmā *(brahmabilam)*,[88] the wise man also extracts the best of *amṛta*s with the tip of his tongue. Truly indeed, o great ascetic lady, he conquers death in a month. Putting the tongue at the root of the palate, he should gently breathe in. He should practise for six months, o goddess; he will be freed from great diseases."

Various benefits arise from the practice: the yogin becomes free of old age and death, he knows the past and future, has long-distance hearing and vision, is not affected by poison and is impervious to attack. Then at 23–26 we read:[89]

> "[The yogin] should recognise that which is in the middle of the uvula in the form of a drop to be *amṛta*, which destroys wrinkles and grey hair. The wise man should put his tongue in the place cool to the touch; he becomes free of wrinkles and grey hair and devoid of all disease. Always devoted to the way of yoga, death cannot happen to him. He should insert his tongue into the base of the palate to destroy disease. Standing, awake, asleep, moving, eating [or] delighting in sexual intercourse, he should curl [back] his tongue constantly, joining it with its own mouth *(svavaktreṇa)*."[90]

The yogin defeats death and becomes free *(svacchandagaḥ)* (vv.27–28).

The final passage describing the conquering of death is from the *Kubjikāmatatantra*:[91]

> "And now I shall teach another practice, which destroys death. [The yogin] should contract the *mūla cakra* situated at the organ of generation and immediately concentrate on it. He should open up the uvula after rubbing and pressing [it]. Satiated by the *amṛta* from the uvula he is sure to conquer death. By carrying out this practice, o beautiful goddess, he destroys fever, consumption, excessive heat or extreme discolouration [of the body].[92] Putting the tongue in the void, without support, not touching the teeth with the teeth nor joining the lips together, eschewing [any] contact of these, [the yogin] is sure to defeat death. This yoga that is the conquest of death has not been [taught] before, nor will it be [taught again]."

As I have said above, these five passages describing techniques for the conquest of death are all from scriptures of possession-based Yoginī cults or their Kaula derivatives. They contain the first references to practices in which the tongue enters the hollow above the palate, so it seems likely that the technique has its roots in rites of possession. The tongue's entry into the cavity above the palate has been reported to occur spontaneously as a result of altered mental states which themselves can be precipitated by breathing practices and drugs.[93] In the above passages the yogin is instructed to put his tongue into the cavity; there is no suggestion of spontaneity. Thus these techniques may be attempts to recreate a state of possession.[94] With the tongue inserted in the cavity, it is difficult for the yogin to swallow and saliva/*amṛta* collects in the mouth.

The last passage from the texts of tantric Śaivism that I shall examine is found in the *Kularatnoddyota*, a work of the Paścimāmnāya's Kubjikā cult. It is the earliest example, that I have located, of a practice involving the tongue being called *khecarīmudrā*.[95] This *khecarīmudrā* is the first of eight *mudrā*s described in the text:[96]

> "[The yogin] should block all the doors of the body and restrain the breath. The tongue should be placed at the tip of the uvula, blocking the internal channel. Tensing the hands and feet, with clenched fists, o great ascetic lady, raising the face upwards, half-stretched out into space, and fixing the pupils [of the eyes], contracting the base region, fixing the gaze in the way of the ether and making the mind have me as its support at the crossroads *(catvarastham)*,[97] o beautiful lady: the technique is considered to be like this. This *mudrā* is called *khecarī* and is the queen of all the *mudrā*-kings."

This practice is in the tradition of the pre-āgamic tongue practices cited earlier rather than those of the tantric Śaiva passages above. Here and in the passages from the Pali canon, the *Viṣṇusmṛti* and the *Maitrāyaṇīyopaniṣad*, the yogin is to exert himself, straining to hold his breath and tensing the body, whereas in the other āgamic passages (and in the *Khecarīvidyā*) the yogin is to relax,[98] breathing freely,[99] as his body is flooded with *amṛta*. The absence of *amṛta* in the *Kularatnoddyota* passage and the description of the tongue as *ghaṇṭikāntasthā*, "at the tip of the uvula", make it likely that the tongue was to be held at the uvula rather than inserted into the cavity above it. The absence of *amṛta* is all the more striking in the light of the third *mudrā* described in the passage, the *śaśinī*, "lunar", *mudrā*:[100]

> "Placing his mind at the left side of the Svādhiṣṭhāna, o queen of the gods, [the yogin] should visualise the Sahasrāra *cakra* as spotless and full of the supreme *amṛta*, o great goddess of illusion. Flooding [it] with a stream of *amṛta* he should visualise his entire body as joined with the Vidyāyoginī. This *mudrā* is called *śaśinī* and accomplishes all ends."

Khecarīmudrā in tantric texts

The passages cited above that describe the conquest of death indicate that physical practices very similar to the *Khecarīvidyā*'s *khecarīmudrā* were used by *sādhaka*s of various tantric traditions before the composition of the *Khecarīvidyā*. Like the *Khecarīvidyā*'s *khecarīmudrā* these practices were connected with the raising of breath/Kuṇḍalinī and enabled the yogin to drink *amṛta* and thereby be free of old age, disease and death. However, despite there being descriptions of many different *khecarīmudrā*s in the texts of tantric Śaivism, it is not until the relatively late *Kularatnoddyota* that we find the first instance of a practice involving the tongue being called by that name, and even then that practice is somewhat different from the *Khecarīvidyā*'s *khecarīmudrā*.[101]

Mudrā in tantric Śaivism is a large and complex subject and I shall not attempt to explore it in detail here.[102] Instead I shall examine only the *khecarīmudrā* in tantric Śaiva texts and in particular those *khecarīmudrā*s which are in some way related to the haṭhayogic *khecarīmudrā*, in order to help explain the adoption of the name for the haṭhayogic practice.

In the texts of tantric Śaivism, a Khecarī is a particular type of Yoginī,[103] and she lives among the Khecaras, "sky-dwellers". Becoming a Khecara, sporting with them, being worshipped by them and reaching their abode *(khecarapada)* are mentioned throughout the Bhairavāgama as goals of *sādhana*, and *khecarīmudrā* is often the means.[104]

The *Kubjikāmatatantra* (*paṭala*s 14–16) describes a hierarchy of five groups of feminine deities: Devīs, Dūtīs, Mātṛs, Yoginīs and Khecarīs, among whom the Khecarīs are the highest, distinguished from Yoginīs. In the *Kaulajñānanirṇaya* Khecarī is described as the overall mother of all *siddhiyoginī*s.[105] The same verse of the *Kaulajñānanirṇaya* lists two other types of Yoginī: Bhūcarī and Gocarī.[106]

Kṣemarāja describes four groups of deities *(devatācakrāṇi)* in the sequence of manifestation of *śakti* at *Spandanirṇaya* 1.20: Khecarī, Gocarī, Dikcarī and Bhūcarī, of which the most refined is Khecarī.[107] In his *Śivasūtravimarśinī* (2.5), the same author describes Khecarī as *°parasaṃvitsvarūpā*, "having the form of the highest consciousness". Kṣemarāja's formulations are sophisticated interpretations of the less metaphysically refined Yoginī cult. In both systems Khecarī, however she is understood, occupies an exalted position, and the same is true of her *mudrā*. Thus, in the 32nd *āhnika* of the *Tantrāloka*, which is devoted to *mudrā*, we read:[108]

> "Among these (i.e. the *mudrā*s taught in the *Mālinīvijayottaratantra*) the most important is *khecarī* [since it is the one] whose essence is a deity."

The importance of *khecarīmudrā* is stressed again later in the same chapter:[109]

> "There is one seed-syllable, that of emission, whose power resides in all mantras; and there is one *mudrā*, *khecarī*, which animates all *mudrā*s."

Similarly, at *Jayadrathayāmala* 4.2.645c *khecarīmudrā* is described as "the queen amongst all *mudrā*s" *(sarvamudrāsu rājeśī)*, and we saw above how *Kularatnoddyota* 3.108d calls *khecarīmudrā* "the queen of all *mudrā*-kings" *(sarvamudreśvareśvarī)*.

Thus *khecarīmudrā* is a key component of tantric practice. But what is it? In his analysis of the *mudrā*s of the *Mālinīvijayottaratantra*, VASUDEVA (1997:15–20) follows the divisions found in the text in identifying three types of *mudrā*: liturgical, iconic and yogic. Yogic *mudrā*s are so called "not because they are primarily employed in yoga but rather because their practice involves yogic principles" (ibid.:18).

The *khecarīmudrā*s of tantric Śaivism fall into this yogic category. In the 32nd *āhnika* of his *Tantrāloka*, Abhinavagupta describes nine variants of the *khecarīmudrā*. These involve esoteric yogic techniques and require the yogin to assume bizarre physical attitudes in imitation of the *mudrā*-deities that he seeks to propitiate.[110] At the beginning of the chapter he cites the *Devyāyāmala*'s definition of *mudrā* as *bimbodayā* and analyses the compound in two ways: either *mudrā* is "that which arises from the original" or "that from which the original arises". As VASUDEVA says (ibid.:19):

> ... these extreme Khecarīmudrās are reflections, imprints or replications *(pratibimba)* of the dynamism of consciousness (Khecarī). The corollary is... the direct experience of Khecarī, or to use different terminology the possession by the goddess Khecarī, manifests itself in the practitioner with these bizarre symptoms.

Thus the two levels of sophistication possible in the interpretation of Khecarī mentioned above are also possible in her *mudrā*. On the level of Khecarī as etheric Yoginī, *khecarīmudrā* brings about possession by her; on the level of Khecarī as supreme consciousness, *khecarīmudrā* brings about experience of that consciousness. In the *Jayadrathayāmala* the *lelihānā mudrā* (one of the nine types of *khecarīmudrā* described by Abhinavagupta) is said to be *sarvadāveśakārikā*, "always effecting possession";[111] Kṣemarāja says that *khecarīmudrā* is so called "because [it brings about] movement in the ether, i.e. the sky of awakened consciousness" *(khe bodhagagane caraṇāt)*.[112]

The *khecarīmudrā* of the *Khecarīvidyā* has many of the attributes of the possession-oriented *mudrā*s of the Bhairavāgama, and these are the key to its understanding rather than the sophisticated interpretations of the Kashmiri exegetes. The *Jayadrathayāmala*'s *mudrāṣaṭka* describes several extremely bizarre *mudrā*s and many of these result in *yoginīmelaka* and *khecaratva*, the aims of *khecarīmudrā* as described in the earliest layer of the *Khecarīvidyā*.[113]

Why was the haṭhayogic practice called *khecarīmudrā*?

The purpose of *mudrā*s in *haṭhayoga* is to awaken Kuṇḍalinī.[114] As we have seen above, causing breath or Kuṇḍalinī to rise up the central channel is mentioned as an aim of many of the practices described in the *śaivāgama* in which the tongue enters the cavity above the palate. Thus it is appropriate that such a practice should be called *mudrā* in the texts of *haṭhayoga*. But why should it be called *khecarīmudrā*?[115]

Many of the practices of *haṭhayoga* can be understood as tantric ritual within the realm of the yogin's own body.[116] The *haṭhayogin* can accomplish the ends of tantric practice without external ritual or a consort with whom to engage in sexual rites. *Gorakṣaśataka* 72–75 locates both *bindu*, sperm, and *rajas*, menstrual fluid, in the body of the yogin. By combining the two, the *haṭhayogin* can produce within his own body the supreme *tattva* of the tantric sexual rite.[117] There are two processes at work in this interiorisation of tantric ritual. Firstly, it is a way of effecting independence similar in some ways to both the vedic renouncer's internalisation of the sacrifice[118] and the Kashmiri Śaiva exegetes' transformation of tantric ritual into a mental process. Secondly, it is the result of a deliberate strategy of the redactors of the texts of *haṭhayoga*. By adopting the terminology of tantric works the writers of these texts would have lent them the authority of the *āgamas*. As we have seen above, *khecarīmudrā* was a highly esteemed part of tantric ritual, and its accommodation within the practices of *haṭhayoga* would have brought that esteem with it. A contraction of *Tantrāloka* 32.64 (which was cited above, on page 25) is found at *Haṭhapradīpikā* 3.53ab:[119]

> "There is one seed-syllable, that of emission, and one *mudrā*, *khecarī*."

Parallel to the interiorisation of tantric ritual is a process in which practices of tantric Śaivism are transformed into techniques that work on the human body. I call this process "corporealisation". Although the techniques of *haṭhayoga* are the richest source of examples of this process, it began long before any haṭhayogic texts had been composed, as is evinced by the five passages describing the conquest of death by drinking *amṛta* cited earlier in this chapter.[120]

Besides *khecarīmudrā*, the *Khecarīvidyā* describes two more corporealised techniques. The first is the bizarre practice of *mathana*, "churning" or "kindling", described at 1.57c–64d, which involves inserting a probe into the nasal cavity and churning it about. At *Kubjikāmatatantra* 12.60–65 a subtler *mathana* is described which combines yogic techniques and visualisation, using sexual intercourse as its explanatory paradigm. This in turn can be seen as a grosser form of a visualisation given in the *Tantrāloka* which, although not called *mathana*, describes the meditation on the rubbing together of Soma, Sūrya and Agni as the *araṇi*, "the kindling stick", by the agitation of which, the meditator, "burning brightly, becomes full by enjoying the oblation of Mahābhairava in the great sacrificial fire which is called the heart".[121] Jayaratha gives a yogic interpretation of this passage which is similar in some ways to the technique of *mathana* described in the *Kubjikāmatatantra*.

The second corporealised technique in the *Khecarīvidyā* is the practice of massaging the body with various bodily fluids described at 2.72–79. This technique appears to be a corporealisation of alchemical practices in which various substances are rubbed into mercury in order to fix it.[122]

An example of corporealisation from elsewhere in the haṭhayogic corpus is the *mudrā* called *mahāvedha*, "the great piercing", described at *Haṭhapradīpikā* 3.25–28. The yogin is to sit cross-legged with his left heel under his perineum. Putting his hands flat on the ground, he should raise his body and then gently drop it, thus making his heel tap against the perineum, forcing the breath or Kuṇḍalinī into the central channel. This is a corporealisation of the tantric *vedhadīkṣā*, "piercing initiation". *TĀ* 29.236–281 describes several different types of *vedhadīkṣā*. Using mantras and visualisations, the guru causes *śakti* to rise up the pupil's middle path and pierce the *cakras* and *ādhāras* stationed along it.

The haṭhayogic *khecarīmudrā* can be seen as a corporealisation of tantric techniques of cheating death in which the head is visualised as containing a store of lunar *amṛta* which, when accessed by means of the breath or Kuṇḍalinī, pours out into the rest of the body, nourishing and immortalising it. The subtle practice is described in many tantric works.[123] The haṭhayogic *khecarīmudrā* (as well as its tantric predecessors) bestows a concrete ontological status on the *amṛta*. In the descriptions of the subtle technique the yogin is to visualise it (verb forms from √*smṛ* are used); in the corporealised technique the tongue is inserted into the cavity above the palate and the yogin drinks the *amṛta*.

The haṭhayogic *khecarīmudrā* is also a corporealisation of the tantric ritual practices of eating meat and drinking wine: the tongue is meat and *amṛta* is wine. This is explicitly stated in the *Haṭhapradīpikā*:[124]

> "[The yogin] should constantly eat the meat of the cow and drink the liquor of the gods. I reckon him to be a Kaula; the others are destroyers of the *kula*. By the word 'cow' the tongue is meant, because the insertion of [the tongue] at the palate is the eating of the meat of the cow, which destroys great sins. The essence that flows from the moon, brought about by the fire generated by the tongue's insertion, is the liquor of the gods."

The name *khecarī*, "[she who] moves in the ether", is particularly appropriate for a practice in which the tongue enters a hollow space.[125] In the *Gorakṣaśataka* the name *khecarī* is explained thus:[126]

> "The mind moves in the ether *(khe)* because the tongue moves in the void *(khe)*; thus there is this *khecarīmudrā* worshipped by all the *siddhas*."

This explanation neatly connects the insertion of the tongue above the palate with a sophisticated interpretation of *khecarīmudrā* similar to that given by the Kashmiri exegetes.[127]

Khecarīmudrā in haṭhayogic texts

If one examines the early texts of *haṭhayoga* different approaches to its practice become apparent.[128] At one end of the spectrum is the *Khecarīvidyā*, with its roots in Yoginī-cults and Kaulism. At the other end is the *Dattātreyayogaśāstra* which, while still far from the realm of orthodoxy, is a product of a more renunciatory and ascetic tradition.[129] The two different approaches are summarised succinctly in the *Śārṅgadharapaddhati* (the *Dattātreyayogaśāstra* practice is given first):[130]

> "[The yogin] should insert the previously trained mind and breath into the *śaṅkhinī [nāḍī]*[131] in the rod[-like] pathway at the rear by contracting the *mūlādhāra*. Breaking the three knots he should lead [mind and breath] to the bee-cave. Then the *bindu* born of *nāda* goes from there to dissolution *(layam)* in the void.[132]Through training the yogin becomes one whose destiny is assured, chaste *(ūrdhvaretāḥ)*, supremely blissful, and free of old age and death.

> Or, by upward impulses of the breath *(udghātaiḥ)*[133] [the yogin] should awaken the sleeping goddess Kuṇḍalinī whose abode is the Base [and] whose form is like a lotus fibre. Inserting her into the Suṣumṇā *[nāḍī]* he should pierce the five *cakras*. Then he should insert the goddess into Śiva, who has the radiance of the moon, a shining faultless light, in the thousand-petalled lotus, and flood his entire body, inside and out, with the nectar there. Then the yogin should think of nothing."

The practices that are taught in the *Khecarīvidyā* can be understood in the terms of the second paradigm. The language and ideas of the first are almost entirely absent, with just a brief appearance at 2.107–115.

Of all the texts of *haṭhayoga* only the *Dattātreyayogaśāstra* describes practices which conform exactly to the first paradigm. The *Dattātreyayogaśāstra* mentions neither Kuṇḍalinī nor *cakras*. Closest to this position are the original *Gorakṣaśataka*[134] and the *Yogabīja*, whose descriptions of *sādhana* match that described in the first alternative but also include *śakticālana*, a technique for awakening Kuṇḍalinī that involves pulling on the tongue.[135] Only the *Khecarīvidyā* and the *Vasiṣṭhasaṃhitā* adhere closely to the second alternative. All other haṭhayogic texts teach both approaches and, as we shall see below, this results in some inconsistencies.

The standpoint of any particular text can be seen in how it understands the purpose of *khecarīmudrā*. In the *Khecarīvidyā*, as we have seen, *khecarīmudrā* is used to raise Kuṇḍalinī and access the store of *amṛta* in the head in order to flood the entire body, rejuvenating and nourishing it. In the *Dattātreyayogaśāstra* the purpose of *khecarīmudrā* is not explicitly stated, but the practice is grouped with *jālandharabandha*, the chin-lock, which is said to prevent the lunar *amṛta* from being consumed by the solar fire in the stomach, thereby rendering the body immortal.[136] This aim of *khecarīmudrā*, for which the name *mudrā*, in its meaning of "seal", is particularly appropriate, is explained in the *Gorakṣaśataka*$_N$:[137]

> "The *bindu*[138] of [the yogin] who has sealed the hollow above the uvula by means of *khecarī* does not fall [even] when he is embraced by an amorous woman. As long as *bindu* is in the body where is the danger of death?"

Thus there are two contradictory aims of *khecarīmudrā* in the texts of *haṭhayoga*. In one, *amṛtaplāvana*, the store of *amṛta* is to be accessed and used to flood the body; in the other, *bindudhāraṇa*, *amṛta* (or *bindu*) is to be kept where it is.[139] Many texts describe both aims. In contrast to the verse cited above, at *Gorakṣaśataka*$_N$ 149–152 the body is to be filled with *amṛta*; the first two lines of the *Gorakṣaśataka*$_N$ passage cited above are also found at *Haṭhapradīpikā* 3.41, while at *Haṭhapradīpikā* 4.53ab in another description of *khecarīmudrā* we read *amṛtaiḥ plāvayed deham āpādatalamastakam*, "[the yogin] should inundate his body from top to toe with the *amṛtas*".[140]

The existence of both ideas in these texts shows how the early manuals of *haṭhayoga* were attempting to syncretise the practices of different schools. None of the texts that attempt to describe a complete system of yoga (e.g. the *Dattātreyayogaśāstra*, *Gorakṣaśataka*$_N$ or *Haṭhapradīpikā*) is entirely coherent. Only the more specialist treatises such as the *Amanaskayoga* and the original *Gorakṣaśataka* present an uncontradictory whole. As mentioned above, the *Khecarīvidyā* has not entirely escaped this syncretism: 2.107–115 is more in keeping with the idea of *bindudhāraṇa* than *amṛtaplāvana*.[141]

The *Khecarīvidyā* seems to be an attempt by a school of yogins whose roots lay in Kaula tantrism at reclaiming the haṭhayogic *khecarīmudrā* from more orthodox *bindudhāraṇa*-oriented schools of *haṭhayoga*.[142] The *Dattātreyayogaśāstra*, which almost certainly predates the *Khecarīvidyā*, teaches a *bindudhāraṇa*-oriented *khecarīmudrā*. The practice as described in the *Gorakṣaśataka*$_N$ is for the most part a technique of *bindudhāraṇa* and may derive from the *khecarīmudrā* described in the *Kularatnoddyota* (see note 96). The compilers of the *Khecarīvidyā* knew the *Gorakṣaśataka*$_N$ and pay it respect at *Khecarīvidyā* 1.16, but give a very different interpretation of the haṭhayogic *khecarīmudrā*.

Of all haṭhayogic works, the most eclectic is the *Haṭhapradīpikā*, which borrows verses from almost every haṭhayogic text that we know existed before its compilation. The *Haṭhapradīpikā* is the second work (after the *Yogabīja*) that claims to belong to the Nātha school and it is the founding of this most eclectic of orders that resulted in its composition.[143]

After the composition of the *Haṭhapradīpikā*, we find a proliferation in the number of haṭhayogic texts and commentaries.[144] The main reason for this increase is the interest in *haṭhayoga* taken by Advaita Vedāntins. Bouy (1994) examines the textual evidence for this interest in detail. He summarises the situation thus (ibid.:5):

> The *Haṭhapradīpikā*, which is nothing more than an anthology, was compiled by Svātmārāma during the XVth century. This Haṭha-yogic work aroused great interest, especially among followers of Śaṃkara's Advaita philosophy. As early as the XVIth–XVIIth centuries, works written by Advaita Vedāntins, such as Nārāyaṇa's *Dīpikā* on a collection of Ātharvaṇa Upaniṣads, Śivānanda Sarasvatī's *Yogacintāmaṇi*, and Nārāyaṇa Tīrtha's commentary on the *Yogasūtra*, entitled the *Yogasiddhāntacandrikā*, referred to Gorakṣa, i.e. the author of the *Gorakṣaśataka*, and quoted from the *Haṭhapradīpikā* and Nātha treatises on *haṭhayoga*. In other words, from that time a number of Sanskrit texts belonging to Nātha literature were considered by Advaita adepts to be authoritative on *yoga*.

The texts of *haṭhayoga* provided material for part of a corpus of one hundred and eight *upaniṣad*s that was compiled in the first half of the eighteenth century. Works on *haṭhayoga* were used to create new recensions of old Upaniṣads and to compose entirely new ones (including the *Yogakuṇḍalyupaniṣad* whose second *adhyāya* contains 49 of the *Khecarīvidyā*'s first 65 verses). This is well documented by Bouy (for a summary see ibid.:6).

What effect did the Advaita interest have on the understanding and practice of *khecarīmudrā*? We may assume that the Nāthas continued to practise it as before: few new Sanskrit Nātha texts appear after the *Haṭhapradīpikā* yet we know that the Nāthas attracted considerable patronage until at least the beginning of the nineteenth century and for a long period were probably the largest ascetic order in North India.[145] It seems that, textually speaking, they could rest on their laurels with an established corpus of works, while the Vedāntins sought to accommodate the newly fashionable practices of *haṭhayoga* within their soteriology.[146] Other than the *Yogakuṇḍalyupaniṣad*'s second *adhyāya* the upaniṣadic passages that mention *khecarīmudrā* are all taken from *Gorakṣaśataka*$_N$ 64–71 and thus describe it as a method of *bindudhāraṇa*.[147] The verses in the *Yogakuṇḍalyupaniṣad* taken from the *Khecarīvidyā* describe the *khecarīmantra* and the mechanics of the practice without mentioning *amṛtaplāvana*. In the *Yogacintāmaṇi* of Śivānanda Sarasvatī (c.1600 CE; see Bouy 1994:119), *khecarīmudrā* is said to be useful in holding *prāṇa* in the head; *bindu* is not mentioned (f. 6r$^{4-7}$). The Advaita Saṃnyāsins, intent on liberation, concentrated on the renunciatory and controlling aspect of *khecarīmudrā*, playing down its *siddhi*-oriented tantric heritage. They added little but a shift of emphasis to the nexus of ideas surrounding the practice.

A late Vaiṣṇava manual of *haṭhayoga*, the *Gheraṇḍasaṃhitā*, makes no mention of *amṛta* when describing the practice, but describes the variously flavoured *rasas* that the tongue will taste (3.27c–28d).[148] The benefits of *khecarīmudrā* listed at 3.24a–26b and 7.11 are purely physical except for *samādhi*. As the orthodox ideologies of Vedānta and Bhakti increased their grip on yoga, tantric ideas were slowly squeezed out. The *khecarīmudrā* of later haṭhayogic works has little connection with tantra; indeed it has more in common with the practice that was current at the time of the composition of the Pali canon.[149]

Khecarīmudrā in modern India

My ethnographic fieldwork in India has focussed on traditional *haṭhayoga*, by which I mean *haṭhayoga* that has not been shaped by the developments which started in the late nineteenth century and which have helped to make yoga the global phenomenon it is today.[150] *Khecarīmudrā* appears to play little part in this modern *haṭhayoga*: Iyengar, perhaps the most influential of all modern teachers of *haṭhayoga*, mentions it only in passing (1977:118-9) and neither Alter (2004) nor De Michelis (2004), who examine the development of modern yoga in India and abroad, mention it at all.

Haṭhayogic texts talk of four types of yoga: *mantra, laya, haṭha* and *rāja*. *Rājayoga* is usually said to be the best and often equated with *samādhi*.[151] Some traditional *haṭhayogins* in India today have adopted the modern yogic understanding of *haṭhayoga* as denoting physical practices and *rājayoga* mental ones. *Haṭha* is seen as a preliminary for *rāja*. Some practices are deemed to have two varieties, one *haṭha* and one *rāja*. Thus the *bindudhāraṇa*-oriented *khecarīmudrā* described at *Haṭhapradīpikā* 3.31–53 is the physical *haṭhayoga* practice, while the *samādhi*-oriented *khecarīmudrā* of 4.42–55, in which the tongue is not explicitly mentioned, is the purely mental, and therefore superior, *rājayoga* practice. This is how *khecarīmudrā* was explained to me by Raghuvara Dās Yogīrāj of Jaipur and he assured me that the *rājayoga* variety was much more important than that of *haṭhayoga*, about which he was somewhat dismissive. Satyānanda SARASVATĪ distinguishes between two types of *khecarīmudrā* in his commentary on the *Haṭhapradīpikā* (1993:279): a *haṭhayoga khecarīmudrā*, in which the tongue is inserted into the cavity above the palate, and an implicitly superior, *samādhi*-oriented *rājayoga khecarīmudrā*, in which the tongue is pressed against the palate in the manner of the practices described in the Pali canon and early Sanskrit works. The majority of the *khecarīmudrā*-practising yogins that I met during my fieldwork emphasised the practice's importance for entering a state of *samādhi*. Paraśurām Dās Yogīrāj of Kota called it *samādhi kā aṅg*, "a limb of *samādhi*". By *samādhi*, most of my informants meant simply a trance-like meditation carried out for long periods of time rather than the specific state of absorption described in the *Yogasūtra* and its commentaries.[152]

Only two of my informants (Dr. Tripāṭhī of Varanasi and Svāmī Praṇavānand Sarasvatī of Rishikesh) mentioned *bindudhāraṇa* as an aim of *khecarīmudrā* and I suspect that this is at least partly due to their having read haṭhayogic texts. Both associated *bindudhāraṇa* with the raising of Kuṇḍalinī. They did not mention the drinking or tasting of *amṛta*. In contrast, all my other informants said that the main aim of the practice is the drinking of *amṛta* and associated it with the ability to fly.[153] Lāl Jī Bhāī of Rishikesh practises *khecarīmudrā* for at least two to three hours every day in order to drink *amṛta*, which, he said, brings about *naśā*, "intoxication", like whisky. If he doesn't drink it every day he feels out of sorts and cannot apply himself to anything. Govind Dās Yogīrāj said that *amṛta* has a taste *jiskā varṇan kiyā nahīṃ jāyega*, "whose taste cannot be described". Similarly, Nainā Dās Yogīrāj said that the goal of the practice is the drinking of *amṛta* and that its rewards could not be described but had to be experienced.[154]

Thus, while all are agreed that *khecarīmudrā* is an important means to *samādhi*, the more educated practitioners of *haṭhayoga* frame their understanding of its aims in the terms of the prevalent ideology of orthodox asceticism (i.e. *samādhi* by means of *bindudhāraṇa* and the raising of Kuṇḍalinī), but those whose understanding derives from non-textual sources see it to be also a means of attaining such *siddhi*s as the drinking of *amṛta*, the power of flight and the ability to remain in meditation without food or water for extended periods. Despite the orthodox elite's attempts to remove or ignore the power-seeking, *siddhi*-oriented heritage of the practice (and of *haṭhayoga* in general), it lives on in the oral tradition of the *haṭhayogin*s of today.

Practitioners of *khecarīmudrā*

What can be said about ascetics who use or have used techniques involving the tongue? Apart from the passage from the *Viṣṇusmṛti*, the evidence from works prior to the haṭhayogic corpus seems to indicate that it was the preserve of unorthodox yogins. In the *Mahāsaccakasutta* the Buddha includes the technique of pressing the tongue against the palate amongst extreme ascetic disciplines, such as extended breath-retention and fasting, that were practised by Jainas and Ājīvikas. SANDERSON (1986:211) has pointed out that the *Jayadrathayāmala* preserves elements of Kāpālika practice. The descriptions of ascetics in the *Kaulajñānanirṇaya* and *Matsyendrasaṃhitā* indicate their Pāśupata and Kāpālika heritage.[155]

Khecarīmudrā gained fame as part of the *sādhana* of the Nāthas who continued this tradition of antinomian asceticism. The long version of the *Haṭhapradīpikā* calls the practitoner of *khecarīmudrā* an *avadhūta*.[156] The Nātha order was open to anyone, regardless of caste or sex and the same text says, "Pure or impure or in any state, he who practises *khecarī* is assuredly an adept", adding that both outcastes and brahmins can quickly attain *mokṣa* through the practice.[157]

The popularity of the Nāthas led to other orders adopting their appearance and practices (and, in the case of the Vedāntins, their texts). With their monopoly on the magical asceticism that so appeals to the Indian public broken, the Nāthas found it hard to compete for patronage. ELIADE (1969:302) described them as showing "all the signs of a sect in decomposition". Meanwhile, the numerically strongest ascetic orders in India today all have suborders that closely resemble the Nāthas, and some of their members practise *haṭhayoga*.[158] In my fieldwork in India I found that among *haṭhayogins* of all sects, those who practise *khecarīmudrā* are rare and are held in respect by their peers. Although the practice has a long pedigree, I doubt that it has ever been very popular.

As indicated by the inclusion of two householders among my ethnographic informants, the practice is not nowadays restricted to ascetics.[159] Whether this is because of the advent of printing having increased awareness of haṭhayogic practices or whether ascetic gurus have always initiated lay disciples into such techniques is impossible for me to say. Both the lay practitioners of *khecarīmudrā* that I met during my fieldwork were acqainted with the texts of *haṭhayoga*, but both had been initiated into the practice by ascetic gurus.

Sources

Manuscript sources of the *Khecarīvidyā*

In this chapter I first list the sources that have been collated as the basis of the critical edition of the *Khecarīvidyā*. These sources are presented here in the order in which they are reported in the apparatus. Their order reflects the age of their archetypes.[160] Thus the manuscripts that make up the group μ are given first because the archetype of μ is the earliest witness of the *Khecarīvidyā* of which we have evidence.

- A (Amritsar)

  Matsyendrasaṃhitā. Paper. Devanāgarī. Good condition. c. 1850 CE. 120 folios, numbered at top left and bottom right of verso. 30 × 14 cm. with 11 lines to a side. The text consists of 55 *paṭala*s with 14.1 to 17.1 (inclusive) corresponding to the first three *paṭala*s of the *Khecarīvidyā*. These are found at ff. 39r-49v. *Paṭala* 14 (f. $39r^{4}$–f. $41v^{5}$) corresponds to the *Khecarīvidyā*'s first *paṭala*. *Paṭala* 15 (f. $41v^{5}$–f. $45r^{7}$) ends at verse 83 (= *KhV* 2.81). *Paṭala* 16 (f. $45r^{7}$–f. $49v^{3}$) consists of 114 verses (= *KhV* 2.82–3.68b). The *Matsyendrasaṃhitā*'s *paṭala* 28 (f. $69v^{10}$–f. $70v^{5}$) corresponds to the *Khecarīvidyā*'s *paṭala* 4. There is a title page consisting of a label from "Bhajan Lal Mss Dealer and Bookseller, Gali Tokrian, Katra Safaid, Amritsar". The label has the number 64657 in arabic numerals written at the top. In addition to the information given above it states that the author of the manuscript is "Matsya Nātha", the "Recension" is "Kasmir" and it was written "Near 1900 V.S.". The "Where from obtained" section has been left blank.

  The readings of A are very close to those of J_6 and J_7 but include more careless errors. A appears to derive from J_7 which in turn derives from J_6.

  Beginning (f. $1r^{1}$):

  > oṃ śrīgaṇeśāya namaḥ śrīnāthāya namaḥ

  End (f. $120r^{1}$):

  > iti śrīmatsyendrasaṃhitāyāṃ paṃcapaṃcāśaḥtpaṭalaḥ samāptasaṃpūrṇam // oṃ yādṛśaṃ pustakaṃ dṛṣṭvā tādṛśaṃ likhitaṃ

mayā yadi śuddhaḥm aśudhaṃ vā / mama doṣa na dīyate // 1
//⊛//⊛//⊛// × // × // × //⊛//⊛//⊛//⊛//

Uncatalogued.

The Wellcome Institute for the History of Medicine, London. MS Sansk. β 1115.

- J6 (Jodhpur)

Matsyendrasaṃhitā. Paper. Devanāgarī. Complete and good condition. c. 19th century. 83 folios, numbered at top left and bottom right of verso. 26 × 10.5 cm. with 11 lines to a side. The *paṭala* and verse numbers correspond to those of the *KhV* in the same way as those of witness A described above. 14.1 (=*KhV* 1.1) is at f. 26v[4], 17.1 (=*KhV* 3.68) is at f. 34r[1] and *paṭala* 28 (=*KhV paṭala* 4) is at f. 48v[2]–f. 49r[3].

I am grateful to David WHITE for providing me with xerox copies of f. 1v, ff. 26v–49r (*paṭalas* 14–28) and f. 83v.

The readings of J6 are very close to those of A and J7. J6 appears to be the source of the readings of J7, and J7 the source of those of A.

Beginning (f. 1v[1]):

śrīgaṇeśaśāradāgurubhyo namaḥ

End (f. 83v[11]):

iti śrīmatsyendrasaṃhitāyāṃ *paṃcapaṃcāśaḥ paṭalaḥ samāptaḥ*

Described by VYAS & KSHIRSAGAR (1986:184–5).

MMSL, Mehrangarh Fort, Jodhpur. MS No. 1784.

- J7 (Jodhpur)

Matsyendrasaṃhitā. Paper. Devanāgarī. Complete. c. 19th century. 179 folios, numbered at top left and bottom right of verso. 27.5 × 12.5 cm. with 10 lines to a side. 14.1 (=*KhV* 1.1) is at f. 55r[8], 17.1 (=*KhV* 3.68) is at f. 71r[1] and *paṭala* 28 (=*KhV paṭala* 4) is at f. 102r[2]–f. 103r[7].

I am grateful to David WHITE for providing me with xerox copies of f. 1v, ff. 55r–f. 78v (*paṭalas* 14–18), ff. 100r–103r (*paṭalas* 27 and 28) and f. 179v.

The readings of J7 are very close to those of A and J6. They appear to derive from those of J6 and to be the source of those of A.

Beginning (f. 1v[1]):

śrīnāthāya namaḥ

End (f. 179v[9]):

iti śrīmatsyendrasaṃhitāyāṃ paṃcapaṃcāśaḥ paṭalaḥ samāptaḥ

Described by VYAS & KSHIRSAGAR (1986:184–5).

MMSL, Mehrangarh Fort, Jodhpur. MS No. 1782.

- G (Grantha)

Khecarīvidyā. Palm Leaf. Grantha. Incomplete, starting with 1.20a at the beginning of f. 18r.[161] At the right hand edge of f. 18r is written "Fol. 16–17 missing". 9 folios, numbered at bottom left of recto. 22.5 × 4.0 cm. with 12 lines to a side. Condition good, but occasionally worm-eaten, and worn at tops of ff. 18v, 19v, 20v and 21v. The text is not divided into *paṭala*s but is numbered intermittently (usually at every fifth verse) from 30 (at the edition's 1.29) to 48 (i.e. 248, at the edition's 3.45c). The fourth *paṭala* of the edition is not found in this manuscript. Following the text of the *KhV* is a work whose colophon (end of f. 29r) reads *iti gorakṣabodha nāma yogaśāstram.* Dominic GOODALL, who had the manuscript photocopied, reported that the rest of the codex is made up of short works on Advaita.

Colophon (f. $26r^{6}$):

> śrīmadādināthaviracite mahākāḷayogaśāstre umāmaheśvarasaṃvāde khecarīvidyāyāṃ prathamaḥ paṭalaḥ —— śivamayam —— nityakalyāṇisahāyya —— gurave namaḥ

Described by RAGHAVAN (1969b:188).

Institut français de Pondichéry. MS RE 12663.

- R_2 (Royal Asiatic Society of Bengal)[162]

Khecarīvidyā. Paper. Devanāgarī. 11 folios. Complete in three *paṭalas*.[163] Torn and badly pasted together, resulting in several lacunae. c. 18th century. Many trivial errors. Its readings show conflation with almost all the other manuscript traditions. The cover page reads *"khecarīvidyā 11 mālavīyaraghunātharāmaśarmmaṇaḥ".*

Beginning (f. $1v^{1}$):

> śrīgaṇeśāya namaḥ

End (f. $1v^{1}1$):

> iti śrīmatādināthaviṃsacite mahākālayogaśāstre umāmaheśvarasaṃvā[....]ḥ samāpto ya graṃthaḥ // //cha // cha // cha // yeṣāṃ na vidyā na tapo na dānaṃ [....] mṛtyuloke bhuvi bhārabhutā mānuṣyarūpeṇa mṛgā caranti // 1 //[164] śrīrāmasahādraḥ gaṇapa[.....]

Described by SHASTRI (1939:303).

Library of the Asiatic Society of Bengal, Kolkata. MS No. 8409.

- *U* (Upaniṣad)

Yogakuṇḍalyupaniṣad. Edited by Mahādev Śāstrī, in *The Yoga Upaniṣads* (Adyar Library 1920). *Adhyāya* 2 (pp. 321–328) consists of 49 of the first 64 *śloka*s of the first *paṭala* of the *Khecarīvidyā*. According to the preface (pp. v–vi), seven sources were used for the edition of the twenty "Yoga Upaniṣads":

1. Adyar Library TR 34. Contains "Minor Upaniṣad-s with Appayācārya's commentary". Devanāgarī.
2. Adyar Library 75883–5. Contains 108 Upaniṣads. Grantha.
3. Adyar Library 75217. Contains 108 Upaniṣads. Grantha.
4. "A Grantha MS. of 108 Upaniṣad-s lent by Mr. V. Kachchapesvara Iyer, B.A., B.L., of Vellore."
5. Adyar Library PM 211. 108 Upaniṣads with Upaniṣadbrahmayogin's commentary. Devanāgarī.
6. Adyar Library 75709–10. 108 Upaniṣads with Upaniṣadbrahmayogin's commentary. Grantha.
7. "The printed edition of 108 Upaniṣad-s published by Tukaram Javaji, Bombay, 1913, based on a South Indian MS."

Upaniṣadbrahmayogin's commentary is given at four places in the edited text:

1. after 17b (=*KhV* 1.32b):

   jñānasahitahaṭhayogasarvasvaṃ pratipādya saprapañcaṃ lambikāyogam ācaṣṭe – atheti / yathā yathāvat // 1-12 // mahyaṃ mattaḥ // 13-15 // hrīm ityādikhecarībījapūrayā
   "antarlakṣyavilīnacittapavano yogī sadā vartate
   dṛṣṭyā niścalatārayā bahir adhaḥ paśyann apaśyann api /
   mudreyaṃ khalu khecarī bhavati sā lakṣyaikatānā śivā
   śūnyāśūnyavivarjitaṃ sphurati sā tattvaṃ padaṃ vaiṣṇavi //"
   iti śrutisiddhakhecarīmudrayā khecarīyogaṃ yuñjan yaḥ kālaṃ nayati // 16 // sa yogī dehānte khecarādhipatiḥ sūryo bhūtvā khecareṣu khecaraṇīyalokeṣu sadā vaset //

2. after 20d (=*KhV* 1.35d):

   melanamantrarājam uddharati—khecareti / khavācakatayā caratīti khecaraḥ hakāraḥ āvasatham iti dhāraṇāśaktir īkāraḥ reti vahniḥ ambumaṇḍalam iti binduḥ / etat sarvaṃ militvā bhūṣitaṃ hrīm iti // 17 // khecarībījam ākhyātam / tenaiva lambikāyogaḥ prasidhyati / śiṣṭabījaṣaṭkam apy ambumaṇḍalabhūṣitam iti jñeyam / somāṃśaḥ sakāraḥ candrabījaṃ tatpratilomena tannavakaṃ varṇam uddharet bham iti // 18 // tasmāt bhakārād anulomena tryaṃśakaṃ candrabījam ākhyātaṃ sam iti / tasmāt sakārāt vilomena aparam aṣṭamaṃ varṇam uddharet mam (ṣam U^{vl}) iti // 19 // tathā makārāt vilomena aparaṃ pañcamavarṇaṃ pam (tham U^{vl}) iti viddhi / punar indoś ca bījaṃ sam ity uddharet / bahubhiḥ kakāraṣakārabindubhiḥ yukto 'yaṃ kūṭaḥ kṣam iti / āhatya bījāni sapta—hrīṃ, bhaṃ, saṃ, maṃ, paṃ, saṃ, kṣaṃ, iti // 20–21 //

3. after 27d (=*KhV* 1.42d):

   nityaṃ dvādaśavāraṃ yo japati sa māyātīto bhavatīty arthaḥ // 22–27 //

4. after the last verse, 49d (=*KhV* 1.65b):

   abhyāsakramam āha—tālv iti // 28–29 // kāryāntaraṃ hitveti / harītakī pathyāśabdārthaḥ // 30–31 // vāgīśvarīdhāmaśiraḥ jihvāgram // 32–34 // tiryak cchākāvadhiḥ śikhāmūlam ity arthaḥ // 35–36 // durlabhāṃ durlabhatām // 37 // ṣaṭsvarabhinnayā hrāṃ hrīṃ ityādinety arthaḥ // 38–40 // brahmārgalam antarjihvāsuṣiram // 41–47 // evaṃ gurumukhāt lambikāvidyām abhyasya dvādaśavarṣānuṣṭhānāt lambikāyogasiddhiḥ bhavati // 48 // śarīre sakalaṃ viśvaṃ paśyatīty anena virāṭ sūtrabījaturyarūpaṃ krameṇa pratipadyate / yatra sahasrāre rājadantordhvakuṇḍalī jihvā prasarati so 'yaṃ mārgaḥ brahmāṇḍanibho bhavati, supathyatvāt / itiśabdaḥ lambikāyogasamāptyarthaḥ, dvitīyādhyāyasamāptyarthaś ca bhavati // 49 //

Section headings are found at four places in the text:

1. at the beginning:

   khecarīvidyā

2. before 17c (*KhV* 1.32c):

   khecarīmantrarājoddhāraḥ

3. before 21a (*KhV* 1.36a):

   mantrajapāt khecarīsiddhiḥ

4. before 28a (*KhV* 1.43a):

   khecaryabhyāsakramaḥ

- T (Madras, Tamil Nadu)

  Khecarīvidyā. Paper transcription in Devanāgarī from a Kannada manuscript in bad condition. It was transcribed on 4th May 1947 from folios 80r–84r of an uncatalogued manuscript R2831(e) into a bound book, and covers seven pages of the book with 20 lines per page. It consists of the first 64 *ślokas* of *paṭala* 1 of the edited *KhV* and contains several careless errors.

Beginning:

> khecarīvidyā

End (p.7):

> iti khecarīvidyā saṃpūrṇam //
> iti śrīmaś śaṃkarācāryapadāraviṃdābhyāṃ namaḥ
> hariḥ oṃ
> kṛṣṇārpaṇam astu
> Copied By S.R.Raghuthanachar *[sic]*
> Darsanakovida 4/5/47
> Restored in 1947-48 from a library ms. R2831

Uncatalogued.

Government Oriental Manuscripts Library, Madras. MS R7878.

- S (Scindia Oriental Research Institute, Ujjain)

Bṛhatkhecarīprakāśa. Paper. Devanāgarī. Complete. 117 folios, numbered at top left of verso up to only 112 because there are two folios numbered 13, three numbered 42 and three numbered 86. I refer to these folios as 13(1), 13(2), 42(1), 42(2),[165] 42(3),[166] 86(1), 86(2) and 86(3) and thus adhere to the numbering found in the manuscript. 31.5 × 13.0 cm. with 9 or 10 lines to a side. Good condition. c. 1750–1800 CE.[167] The manuscript consists of the text of the *Khecarīvidyā*, the verses of which are written in the middle of each folio, with a *ṭīkā* by Ballāla. Sometimes the text of the *ṭīkā*, having filled up the page, runs from the bottom right of the page up the right hand margin, occasionally running around the top of the folio upside down relative to the main body of text. At many places in the manuscript comments, corrections, and additions have been made in the margins by later hands. There are very few errors in the text of the commentary. From variant readings given in the commentary it is clear that Ballāla had access to manuscripts in the traditions of groups α and β.[168]

Beginning (f. 1v[1], after a *maṅgala* invoking Hanumān written in the top margin of f. 1v by a later hand):

> śrīgaṇeśāya namaḥ // oṃ namaḥ śivāya // namaḥ sarasvatyai // gaṇādhyakṣaṃ namaskṛtya śivam aṃbāṃ sarasvatīṃ // prakāśaṃ khecarīnāmnyā bruve ballāḷanāmakaḥ //1// jayati sadā śivatīrthaḥ kāśyāṃ yasmād avāptavān eṣaḥ // vidyāṃ khecarasaṃjñāṃ sābhyāsāṃ suhitapustakāṃ sāṃgāṃ //2// ataḥ sāraṃ samālocya graṃthe⌈bhya⌉s tatvato mayā ⌈śaktye⌉ // vyākhyāsye khecarīvidyāpaṭalam iti śabdataḥ //3// ādināthaṃ ca matsyeṃdraṃ gorakṣaṃ cānyayoginaḥ // namaskurmo haṭhasyāsya rājayogasya cāptaye // 4// guror ājñāṃ samālaṃbya durbodhām api khecarīṃ // apūrvaṭīkāṃ savyākhyāṃ kurve yogijanapriyāṃ //5//

Then follows the commentary on the first verse of the *Khecarīvidyā*.

End of commentary on the first *paṭala* (f. 28v^{9}):

> iti śrīmajjāmadagnyagotra⌈bābūbhaṭṭātmaja śrī⌉rudrabhaṭṭ[...] sarvavidyānidhānayogataṃtrapravīṇaśrīballāḷaviracite khecarīpaṭalaprakāśe upodghātādidvādaśavārṣikābhyāsanirūpaṇaṃ nāma prathama udyotaḥ ⌈saṃpūrṇaḥ⌉ // cha

End of *KhV* (f. 112r^{8}):

> iti śrīmadādināthanirūpite mahākālopavartini umāmaheśvarasaṃvāde khecarīvidyāyāṃ caturthaḥ paṭalaḥ saṃpūrṇaḥ // ccha //

End of *ṭīkā* (f. 112r^{5}):

> bābūbhaṭṭatanūjarudratanujaḥ sāṃbe śive bhaktimān evaṃ sadgurupādayor atha janitror anyasādhuṣv api ballāḷo 'racayat prakāśam atulaṃ śāstraikasiddhāṃtajaṃ khecaryās tam imaṃ vibhāvanaparā gṛh*ṇ*aṃtv aho bhāvakāḥ //1// muktāphalāṃtararasagrahaṇā hi haṃsā āraktacaṃcucaraṇā madhurāsadacchāḥ // śuktyāratās taditare *'*rasamāṃsabhāvā ekākṣavṛṣṇatanavo vicaraṃti loke //2// sādhvī mātā pārvatī ∗yadbharyā rukmiṇī tathā // vāsudevaḥ somanātho putraugadhe pi nāma ca // ⌈3⌉ tenātra sad asat proktaṃ kṣaṃtavyaṃ tan mahātmabhiḥ // bālakasya pralāpo hi kṣamyate gurubhiḥ kila //4// prakāśanāt kalādīnāṃ pāṃḍityasya parasya ca // jñānaikarūpī sarvātmā śivaḥ prīṇātu kevalaḥ //5// ⌈saṃkarṣaṇo mahābuddhir brāhmaṇo hi janārdanaḥ tadannāśrayato nūnaṃ vyekaṭāṃṇṇā sahāyataḥ //⌈6⌉ agāṃka*maja* ⌈1897⌉caṃdrākhye vatsare vyaṃgatas tathā // śake saptemduke ⌈176*2*⌉ pūrṇaḥ paurṇamāsyāṃ śucer bhuvi //7//⌉ iti śrīmajjāmadagnyagotrabābūbhaṭṭātmajaśrīru drabhaṭṭasūnusarvavidyānidhānayogataṃtrapra -vīṇaśrīgoviṃdāparanāmaśrīballāḷaviracite śrīkhecarī⌈vidyāpaṭala⌉∗śe yogopayuktauṣadhīvyākhyāne ⌈caturthaṃ paṭalaṃ⌉ saṃpūrṇatām agamad iti //1//(**f. 112v**) iti bṛhatkhecarīprakāśaḥ saṃpūrṇaḥ //

At f. 1v^{2} there is a benediction to "Sadāśivatīrtha" from whom the commentator obtained the text of the *Khecarīvidyā*. In the margin, the note *saṃnyāsīty arthaḥ* has been added by a later hand confirming that the name refers to a Daśanāmī ascetic (*saṃnyāsī*). The Tīrtha suborder of the Daśanāmīs consists of Daṇḍī *saṃnyāsī*s of Brahmin birth. We thus have some indication of the milieu in which the commentary was composed. Ballāla, however, appears to have no particular axe to grind, be it that of *advaitavedānta* or brahmanic orthodoxy and describes extreme ascetic practices that go far beyond those found in other haṭhayogic texts and commentaries.[169]

Ballāla mentions and quotes from several works in his commentary (a list of all the works cited and the location(s) in the manuscript of their citations is found in the appendices, pp. 157–162). I have quoted from the commentary extensively in the notes to the translation. Unless indicated otherwise, the quotations are exactly as found in the manuscript.

Described by Raghavan (1969b:188).

Scindia Oriental Research Institute Library, Ujjain. MS 14575.

- N (Nasik)

Khecarīvidyā. Paper. Devanāgarī. Complete and in good condition. c. 20th century. 42 folios, numbered at bottom right of verso. Approximately 18 × 9 cm. 5 lines to a side.

Beginning (f. $1v^1$):

> śrīgaṇeśāya namaḥ // śrīgurubhyo namaḥ //

After the edition's final verse N has (f. $42r^5$):

> / cha // yāvaṃ naiva praviśati caranmāruto madhyamārgaṃ yāvad viṃdur na bhavati dṛḍhaḥ prāṇavātapraba(**f. 43v**)ddhaḥ // yāvat vyomnā sahajasadṛśaṃ jāyate naiva cittaṃ yāvaj jñānaṃ vadati manujo daṃbhamithyāpralāpaḥ //1// śrībhavānīśaṃkarārpaṇam astu // cha

N and W_1 are very similar. At 2.110c both contain an extra section consisting of *Gorakṣaśataka*$_N$ 184–90, 192 and 197–8. N concludes the second *paṭala* after this section; W_1 has the final 14 *ślokas* of the *KhV*'s second *paṭala*. The passage in N runs as follows (f. $28r^2$–f. $29v^5$):

> dhāraṇā paṃcanāḍīṣu dhyāna dvisaptanāḍikaṃ
> dinadvādaśakenaiva samādhi prāṇasaṃyamāt
> anasaṃdhāna yo yogai soḍaṃlasatināṃgināṃ
> tathātmanasayor aikyaṃ samādhiḥ so bhidhīyate
> tathā saṃkṣīyate prāṇo mānasaṃ ca pralīyate
> tathā (**f. 28v**) samarasatvaṃ ca samādhiḥ so bhidhīyate
> yat samatvaṃ dvayor atra jīvātmāparamātmanoḥ
> naṣṭasamastasaṃkalpa samādhiḥ so bhidhīyate
> iṃdriyāṇi manovṛtti sarvajīvāśrayaṃ bhavet
> atha yat tad gate jīve na mano neṃdriyāṇi ca
> na gaṃdho na raso rūpaṃ na sparśaḥ śabdatanmayaṃ
> nātmānaṃ na paraṃ vetti yogī yuktiṃ samādhi(**f. 29r**)na
> khādyate na sa kālena bādhyate na sa karmaṇā
> bādhyate na sa kenāpi yogī yuktisamādhitaḥ
> na ca jānāti śītoṣṇaṃ na duḥkhaṃ na sukhaṃ tathā
> na mānaṃ nāvamānaṃ ca yogī yuktasamādhitaḥ
> avadhya sarvaśāstrāṇām abādhyaḥ sarvadehināṃ
> agrāhyo maṃtrataṃtrāṇāṃ yogī yuktasamādhitaḥ
> nirādyaṃ ca nirālaṃbaṃ niḥprapaṃcaṃ nirāśra(**f. 29v**)yaṃ

nirāya ca nirākāraṃ tatvaṃ tatvavido viduḥ
dugdhe kṣīraṃ ghṛte sarpir agnau vahnir ivārpayet
tanmayatvaṃ vraje yogī sa līnaḥ parame pade
sakāra sarvavarṇeṣu yuktaceṣṭas tu sarvataḥ
yuktāni drāvabodhas tu yas tatvaṃ sa ca viṃdati
bhavabhaya bhavavahnir muktisopānapaṃktiḥ
prakaṭitaparamārthe yāni guhyaṃ

The P.D. Chandratre mentioned as the owner of a manuscript of the *Khecarīvidyā* in the NCC (RAGHAVAN 1969b:188) gave all his manuscripts to the Sarvajanik Library, Nasik. The *Khecarīvidyā* MS is No. 1973; acc. No. 5/3 in the library hand-list.

- W_1 (Wai Prajñāpāṭhaśālā)

Yogaśāstrakhecarīmudrāpaṭala. Devanāgarī. Paper. Complete and in good condition. Dated Śaka 1777 (1855 CE). 25 folios numbered at bottom right of verso. 21.5 × 15.0 cm. 10 lines to a side. On the front cover is written:

// atha yogaśāstrakhecarīmudrāpaṭalaprāraṃbhaḥ //

On the back (f. 25v) is written:

// iti yogaśāstrakhecarīmudrāpaṭalasamāptaḥ //

Beginning (f. $1v^1$):

śrīgaṇeśāya namaḥ // śrīsarasvatyai namaḥ // śrīgurubhyo namaḥ

End (f. $24v^9$):

iti śrī ādināthanirūpite mahākālayogaśāstre umāmaheśvarasaṃvāde (**f. 25r**) khecarīmudrābījaṃ nāma caturthapaṭalaṃ saṃpūrṇaṃ // // śrīkṛṣṇārpanam astu // // śake 1777 rākṣasanāmasaṃvatsare bhādrapadakṛṣṇaṣaṣṭhyāṃ tithau iṃduvāsare taddine pustakaṃ samāptaḥ // // śubhaṃ bhavatu // // cha // //

As mentioned above, both N and W_1 contain an extra section of 12 *śloka*s, consisting of *Gorakṣaśataka*$_N$ 184–90, 192 and 197–8, at 2.111c. N concludes the second *paṭala* after this section; W_1 has the usual last 14 verses. In W_1 this section is as follows (f. $15r^3$–f. $16r^2$):

satatadhyānataḥ paraṃ //
dhāraṇā paṃcanāḍīṣu dhyānaṃ dviḥsaptanāḍikaṃ //
dinadvādaśakenaiva sadhiḥ prāṇasaṃtramāt //
anusaṃdhāna yo yogai sohaṃ lasatināṃgināṃ //
tathātmamanasayor aikyaṃ samādhiḥ so bhidhīyate //
yathā saṃkṣīyate prāṇo mānasaṃ ca pralīyate //
tathā samarasatvaṃ ca samādhiḥ so bhidhīyate //

yat samatvaṃ dvayor atra jīvātmāparamātmanoḥ //
naṣṭaḥ samastasaṃkalpaḥ samādhiḥ so bhidhīyate //
iṃdriyāṇi manovṛtti sarvajīvāśrayaṃ bhavet //
atha yat tad ga(f. 15v)te jīve na mano neṃdriyāṇi ca //
na gaṃdho na raso rūpaṃ na sparśaḥ śabdatanmayaṃ //
nātmānaṃ na paraṃ vetti yogī yuktaḥ samādhinā //
khādyate na sa kālena bādhyate na sa karmaṇā //
bādhyate na sa kenāpi yogī yuktaḥ samādhinā //
na ca jānāti śītoṣṇaṃ na duḥkhaṃ na sukhaṃ tathā //
na mānaṃ nāpamānaṃ ca yogī yukta samādhitaḥ //
abadhyaḥ sarvaśāstrāṇām abādhyaḥ sarvadehināṃ //
agrāhyo maṃtrataṃtrāṇāṃ yogī yukta samādhitaḥ //
nirādyaṃ ca nirālaṃbaṃ niṣprapaṃca nirāśrayaṃ //
nirāmayaṃ nirākāraṃ tatvaṃ tatvavido viduḥ //

dugdhe kṣīraṃ ghṛte sarpir agnār agnir ivārpayet //
tanmayatvaṃ vrajet yogī sa līnaḥ parame pade //
sakāra sarvavarṇeṣu yuktaceṣṭas tu sarvataḥ //
yukta(f. 16r)nidrāvabādhas tu yas tatvaṃ sa ca viṃdati //
bhavabhaya va*bhe vahnir muktisopānapaṃktiḥ //
prakaṭitaparamārthe yāni guhyaṃ

W1 also has an additional passage at the end of the text which is not found in N (f. 23v[4]–f. 24v[9]):

śrīsūryaśastra 1 caṃdraśastra 2 rudraśastra 3 bhavānīśastra 4 gaṇapatiśastra 5 iṃdraśastra 6 brahmaśastra 7 cohyāsīsiddhaśastra 8 navanāthaśastra 9 kuṃbhaśastra 10 śvetarajaśastra 11 nakhaśastra 12 romaśastra 13 cāpaśastra 14 kaiṃcaśastra 15 siddhaśastra 16 etāni śastrāṇi khecarīchedanārthaṃ // tena vṛddhigāmī bhavati jihvā etat // [*The next section, up to* khecarīpaṭele, *is also found in the colophon of* K1] // īśvara uvāca // khecarīsamarpaṇaṃ / / sa tu khecarīmaṃtragraṃthokta // someśān navamaṃ varṇam ityādi // gamanasaphalaṃ // ṣaḍākṣarakhecarībījaṃ // hrīṃkārā khecarīpaṭele paśo anekayogeśvarāsādhitale upadeśakramaṃ // [*There follows a ṣaṭkoṇa star with* oṃ *at the top*, sa *to the right*, kha *at the bottom and* phroṃ *to the left. In the points, starting at the top and going clockwise, are* gaṃ, saṃ, na, ma, pha *and* laṃ. *In the centre is* hrīṃ.] asya śrīkhecarīmaṃtrasya // kapila ṛṣiḥ // siddhir anāyāse khecarīmudrāprasādasidhyarthe jape viniyogaḥ // atha nyāsaḥ // gaṃ hṛdayāya namaḥ // saṃ śirase svāhā // naṃ śikhāyai vaṣaṭ // ma kavacāya huṃ // pha netratrayāya vauṣaṭ // laṃ astrāya phaṭ // hrāṃ hrīṃ hrūṃ hraiṃ hrauṃ hraḥ iti ṣaḍaṃgaḥ // ādhārapadmabhavena khecararājahaṃsam atar mahāgaganavāsavibhāpralekhaṃ // ānnaṃdabījakam anaṃgaripoḥ puraṃdhrīm

> ābrahmalokajananīm abhivādaye tvāṃ // mūlālavālakuharād uditā bhavānīṃ // oṃ hrīṃ gasanasaphalaṃ aṃsakhaphroṃ // iti maṃtraḥ //

Throughout the manuscript several incorrect "corrections" have been made in the margin.

Described by RAGHAVAN (1969b:188).

Prajñāpāṭhaśālā, Wai, Maharashtra. List No. 6-4/398.

- M (Mysore)

Khecarīpaṭala. Paper. Devanāgarī. 13 folios, numbered on bottom right of verso. Approximately 22 × 8 cm., with 11 lines to a side. Complete and in good condition. c. 19th century. Untidy hand.

Beginning (f. 1v[1]):

> śrīgaṇeśāya namaḥ // īśvara uvāca //

End (f. 13r[8]):

> iti siddhauṣadhāni //

The first three *paṭala*s end:

> iti śrī ādināthaviracite mahākālayogaśāstre khecaryāṃ [amukaḥ] paṭalaḥ

Described by RAGHAVAN (1969b:188).

Oriental Research Institute, Mysore. MS No. 34979 C170.

- K_1 (Kathmandu)

Catalogued as *Mahākālayogaśāstra*, but the first two folios have *khe paṭ* at top left of verso while subsequent folios have *khe vi*. Devanāgarī. Paper. Complete and in good condition. 13 folios numbered at top left of verso. 28 × 12.5 cm. with 9 lines to a side. c. 19th century. Similar to K_3 and equally full of careless errors, but both K_1 and K_3 often have good readings which they share only with μ. Final -m and homorganic nasals are not written as *anusvāra*.

Beginning (f. 1v[1]):

> oṃ namaḥ śrī gaṇeśāya namaḥ oṃ namaḥ śivāya

End (f. 13r[9]):

> iti śrīmahā(**f. 13v**)ādināthena nirūpite mahākālayogaśāstre khecaryāṃ vidyāyāṃm auṣadhayogo nāma caturtha paṭalaḥ 4 // īśvara uvāca // śrīkhecarīsamarpaṇasatu khecarīmantragranthoktasomemātuvasaṃvarṇamity ādi // gamanasaphalaṃ ṣaḍākṣarakhecarībījam // hrīṃkārā khecarīpaṭalepa

NAK 5-6568. NGMPP Reel A 207/9.

- K_3 (**K**athmandu)

  Mahākālayogaśāstra Khecarīvidyā. Devanāgarī. Paper. 17 folios, numbered at bottom right of verso. 23.1 × 10.5 cm. with 9 lines to a side. Complete and in good condition. c. 20th century. Similar to K_1 and equally full of careless errors. However, as stated above, both K_1 and K_3 often have good readings which they share only with μ.

  Beginning (f. $1v^{1}$):

  > śrīgaṇeśāya namaḥ // // oṃ namaḥ śivāya //

  End (f. $17v^{3}$):

  > iti śrīmahā ādināthena nirūpite mahākālayogaśāstre khecaryāṃ vidyāyām auṣadhyogo nāma caturthaḥ paṭalaḥ // 4 // samāptā // śubhm *[sic]* // o //

  Kesar Library, Kathmandu. MS No. 316. NGMPP Reel C 32/12. (Retake of C86/6).

- J_2 (Jodhpur)

  Khecarīpaṭalaḥ. Devanāgarī. Paper. 19 folios, numbered at bottom right of verso. Approximately 23 × 10 cm. with 8 lines to a side. Complete and in good condition. Untidy hand. Dated Samvat 1783 (1726 CE) and copied in Varanasi. From f. $15v^{7}$ to the end of *paṭala* 4, the verse order is different from that of all other witnesses apart from J_4. 3.27c–55b are found at the end of the manuscript (f. $17v^{8}$ onwards) with just the last 2 *pāda*s of *paṭala* 4 after them. 3.27c–30b can also be found as a marginal insertion on f. 15v, indicating that an attempt at sorting out the order has been made.

  Beginning (f. $1v^{1}$):

  > śrīgaṇeśāya namaḥ

  End (f. $19v^{4}$):

  > iti śrīmahādināthanirupite mahākālayogaḥ caturthaḥ paṭalaḥ samāptāḥ saṃvat 1783 likhitaṃ kāśyāṃ madhye maṇikarṇikāsanīpe // subham astu // śrīrāma // śrī // śrīrāma // śrīrāma // śrīrāma // śrīvisvesvara //

  Described by Vyas & Kshirsagar (1986:168–9).

  MMSL, Jodhpur. MS No. 1375.

- J_4 (Jodhpur)

  Khecarīvidyā. Devanāgarī. Paper. 15 folios, numbered at top left of verso. Approximately 23 × 10.5 cm. with 9 lines to a side. Complete and in good condition. Dated Samvat 1740 (1683 CE) and copied in Varanasi. As in J2, from 3.27b (f. 12v^{1}) the verse order is different from that of other witnesses. 3.27c–3.55c is found at the end of the manuscript (f. 14r^{5} to f. 15v^{5}). 3.27c–29d is also given in its usual position at f. 12v$^{1-3}$. 3.55c to the end of *paṭala* 4 is found after this, at f. 12v^{3}– f. 14r^{5}.

On f. 1r is written twice, in different hands, a *nyāsa* of a six-syllable mantra. The first is in the same hand as the rest of the manuscript and is easy to read:

> anyanyāsa haṃ hṛdayāya namaḥ saṃ sirase svāhā ṣaṃ sikhāya vauṣaṭ phaṃ kavacāya hūṃ raṃ netratrayāya baṣaṭ iṃ strāya phaṭ // hsphrīṃ //

The second is upside-down relative to the first, in a different hand and very unclear, with some parts so faded as to be illegible:

> haṃ *dayāya namaḥ saṃ śirase svāhā // khaṃ *i*āya vauṣaṭ // phaṃ kavacāya hūṃ // raṃ netratrayāya ***īṃ ⌈astrāya phaṭ⌉// 7 // *[Above in a different hand]* hskhphrīṃ

Beginning (f. 1v^{1}):

> śrīgaṇeśāya namaḥ // atha khecarīpaṭala likhyate //

End (f. 15v^{5}):

> iti śrīmadādināthanirūpite mahākālayogaśāstre° *[sic]* caturthaḥ paṭalaḥ // 4 // saṃvat // 1740 // agahanakṛṣṇa ekama ravivāsara likhitaṃ gaṃgānāthena kāsyāṃ madhye svarga⌈dvā⌉rīsiddhipīṭhe maṇikarṇikātārakesvarasamīpe pustakaṃ saṃpūrṇaṃ samāptaṃ lekhakapāṭhakānāṃ subhaṃ bhuyāt // // // śrīādināthāya namaḥ // devyai namaḥ //

Described by VYAS & KSHIRSAGAR (1986:168–9).

MMSL, Jodhpur. MS No. 1377.

- V (Vaḍodarā)

Khecarīvidyā. Devanāgarī. Paper. 20 folios, numbered on bottom right of verso. Approximately 24 × 12 cm. with 9 or 10 lines to a side. Complete and in good condition. c. 19th century. From the beginning of *paṭala* 3 (f. 14v^{8}) to the end of the manuscript another hand has deliberately altered the text to produce nonsense. For example, at 3.2c (f. 14v^{10}) भित्वा रसनया योगी has been altered to भित्वा रेसंमयो योगी. Corrected forms of these alterations have been used in the critical edition; the uncorrected forms are given in the full collation at http://www.khecari.com. Uncorrected readings are marked V^{ae}, corrected readings V^{pe} (V *ante/post emendationem*).

Beginning (f. 1v^{1}):

// śrī gaṇeśāya namaḥ // śrī gurubhyo namaḥ //

End (f. 20v[4]):

iti śrīmadādināthanirūpite mahākālayogaśāstre umāmaheśvarasaṃvāde khecarīvidyāyāṃ caturthaḥ paṭalaḥ // 4 //

After the colophon is written in a different hand from the rest of the manuscript (f. 20v[7]):

oṃ hrīṃ ⌈gaṃ⌉saṃ naṃ maṃ phaṃ laṃ // phreṃ ṣaṭdīrghabhājā // oṃ hrīṃ gaṃ saṃ naṃ maṃ phaṃ laṃ aṃ saṃ khaṃ

Described by RAGHAVAN (1969b:188).

Oriental Institute, Baroda. MS No. 4109.

- K_4 (Kathmandu)

Khecarīvidyā. Paper. Devanāgarī. 11 folios, numbered at top left and bottom right of verso. 27.1 × 12.4 cm. with 10 lines to a side. Complete and in good condition. c. 18th century. K_4 is very similar to J_2 but shows contamination with the manuscript traditions of J_6 (1.18c) and $\mu GS\alpha$ (2.28b). There are some idiosyncracies in writing style: *tu* looks like *nu*, *dhā* is written as *dhya*, *ca* and *ja* in conjunct consonants are written vertically; *-o* is often wrongly written for *-ī* and there are many incorrect *anusvāras*.

Beginning (f. 1v[1]):

śrīgaṇeśāya namaḥ

End (f. 11v[3]):

iti śrīmahādināthanirūpite mahākālayogaśāstre khecarīvidyāyāṃ umāmaheśvarasaṃvāde caturthaḥ paṭalaḥ samāptaḥ

NAK 4-1817. NGMPP Reel A 1289/9.

- K_2 (Kathmandu)

Khecarīvidyā. Paper. Devanāgarī. 15 folios, numbered at top left and bottom right of verso. 28.6 × 12 cm. with 11 lines to a side. Complete and in fair condition. c. 19th century. Full of simple errors and very close to the readings of P but occasionally unique (e.g. 3.31b, 3.59b).

Beginning (f. 1v[1]):

śrīmataṃ rāmānujāya namaḥ oṃ

End (f. 14v[9]):

iti śrīmahākālayogaśāstre umāmaheśvarasamvāde ādināthaviracite caturthapaṭalaḥ 4 ⊛

After the *Khecarīvidyā* the codex has two short works: from f. $14v^{9}$–f. $15v^{10}$ is a work describing a mantra and its effects whose colophon reads:

> itty ātharvaṇavede upaniṣadaḥ prātemṛttyulāṃgūlaṃ (**f. 15v**) samāptam ❀

The second work (f. $15v^{1-10}$) has the following colophon:

> iti śrī atharvaṇavedokta allopaniṣat samāptā ❀ ❀ ❀ ❀ ❀ ❀

Found in Janakpur. From the private collection of Rāmakṛpālaśaraṇa. NGMPP Reel M 23/10.

- P (Pune)

Khecarīvidyā. Paper. Devanāgarī. 15 folios, numbered at top left and bottom right of verso. Approximately 22 × 11 cm. with 9 lines to a side. Complete and in good condition. Dated Samvat 1805 (1748 CE) and copied in Varanasi.

Beginning (f. $1v^{1}$):

> śrīgaṇeśāya namaḥ

End (f. $15v^{3}$):

> iti śrīmadināthanirupite mahākālayogaśāstre khecarīvidyāyāṃ umāmaheśvarasaṃvāde caturthaṃḥ paṭalaḥ saṃpūrṇaṃ saṃvat 1805 śamai nāma agahanamāse śuklu pakṣe ca paṃcamīyāṃ ravīvāśare // liḥ kāśyā madhye kedāraghāṭanyāre hanumānaghāṭa /

Described by RAGHAVAN (1969b:188).

Bhandarkar Oriental Research Institute, Pune. MS 129 of A1882–3.[170]

- J3 (Jodhpur)

Khecarīvidyā. Devanāgarī. Paper. 23 folios, numbered at bottom right of verso. The sixth and seventh folios are both numbered 6; all subsequent folios are thus numbered one less than they should be. Approximately 25 × 11 cm. with 7 lines to a side. Complete and in good condition. c. 18th century.

Beginning (f. $1v^{1}$):

> śrīgaṇeśāya namaḥ // atha khecarīpaṭa likhyate // śrīśiva uvāca //

End (f. $23v^{3}$):

> iti śrīmadādinātheprokte mahākālayogaśāstre umāmaheśvarasaṃvade khecarīvidyāyāṃ caturthapaṭalaḥ // samāptaṃ // hasta akṣa viśvanāthena likhitaṃ // cha // cha // cha // cha // cha // cha // cha //

Described by VYAS & KSHIRSAGAR (1986:168–9).

MMSL, Jodhpur. MS No. 1376.

- F (Institut Français de Pondichéry)

Khecarīvidyā. Telugu. Paper. 37 pages, numbered in arabic numerals at the top of each page. 17.5 × 22 cm. with 19 lines to a side. c. 1850 CE. *Paṭala* 1 is written in a neat hand. *Paṭala* 2 onwards (from p. 9 l. 8) is written in a less tidy hand which becomes progressively untidier. This second hand has also made some corrections to *paṭala* 1. Aspirated and unaspirated consonants are often confused. In sandhi final *-ḥ* assumes the form of a following sibilant. Initial *e-* is written *ye-*.

Beginning (p.1 l.2):

> śrīmātre namaḥ śrīsaccidānandasadguruparabrahmane namaḥ śrī mahāgaṇādhipataye namaḥ
>
> > śuklāmbaradharaṃ viṣṇuṃ śaśivarṇaṃ caturbhujaṃ
> > prasannavadanaṃ dhyāyet sarvavighnopaśāntaye

End (p.37 l.4):

> iti śrīmadādināthanirūpite mahākālayogaśāstre khecarīvidyāyāṃ caturthaḥ paṭalaḥ hariḥ oṃ tat sat sarvaṃ śrī kṛṣṇārpaṇam astu

Described by RAGHAVAN (1969b:188).

Institut français de Pondichéry. MS RE 19027.

- K5 (Kathmandu)

Khecarīvidyā. Devanāgarī. Good condition. 14 folios numbered 1 to 15 with folio 11 missing. Numbered at top left and bottom right of verso. 27 × 11.7 cm. with 9 lines to a side. Dated 1813 CE. Readings generally match β but are occasionally unique (e.g. *śaṃkarapūjanāt* at 1.22d) and in *paṭala* 4 show conflation with witnesses of α, especially M (see e.g. 4.3c).

Beginning (f. 1v[1]):

> śrīkṛṣṇāya namaḥ

End (f. 15r[2]):

> iti śrīmadādināthanirūpite mahākālayogaśāstre umāmaheśvarasaṃvāde khecarīvidyāyāṃ caturthaḥ paṭalaḥ //4// // // śubham astu // //graṃthasaṃkhyā//285//oṃ maṅgalam maṅgalanātho maṅgalam maṅgalā sutaḥ//maṅgalam maṅgalā nityaṅ karotu mama maṃdire //1//oṃ maṅgalam bhagavān viṣṇur maṅgalaṅ garuḍadhvajaḥ//maṅgalaṃ puṇḍarikākṣo maṅgalāyatano hariḥ//2// //yādṛśaṃ pustakaṃ dṛṣṭvā tādṛśaṃ likhitaṃ mayā//yadi śuddham

aśuddhaṃ vā śodhanīyā mahajjanaiḥ//3// //idaṃ pustakaṃ śrī-******** *(these syllables have been deliberately obscured)* sya//śrīḥ/ / //śrīvikramādityasaṃvat 1870//śrīśalivāhanīyaśāke 1735//śrīnaipālāvde 933//vaiśākhamāsi sitetaradale vyālatithau vudhavāsare likhitam idam pustakam pāśu[pata]kṣatre śubham bhūyāt // // //

MS No. 6-1636 from the Rāṣṭrīyābhilekhālaya. NGMPP Reel A 999/7.

- K_6 (Kathmandu)

  Khecarīvidyā. Paper. Devanāgarī and Nevārī. 20 folios numbered 2–21 with 1 and 22 missing due to damage. Numbered at bottom right of verso. c. 19th century. Starts in reasonably tidy Devanāgarī but at f. $5r^2$ becomes Nevārī with occasional reversions to Devanāgarī, giving the impression that the scribe was copying from a Devanāgarī witness but slipped into his native hand. Readings generally tally with those of β but some contamination is evident, e.g. with α_1 at 3.65b. Nasals are usually assimilated with following consonants and not written as *anusvāras*; *sch* is written for *sth*. Neither of these idiosyncracies is reported in the collations.

  NGMPP Reel No. E1145/12.

- C (Chandra Shum Shere)

  Khecarīvidhāna. Paper. Devanāgarī. 7 folios. Good condition. Incomplete, ending at 2.14d. c. 19th century.

  Beginning (f. $1v^1$):

  > śrīgaṇeśāya namaḥ

  Uncatalogued.

  Bodleian Library, Oxford. MS e.155(5) in the Chandra Shum Shere collection.

- J_1 (Jodhpur)

  Khecarīvidyā. Devanāgarī. Paper. 16 folios, numbered at bottom right of verso. 27 × 13 cm. with 9 lines to a side. Complete and in good condition. c. 18th century.

  Beginning (f. $1r^1$):

  > śrīnāthāya namaḥ

  End (f. $16r^8$):

  > iti śrīmadādināthaniropite mahākālayogaśāstre khecarīvidyāyāṃ umāmaheśvarasaṃvāde caturthaḥ paṭalaṃ samāptam iti // // śrīkalyāṇam astu

Described by VYAS & KSHIRSAGAR (1986:168–9).

MMSL, Jodhpur. MS No. 1374.

- J5 (Jodhpur)

Khecarīvidyā. Devanāgarī. Paper. 9 folios, numbered at top left and bottom right of verso. 29.5 × 15.5 cm. with 14 lines to a side. Complete and in good condition. c. 18th century. For *sth* the scribe writes *sch*—this is not reported in the collations.

Beginning (f. 1v[1]):

> śrīyogeśvarāya namaḥ

End (f. 9v[12]):

> iti śrīmadādināthaniropitem mahākālayogaśāstre khecarīvidyāyāṃ umāmaheśvarasaṃvāde caturthaḥ paṭalaṃ // cha // cha // cha //

Described by VYAS & KSHIRSAGAR (1986:170–1).

MMSL, Jodhpur. MS No. 1378.

- W2 (Wai Prajñāpāṭhaśālā)

Khecarīmudrāpaṭala. Paper. Devanāgarī. 18 folios, numbered at bottom right and top left of each folio. 21.5 × 11.5 cm. with 10 lines to a side. Complete and in good condition. c. 19th century. The covering folio has *haṭṭadīpikā* written in its centre and the rest of the codex (ff. 18v–39r) consists of the *Haṭhapradīpikā* of Svātmārāma.

Beginning (f. 1v[1]):

> // śrīgaṇeśāya namaḥ //

End (f. 18r[9]):

> iti śrīmadādināthaniropite mahākālayogaśāstre khecarīvidyāyāṃ umāmaheśvarasaṃvāde caturthapaṭalaṃ // 4 // // gratha // 279 // cha

Described by RAGHAVAN (1969b:188).

Prajñāpāṭhaśālā, Wai, Maharashtra. List No. 6-4/399.

- R1 (Royal Asiatic Society of Bengal)

Khecarīvidyā. Devanāgarī. Paper. 48 folios, numbered at bottom right of verso. 28 × 12.7 cm. 4 or 5 lines to a side. Complete and in good condition. c. 19th century. M. Ram of Marseille kindly provided me with photostat copies of xeroxes from a microfilm of the manuscript. F.17v (2.14d °*śācora*°–2.16c *trikālajñaḥ*) is missing from the copy. Due to a copyist missing a folio and then noticing his mistake, f. 35 is found after f. 39 and 3.16b–17d and

3.19 are found twice, on f. 36r and at f. 37r^{1}–f. 37v^{1} (where 3.18 is also found). The manuscript contains many minor mistakes.[171]

Beginning (f. 1v^{1}):

> oṃ śrīgaṇeśāya namaḥ

End (f. 48r^{3}):

> iti śrīmadādināthaniropite mahākālayogaśāstre khecarīvidyāyāṃ umāmaheśvarasaṃvāde caturthaḥ paṭalaṃ samāptam iti // śrīgurunārāṇa '*syaṇa*

Described by Shastri (1939:302) and Raghavan (1969b:188).

Library of the Asiatic Society of Bengal, Calcutta. MS 5854.

- B (**B**ombay)

Khecarīvidyā. Devanāgarī. Paper. 17 folios, numbered at bottom right of verso. Approximately 21 × 11 cm. with 10 lines to a side. Complete and in good condition. c. 19th century. The codex continues with the *Haṭhapradīpikā* of Svātmārāma. The text often shows signs of scribal emendation and in many places where the other members of γ have corrupt readings a meaningful reading can be found in B which is not found in any other witness.

Beginning (f. 1v^{1}):

> śrīmaṃgalamūrtaye namaḥ // śrīmadavadhūtadigaṃvarāya namaḥ //

End (f. 17r^{4}):

> iti śrīmadādināthaviracite mahākālayogaśāstre umāmaheśvarasaṃvāde khecarīvidyāyāṃ caturthaṃ paṭalaṃ samāptaṃ // 4 //

Described by Raghavan (1969b:188).

Bombay University Library. MS 2016.

There is another manuscript of the *Khecarīvidyā* in the Bombay University Library, No. 2015. It is a xerox copy of a poor reconstruction of a badly damaged paper manuscript and is full of lacunae. The crumbling original is also in the library but is little more than a collection of fragments. Where the reconstruction is legible, it is virtually identical to 2016 and its readings have not been collated. However it seems that neither is a direct copy of the other since the introductory *maṅgala*s are different. 2015 has:

> śrīgaṇeśāya namaḥ // śrīsarasvatyai namaḥ // śrīgurubhyo namaḥ //

Testimonia

- *D* (**D**īpikā)

Nārāyaṇa's *Dīpikā* on one hundred and eight *upaniṣads* cites the *KhV* in three places. Readings from the text have been included in the apparatus of the critical edition and the full collation, for which two editions of the text have been consulted:

1. D_1 : *Śrīnārāyaṇaśaṅkarānandaviracitadīpikāsametānām upaniṣadāṃ samuccayaḥ*. Ānandāśrama Sanskrit Series 29. Poona. 1895.

2. D_2 : *Ātharvvaṇopaniṣadaḥ Nārāyaṇakṛtadīpikāsahitāḥ*, ed. Rāmamaya Tarkaratna. Calcutta: Asiatic Society of Bengal (New Series No. 249). 1872.

Bouy (1994:30), following Gode (1938:128–32), dates Nārāyaṇa to between 1500 CE and 1700 CE. The *KhV* passage cited *ad Brahmavidyopaniṣad* 8 is without the corrupt interpolation of 2.75ab found after 2.72b in S$\alpha\beta\gamma$. The later limit of Nārāyaṇa's dates can thus be put back to before 1683 CE, the date that J_4 was copied.

The passages from the *KhV* which are cited are as follows:

1.45–49, 55c–56d, 64 *ad Kṣurikopaniṣad* 11 *("khecaryām")*. This citation is not found in D_2.

2.72a–73b *ad Brahmavidyopaniṣad* 8 (ascribed with the preceding quotation to Yājñavalkya in D_1; *"khecaryyām"* in D_2.)

3.32c–47d *ad Kṣurikopaniṣad* 12 *("khecarīpaṭale")*.

3.41c–42d *ad Yogaśikhopaniṣad* 2.3 *("khecaryām")*.

- O (Rajasthan **O**riental Research Institute, Jodhpur.)

Khecarīvidyā. Devanāgarī. Paper. 11 folios. Good condition. c. 19th century. Approximately 22 cm. × 10 cm. 7 lines to a side. This manuscript consists of a short treatise on physical yoga, composed mainly of citations (from the *Khecarīvidyā*, the *Śivasaṃhitā*, the *Haṭhapradīpikā*, the *Haṭhasaṃketacandrikā* and the *Yogasaṃgraha*), with sections on the *khecarīmantra*, *turīyāvasthā*, *kuṭīpraveśa*, *auṣadhikalpa* and *śivāmbupāna*. The following three passages from the edited *KhV* are cited:

1. 1.30c–33b, 35c–44d at f. $1v^7$–f. $3v^6$. Introduced with *"yathā coktaṃ khecarīpaṭale"* and closed with *"iti khecarīpaṭalāt khecarīvidyā"*. Between 1.41b and 1.41c is an explanatory section:

prastāraḥ // *h*sphreṃ khecaryai namaḥ // asya śrī khecarīmaṃtrasya bhagavān ādinātho ṛṣiḥ gāyatrī chandaḥ śrīkhecarīsiddhipradā khecarī devatā *oṃ h* sphreṃ vīja namaḥ // śaktiḥ mama yogasiddhyarthaṃ jape viniyogaḥ // oṃ hrāṃ aṃguṣṭhābhyāṃ hṛdayāya namaḥ // oṃ hrīṃ tarjanībhyāṃ śirase svāhā // oṃ hraḥ karatalakarapraṣṭābhyāṃ astrāya phaṭ //

> atha dhyānaṃ
> (**f. 3r**) mūlādibrahmaraṃdhrāṃtavisataṃtunipasīṃ //
> udyatsūryaprabhājālavidyutkoṭisamaṃprabhāṃ //14//
> caṃdrakoṭiprabhād āva trailokyaikaprabhāmayā //
> aśeṣajagadutpatisthitisaṃhārakāriṇīṃ //15//
> dhyāyed yathā mano devi niścalaṃ jāyate tataḥ //
> sahajānaṃdasaṃdohamaṃdiraṃ bhavati kṣaṇāt //16//
> mano niścalatāṃ prāptaṃ śivaśaktiprabhāvataḥ //
> samādhi jāyate tatra saṃjñādvayavijṛṃbhitaḥ //17//
> śaṃbhavena ca vedhena sukhī bhūyān nirantaraṃ //

atra suṣumṇādhyānamahimnā manasthairya svayam eva yātini // śaktiḥ suṣumṇāsarvasṛṣṭimayī mūlaprakṛtiḥ //(**f. 3v**) śivas tadantargatacitrāṃtaḥ *rūpa*paṃcadevātmakaṃ vale // iti dhyātvā japet

2. 3.1cd at f. 4r[1], introduced with *"tad uktaṃ khecarīdhavale"*. There follows a description of Kuṇḍalinī (up to f. 5r[1]) of which only the first two lines are found in the *Khecarīvidyā*.
3. 4.4 at f. 8v[7]–f. 9r[4]. This verse is not introduced as a quotation. It follows a verse about *"muṃḍīkalpa"* and is followed by *"iti vārohīkaṃdakalpaḥ"*.

MS No. 34946 in the collection of the Rajasthan Oriental Research Institute, Jodhpur. Reported as '"Khecarīvidyā" (O)' in the testimonia apparatus.[172]

- *H*1 (Haṭhapradīpikā)

The *Haṭhapradīpikā* includes four verses which it has borrowed from the *Khecarīvidyā*.[173] I have used the edition of Digambarjī & Jhā to note variants from the critical edition of the *Khecarīvidyā*. The passages are *HP* 3.33–35 (= *KhV* 1.44–46) and *HP* 4.42 (= *KhV* 3.19).

- H2 (Haṭhapradīpikā)

Haṭhapradīpikā. Devanāgarī. Paper. 171 folios, numbered at top left and bottom right of verso. 20 cm. × 11 cm. 8 or 9 lines to a side. Complete and in good condition. Copied at the command of King Jayasiṃhadeva of Jodhpur in 1707 CE.

Beginning (f. 1v[1]):

> śrīmānmahāgaṇapataye namaḥ

End (f. 171v[2]):

> iti śrīsahajanāthasiṣyeṇa śrīsvātmārāmayogīṃdreṇa viracitāyāṃ haṭhapradīpikāyāṃ siddhāṃtamuktāvalyāṃ ṣaṣṭhopadeśaḥ // iti //// śrīr astu ///////śrīmanmahārājādhirājajīśrījayasiṃhadevajīkasyājñayā likhitam idaṃ tulārāmeṇa // saṃvat 1765 varṣe caitre māse kṛṣṇe pakṣe 10 //// śrīrāmo jayati //// śrīgaṇapataye namaḥ ///// sarve te sukhinaḥ saṃtu sarveḥ saṃtu nirāmayāḥ // sarve bhadrāṇi

This is the longest version of the *Haṭhapradīpikā* so far discovered (1553 verses in 6 *upadeśas*). The manuscript is described in detail in GHAROTE 1991. In all the chapter colophons the text is called *Siddhāntamuktāvalī* as well as *Haṭhapradīpikā*.

The manuscript has a long passage (vv. 5.93–5.347) on *khecarīmudrā* at f. 95v[4] to f. 119v[1]. Amongst these verses are the following from the *Khecarīvidyā* — *paṭala* 1: 1–4, 6ab, 8–16, 19c–30b, 31c–34d, 35c–44b, 45–52b, 53ab, 54c–55b, 56c-58b, 61ab, 63c-64b, 66c-67b, 68cd, 70ab, 74cd; *paṭala* 2: 78c–81b, 93c–94b, 95cd, 96cd, 105; *paṭala* 3: 15, 18, 21ab, 26, 29cd, 30cd, 31c–32b.[174] Noteworthy features of this passage are the detailed description of the lengthening of the tongue and the division of the practice of *khecarī* into six *aṅgas*: *chedana, cālana, dohana, pāṇigharṣaṇa, praveśa* and *mantrasādhana*. The *Khecarīvidyā* verses have been collated for the critical edition and many of the remaining verses have been adduced in the introduction and notes to the translation. The readings of this witness are very similar to those of the manuscripts of the subgroup α_3.

Rajasthan Oriental Research Institute, Jodhpur. MS No. 6756.

- *H3* (Haṭhapradīpikā)

  There are two manuscripts of a ten chapter *Haṭhapradīpikā* in the MMSL. Its vv. 5.39–41 and 5.43–49 are the *Khecarīvidyā*'s vv. 1.33cd, 1.45–46, 1.48–52b, 1.53ab, 1.54a–55b, 1.56cd and 1.57ab (but not in exactly the same order); its 7.41c–42b is *KhV* 3.19. I have used the edition of GHAROTE & DEVNATH to collate the verses from the *Khecarīvidyā*.

- *Gorakṣasiddhāntasaṃgraha*

  The *Gorakṣasiddhāntasaṃgraha* (pp.10–11) quotes three verses from a *Khecarīsaṃhitā* of which only the first is found in the *Khecarīvidyā*, at 3.15. Its readings have not been collated. The text of the quotation runs as follows:

> utsṛjya sarvaśāstrāṇi japahomādi karma ca /
> dharmādharmavinirmukto yogī yogaṃ samabhyaset //
> varṇāśramābhimānena vartate śrutikiṃkaraḥ /
> abhimānavihīnas tu vartate śrutimūrddhani //

na vedo veda ity āhur vedāvedo nigadyate /
parātmā vidyate yena sa vedo veda ucyate //

Manuscripts consulted but not collated

1. *Mahākālayogaśāstra* MS No. 1794(c) in the collection of the MMSL. Paper. Devanāgarī. Incomplete. c. 19th century. 28 × 19 cm. 5 folios, numbered 2–6 at bottom right of verso. Folio 2r starts with *Khecarīvidyā* 1.43d *(digbhāga [sic] bhavet)*. This verse is numbered 23 in the manuscript. The verses of *paṭala* 1 are all numbered, the last being 57. None of the subsequent verses is numbered. The colophon to *paṭala* 1 is found at f. $3v^{4-6}$ and reads:

   iti śrīmahāādināthena mahākālayogaśāstre umāmaheśvarasaṃvāde prathamaḥ paṭalaḥ samāptaḥ //1

   The text of the *Khecarīvidyā* breaks off abruptly at f. $5r^{8}$, in the middle of *Khecarīvidyā* 2.38d with *āpādatalaryaṃta vyā śrīrāmāya namaḥ // śrīgurave namaḥ //* From here to the end of the codex (f. $6v^{12}$) is a short work on mantras, introduced with *atha japanāmasaṃkhyāṃ*.

   The text as found in this witness is very similar to that in the manuscripts of the subgroup α_3.

2. *Khecarīvidyā*. Rajasthan Oriental Research Institute, Jodhpur MS No. 39873. Paper. Devanāgarī. Incomplete. The first folio is missing; the text starts with 1.39b at f. $2r^{1}$. 10 folios, numbered at top left and bottom right of verso. Many folios are damaged. c. 18th century. 27.5 × 14 cm. In some of the *paṭala* colophons the text is said to be the *mūla* of the *Bṛhatkhecarīprakāśa* (a manuscript of which has been collated as witness S in the critical edition of the *Khecarīvidyā*), but the manuscript does not give Ballāla's commentary. In the top left of each verso is written the abbreviation *khe°rī°kā°* (every other syllable of *khecarīprakāśa*). The *paṭala* colophons are as follows:

   1. iti śrīmadādināthanirūpite mahākālataṃtrāṃtargatayogaśāstre umāmaheśvarasaṃvāde khecarīvidyāyāṃ prathamaḥ paṭalaḥ //1//
   2. iti śrīmadādināthanirūpite mahākālataṃtrāṃtargatayogaśāstre umāmaheśvarasaṃvāde khecarīvidyāyāṃ dvitīyaḥ paṭalaḥ pūrṇaḥ //2//
   3. iti śrī°vṛhatkhecarīprakāśe tṛtīyaḥ paṭalaḥ //3//
   4. iti śrīmadādināthanirūpite mahākālāntarvartiny umāmaheśvarasaṃvāde khecarīvidyāyāṃ caturthaḥ paṭalaḥ saṃpūrṇaḥ //4//iti vṛhatkhecarīmūlasamāptam //śrīḥ//śrīḥ//śrīḥ//śrīḥ//śrīḥ// śrīvedamātāyai namo namaḥ // śubhaṃ bhūyāj janatāyāḥ//

   The text of the *Khecarīvidyā* as given in this manuscript is very similar to that given in witness S.

3. *Khecarīvidyā.* Rajasthan Oriental Research Institute, Jodhpur MS No. 18376. Paper. Devanāgarī. Complete. 14 folios, numbered at the bottom right of each verso. 26.5 × 13 cm. Good condition.

 Beginning (f. 1r¹):

 > //śrīgaṇeśāya namaḥ//śrīnāthāya namaḥ//

 End (f. 14v⁸):

 > iti śrīmadādināthaniropite mahākālayogaśāstre khecarīvidyāyāṃ umāmaheśvarasaṃvāde caturthaḥ paṭalaḥ samāptam//14//

 This manuscript would be in the subgroup γ were it to be collated.

4. *Khecarīvidyā.* Asiatic Society of Bengal MS No. 8827. Paper. Devanāgarī. Incomplete. The first folio is missing; the text starts with 1.9b at f. 2r¹. 13 folios, numbered at the top left and bottom right of verso. Good condition but written in an untidy hand. 24 × 12.5 cm. 1799 CE.

 End (f. 14r⁶):

 > iti śrīmahādināthanirūpite mahākālayogaśāstre khecarīvidyāyāṃ umāmaheśvarasaṃvāde caturtha paṭalaḥ //4//śubham astu samvat 1856 śāke 1721 mārgasīrṣa śukladutiyāyāṃ guruvāsare līṣata durgāprasāda tīvāri śubhaḥ //

 There follows a description of the *khecarīmantra* almost identical to the passage in the colophon of W_1 which starts *śrīkhecarīmantrasya* and finishes *abhivādaye tvāṃ*. In this manuscript it ends with a colophon: *iti khecarīmudrābījayaṃtra nāma pañcamaḥ paṭala*. This is followed by instructions for the *mālakāgulīkalpa*.

 Described by SHASTRI (1939:304).

 This manuscript would be in the subgroup β were it to be collated.

5. *Matsyendrasaṃhitā.* MMSL, Jodhpur MS No. 1783. Paper. Devanāgarī. Complete. Good condition. 172 folios. 11 lines per page. 30 letters per line. 13.3 × 28.5 cm. (VYAS & KSHIRSAGAR 1986:184–5).[175]

 The readings of this manuscript are very similar to those of J_6 but include several careless errors. In a personal communication in August 2005 Csaba KISS pointed out to me that comparison of the readings found in this manuscript with those of J_6 at *Matsyendrasaṃhitā* 13.9 indicates that it is in fact a direct copy of J_6.

Manuscripts not consulted

I have not located the following catalogued manuscripts. I have not tried to find any of them other than the first in the list.

1. *Khecarīpaṭala*. MS No.1279 in the collection of the library of the Maharaja of Bikaner. Paper. Devanāgarī. 19 folios. 12 lines per page. "On secret worship of Piśāchīs or female imps to bring them under subjugation. An extract from a Tantra." (MITRA 1880:589). I was unable to locate this manuscript on a visit to Bikaner in February 2001. It is not mentioned in the Anup Sanskrit Library Catalogue at the Lalgarh Palace nor in the library catalogue at the Bikaner Oriental Research Institute. Dr. Usha GOSWAMI suggested that it may have been moved to Jodhpur since no works on Tantra or Yoga are held in Bikaner.

2. *Khecarīvidyā* by Śiva. 20 folios. 10 lines per page. No date. "In possession of Yajñeśvara Śāstrī, Surat" (BÜHLER 1873: A 2–3.)[176]

3. *Khecarīvidyā*. No. 1131 in HIRALAL 1926 (p. 108). "Author—Ādinātha. Subject—Yoga. Is a part of Mahākāla Yoga Śāstra by Ādinātha. Owner—- Puttelāl Gauriśaṅkar of Valgaon (Amraoti district)."

4. *Khecarīvidyā* of Ādinātha. Reported by WESTERGAARD (1846:9). Codex XII(2). Palm leaf. Telugu. 66 folios. The first 40 folios are of the *Pāṭha*[sic]-*pradīpikā*. The *KhV* is on f. 40r – f. 59v. It is part of the *Kālayogaśāstra*. It opens with *oṃ namaḥ kapileśāya mahādevāya śambhave viśvatattvapa*[sic]*dātre [ca] viśvasiddhipradāyine*. The manuscript is summarised thus: "Śiva expounds to the goddess Uma the magical science of flying through the air".[177]

5. *Khecarīvidyā*. Tantra MS 19 listed by KIELHORN (1874:38) and said to be in the possession of Chāndā Gaḍīpanta Paṭalavāra. Attributed to "Madādi" (presumably Śrīmadādinātha). 19 folios, 9 lines to a side. 342 *śloka*s. c. 1825 CE.[178]

6. *Khecarīvidyā*. MS No. 174 in a list in the Municipal Museum, Allahabad (RAGHAVAN 1969b:188).

7. *Khecarītantra*. No. 1663 A in the collection of Dacca University, Dacca, Bangladesh (RAGHAVAN *loc. cit.*).

8. *Mahākālayogaśāstram*. Oriental Research Institute, Mysore. MS No. 35007 C4063/4. Kannada (RAGHAVAN *loc. cit.).*

9. *Khecarīvidyā*. Incomplete MS listed on p. 30 of the Catalogue of Sanskrit Manuscripts in the Punjab University Library, Lahore Vol. 2 (RAGHAVAN *loc. cit.).*

10. *Khecarīvidyā*. No. 25 in a list of manuscripts belonging to Pt. Radhakrishnan of Lahore (RAGHAVAN *loc. cit.).*

11. *Khecarīvidyā*. No. 41 in the above list.

Ethnographic sources

In the introductory chapters and the notes to the translation I have occasionally used ethnographic data. I have primarily drawn on the experiences of *haṭhayogins* that I met during my fieldwork, but have also used reports of others who have met *haṭhayogins* that practise *khecarīmudrā*, and published accounts.

I met the following *haṭhayogins* during my fieldwork:[179]

Śrī Bālyogī Rām Bālak Dās Jī Though not a practitioner of *khecarīmudrā*, Rām Bālak Dās has been a *haṭhayogin* since early childhood. His insights into haṭhayogic practice have helped me considerably with my research and he introduced me to several of my other informants. He is a Rāmānandī Tyāgī *sādhu* and is for the most part itinerant but has established ashrams near Bharuch and Nasik.

Śrī Paraśurām Dās Jī Yogīrāj Another Rāmānandī Tyāgī, Paraśurām Dās has been practising *khecarīmudrā* for many years. I first met him at the Daśaharā festival in Kullu, Himachal Pradesh in October 1996, where he demonstrated the technique and discussed it with me. He is also mainly itinerant, but has established an ashram near Kota.

Śrī Govind Dās Jī Mahātyāgī Again a Rāmānandī, but of the Mahātyāgī sub-order, Govind Dās showed me *khecarīmudrā* at an ashram near Surat, Gujarat, in November 1996. He had not practised it for some years and had difficulty in doing so when I asked him to demonstrate it.

Dr. K.M.Tripāṭhī I met Dr. Tripāṭhī in December 1996 when he was working at the Yoga Centre at Benares Hindu University. He showed me a *khecarīmudrā* different from that described in haṭhayogic texts and demonstrated to me by other yogins. It involved placing the tip of the tongue behind the upper front teeth and holding it there while opening the mouth as wide as possible. This action was to be repeated at least a thousand times a day. By doing thus, pressure is exerted on the *merudaṇḍa* and Kuṇḍalinī is awakened.

Dr. Ashok Ṭhākur Dr. Ṭhākur is an āyurvedic doctor from Mumbai. I met him in January 1997. He first experienced *khecarīmudrā* when his tongue spontaneously adopted the position while he was practising *prāṇāyāma*. He demonstrated the technique to me and introduced me to his son who rarely practises yoga but is a keen swimmer and has found that his tongue also spontaneously adopts the position when he holds his breath for long periods.

Śrī Nainā Dās Jī Yogīrāj Nainā Dās is a Rāmānandī Nāgā *sādhu* who lives in Delhi. I met him in February 1997. A well-respected ascetic, he had mastered various haṭhayogic techniques, including both *khecarī-* and *vajrolī- mudrā*s but did not practise them any more.

Svāmī Praṇavānand Sarasvatī I met Svāmī Praṇavānand at his ashram in Rishikesh in February 1997. A well-educated Śaiva Dasnāmī Saṃnyāsī, he has been practising *khecarīmudrā* for many years and has written a book called *Jñān Bherī* which includes a chapter on yoga.

ŚRĪ BĀLYOGĪ LĀL JĪ BHĀĪ A neighbour of Svāmī Praṇavānand, I met Lāl Jī Bhāī at his ashram in Rishikesh in February 1997. Initiated a Rāmānandī Tyāgī, he had also studied under Nāthapanthī *sādhus*. Well-read in Sanskrit and Hindī, he has been practising *khecarīmudrā* for many years and is a fount of information on the subject.

ŚRĪ RAGHUVAR DĀS JĪ YOGĪRĀJ A *gurubhāī* of Rām Bālak Dās, Raghuvar Dās lives in Jaipur. I had met him several times before he surprised me by demonstrating *khecarīmudrā* to me at the 1998 Hardwar Kumbh Melā.

I heard accounts of the following practitioners of *khecarīmudrā*:

ŚRĪ PRAHLĀD DĀS JĪ YOGIRĀJ The guru of Rām Bālak Dās and Raghuvar Dās, Prahlād Dās was an itinerant Rāmānandī Tyāgī who had mastered the practices of *haṭhayoga*. A disciple of the famous Devrāhā Bābā, he died in 1991.

ŚRĪ RĀM DĀS JĪ YOGĪRĀJ Another disciple of Prahlād Dās, Rām Dās lives in Jaipur.

SAMPAT NĀTH A Nāthapanthī ascetic living near Ajmer, Rajasthan, Sampat Nāth is said to be an expert practitioner of *khecarīmudrā* whose tongue can reach his forehead.

SVĀMĪ RĀMĀNAND An ascetic of the Caitanya tradition, the late Svāmī Rāmānand lived at the Kaivalya Dhām Yoga Research Institute in Lonavla, Maharashtra.

I have consulted the following published accounts of the practice of *khecarīmudrā*:

BERNARD 1982: 65–69

BRUNTON 1995: 117

GERVIS 1970: 201–202

Praṇavānand SARASVATĪ 1984: 203–204

Satyānanda SARASVATĪ 1993: 278–298, 474–490

SVOBODA 1986: 278–279.

Conventions in the apparatus

There are four registers in the apparatus of the critical edition, of which only the third is found on every page. The first register reports testimonia and parallel passages from other texts. The second is found only on the first page of each *paṭala*. It reports all the witnesses for that *paṭala* and gives the key to the manuscript groups. The third register reports variants from the edited text. The fourth register reports significant omissions and additions in the witnesses and any other comments.[180]

With thirty-one witnesses of the text, a critical edition with a full collation would have an unwieldy and uninviting apparatus. I have therefore presented the text as a critical edition with only significant variants reported in the apparatus. In this case, the criteria for significance are, of course, subjective, so I have put a full collation at http://www.khecari.com for those who want to be sure of having all the available evidence.

In the critical edition, I have reported all variants whenever there is considerable disagreement between the witnesses or if I am at all unsure of which reading to choose for the edited text. If only one or two witnesses differ from the edited text, I have considered the importance of both variant and witness. Thus, if a variant appears insignificant but is from a witness that is often the only one to preserve a good reading (i.e. A, J_6, J_7, G or R_2), then I am much more likely to report it[181] than if it is from a witness that is rarely or never the only one to preserve a good reading[182] or if it is from a witness that is part of a manuscript group and the variant can easily be explained as a corruption of the form found in the other members of that group.[183] However, if one of these less individual witnesses has a variant that is interesting in its own right, then even if I think it unlikely that it might be useful in establishing an older stage of the text, I do report it. Thus I report all the variants found in *U*, the *Yogakuṇḍalyupaniṣad*.

I have composed the following half-verse and hypothetical apparatus to illustrate most of the conventions and abbreviations used in the third register of the apparatus of the critical edition:

शिवोक्ता खेचरीविद्या †कथं† संपादिता मया ॥४७॥

47c शिवोक्ता] *conj.* DEVADATTA; देव्युक्ता *codd.* ◇ खेचरी°] *em.*; ⌈शाम्भ⌉वी° A, शाम्भवी J_6J_7, खेचर° *cett.* *(unm.)* ◇ °विद्या] °∗द्यां A, °*व*द्या G, यथा γ *(unm.)* **47d** †कथं†] μGR_2*U*Tβ_1; परा Sα, साधु K_2P, न सु° J_3FK_5K_6C, तथा γ_1, परि° B^{ac}, यथा B^{pc} ◇ संपादिता मया] *transp.* μ *(unm.)*, संपादिता त्व[.] G, संपादिता ␣या N

The verse number and *pāda* letter precede the apparatus entries for each *pāda*. Entries for different elements within a *pāda* are separated by a diamond (◇). The lemma word or phrase is followed by the lemma sign (]). If the lemma word or phrase is found in the majority of witnesses then the apparatus is negative; if not, or if the distribution of witnesses whose readings match the lemma word is not clearly split within manuscript groups, then the apparatus is positive. When the apparatus is positive, all witnesses whose readings match the lemma word are given after the lemma sign, followed by a semi-colon, after which the readings of the other witnesses are reported, separated by commas. When the apparatus is negative, all the variant readings are separated by commas. The witnesses' readings are always reported in the order in which the witnesses are listed in the description of sources (μGR$_2$ *UT*S$\alpha\beta\gamma$*DH*).

In the above example, in *pāda* 47c, *śivoktā* has been conjectured by Devadatta. All the witnesses ("*codd.*") have the reading *devyuktā*.

In the next entry, that of *khecarī*°, the sign "°" is used to indicate that *khecarī* is part of a longer word or compound. The abbreviation *em.* indicates that I have emended the readings of the witnesses. Where I have emended the text to *khecarī*, witness A has ⌈*śāmbha*⌉*vī*. The "⌈" and "⌉" signs show that *śāmbha* is found in the witness as a *kākapada* or addition in the margin. Witnesses J$_6$ and J$_7$ have *śāmbhavī*. The rest of the witnesses ("*cett.*') have *khecara* which is unmetrical (" *(unm.)*").

At the next entry, for *vidyā*, the apparatus is negative. Thus all witnesses except AGγ have *vidyā*. Witness A has an illegible syllable ("$*$") followed by *dyāṃ*. Witness G has **v** *idyā*, indicating that the letter "v" is written unclearly (the "i" part of the syllable is clear).[184] The manuscript group γ has *yathā* which is unmetrical.

In *pāda* 47d, the reading *kathaṃ* is marked with crux marks ("†") because it is spurious and I have been unable to conjecture anything better. It is found in witnesses μGR$_2$ *UT*β_1; Sα have *parā*; K$_2$ and P have *sādhu*; J$_3$FK$_5$K$_6$ and C have *na su*°, with the "°" sign indicating that I think that *su* should be construed with the following word; γ_1 has *tathā*; B originally (B^{ac}, i.e. B before correction, "*ante correctionem*") had *pari* (with the "°" sign again indicating that *pari* is to be read with the following word); B has been corrected (B^{pc}, "*post correctionem*") to read *yathā*.

All the witnesses except μGN have the reading *saṃpāditā mayā*. μ has *mayā saṃpāditā* which is unmetrical. G has *saṃpāditā tva* followed by a syllable missing due to damage to the manuscript ("[.]"—the number of full stops indicates the number of syllables omitted). In N the scribe has deliberately left a gap before the syllable *yā* ("⊔yā").

A word or phrase not reported in the apparatus of the critical edition has no significant variants.

There is some misrepresentation of the witnesses' readings in the apparatus of the critical edition. I have reported neither the punctuation nor the verse numbering of any of the witnesses. Neither has been helpful in establishing the text (in *paṭala* 4 the punctuation of some witnesses only added to the confusion caused by the different metres). Where the apparatus is positive and I have reported that readings match the lemmata, they often do not match them exactly. This is because the lemmata are reproduced as they are found in the edited text and the Sanskrit of the edited text has been standardised: *-m* at the end of a half-verse is written as such but is found as *-ṃ* in almost all the witnesses; homorganic nasals have been written in full in the edited text while again almost all the witnesses use only *anusvāra*.

In order to keep the apparatus to a manageable size, I have occasionally sacrificed veracity for economy of space. When grouping readings together, I have ignored gemination and degemination of consonants in ligature with semivowels,[185] variant spellings,[186] and confusion of *v* with *b* and *s* with *ś*. I do not report variants that are the result of different effects of *sandhi* caused by variants that I do report.[187] When the reading of one or two members of a manuscript group differs from the rest of the group in a way that I consider insignificant, I ignore the variant and report that the group agrees on that reading.[188] Occasionally I report a variant in a corrected form.[189] I have only corrected readings in this way when I am confident that I am not obscuring any important detail. If I am unsure of the reading adopted in the edited text then I include all available information.

खेचरीविद्या

प्रथमः पटलः

ईश्वर उवाच
अथ देवि प्रवक्ष्यामि विद्यां खेचरिसंज्ञिताम् ।
यया विज्ञातया च स्याल्लोके ऽस्मिन्नजरामरः ॥१॥
मृत्युव्याधिजराग्रस्तं दृष्ट्वा विश्वमिदं प्रिये ।
बुद्धिं दृढतरां कृत्वा खेचरीं तु समाश्रयेत् ॥२॥
जरामृत्युगदघ्नीं यः खेचरीं वेत्ति भूतले ।
ग्रन्थतश्चार्थतश्चैव तदभ्यासप्रयोगतः ॥३॥
[मेलकम्]
तं देवि सर्वभावेन गुरुं नत्वा समाश्रयेत् ।
दुर्लभा खेचरीविद्या तदभ्यासश्च दुर्लभः ॥४॥
अभ्यासो मेलकं चैव युगपन्नैव सिध्यति ।

Witnesses for the first paṭala:
$\mathrm{AJ_6J_7R_2SNW_1MK_1K_3J_2J_4VK_4K_2PJ_3FK_5CJ_1J_5W_2R_1B}$; G *from* 20b; *U* (1–13b, 20cd, 26ab, 29–30b, 31–61d, 62c–65b); T (1–10c, 13b–65b); K_6 *from* 8a; O (30c–33b, 35c–44d); *D* (45–49, 55c–56d, 64); H_1H_3 (46–48); $\mathrm{H_2}$ (1–4, 6ab, 8–16, 19c–30b, 31c–34d, 35c–44b, 45–52b, 53ab, 54c–55b, 56c-58b, 61ab, 63c-64b, 66c-67b, 68cd, 70ab, 74cd).
$\mu=\mathrm{AJ_6J_7}$ ◇ $\alpha=\mathrm{NW_1MK_1K_3}$ $\alpha_1=\mathrm{NW_1M}$ $\alpha_2=\mathrm{NW_1}$ $\alpha_3=\mathrm{K_1K_3}$ ◇
$\beta=\mathrm{J_2J_4VK_4K_2PJ_3FK_5K_6C}$ $\beta_1=\mathrm{J_2J_4VK_4}$ ◇ $\gamma=\mathrm{J_1J_5W_2R_1B}$ $\gamma_1=\mathrm{J_1J_5W_2R_1}$ $\gamma_2=\mathrm{J_1J_5}$

1a अथ देवि] शृणु देवि $\mathrm{R_2}$, अथाह सं° *U*, अथ देवीं α_3, अथातः सं° $\mathrm{H_2}$ **1b** खेचरि°] खेचर° $\mu\mathrm{MK_2}$, खेचरी° VF *(unm.)* ◇ °संज्ञिताम्] °संहितां μ, °संज्ञिकां $\mathrm{R_2}$, °संज्ञिकाम् *U*, °संज्ञकं $\mathrm{J_3}$ **1c** यया] $\mu\alpha_3\beta_1\mathrm{H_2}$; यथा $\mathrm{R_2}$*U*$\mathrm{TPJ_3C}$, यस्या $\mathrm{S}\alpha_1\mathrm{FK_5}\gamma_1$, यस्याः B ◇ विज्ञातया च स्याल्] $\beta_1\mathrm{K_5C}$; विज्ञायते भ्यासात् μ, विज्ञाय पुंस स्या $\mathrm{R_2}$, विज्ञातवानस्य *U*T, विज्ञानवानस्य U^{vl}, विज्ञानमात्रेण $\mathrm{S}\alpha\mathrm{K_2J_3FH_2}$, विज्ञातयां च स्या P, संज्ञानमात्रेण γ **1d** लोके ऽस्मिन्न°] त्रैलोक्ये स्मिन्न° α_3 *(unm.)*, त्रैलोक्ये स्मिन् $\mathrm{H_2}$ **2a** °ग्रस्तं] °ग्रस्तो *U*, °ग्रस्ता T **2b** विश्वमिदं प्रिये] लोकमिमं प्रिये $\mathrm{R_2}$, विद्यामिमां मुने *U* **2d** खेचरीं तु समाश्रयेत्] $\mu\mathrm{R_2NM}\alpha_3\mathrm{H_2}$; खेचरीं तु सम्अभ्यसेत् *U*T, खेचरीं च समाश्रयेत् $\mathrm{SW_1}$, खेचरीं च समाचरेत् $\beta\gamma_2$, खेचरीचरमाचरेत् $\mathrm{W_2}$, खेचरी च समाचरेत् $\mathrm{R_1}$, खेचरीवरमाप्नुयात् B **3a** °घ्नीं] $\mathrm{R_2S}\alpha_1\mathrm{K_1}\beta_1\mathrm{CBH_2}$; °घ्नी $\mu\mathrm{K_3K_2PJ_3}\gamma_1$, °घ्नो *U*T ◇ यः] $\mathrm{R_2}$*U*$\mathrm{TS}\alpha_1\mathrm{K_5}$; या $\mu\mathrm{K_3H_2}$, यां $\mathrm{K_1}$, यो $\beta_1\mathrm{K_2PJ_3FC}\gamma$ **3c** ग्रन्थतश्चार्थतश्] $\mu\mathrm{R_2}$*U*$\mathrm{T}\alpha_3\mathrm{H_2}$; ग्रंथादाचार्यतश् $\mathrm{S}\alpha_1\beta\gamma$ ◇ चैव] चापि μ **3d** तदभ्यास°] तच्चयास° A **4a** तं देवि] $\mu\mathrm{TS}\alpha_1\mathrm{J_2J_4K_4}$; तां देवीं $\mathrm{R_2K_2}$, तं मुने *U*, तां सर्व° α_3, तं देवी $\mathrm{VPCH_2}$, तां देवी $\mathrm{J_3F}$, तन् देवं $\mathrm{K_5}$, तां देवि γ ◇ सर्वभावेन] °भावेन गुरुं α_3 **4b** गुरुं] तां च $\mathrm{K_1}$, तां व $\mathrm{K_3}$ ◇ नत्वा] $\mathrm{R_2SMVK_2K_5}\gamma$; मत्वा μ*U*$\mathrm{T}\alpha_2\mathrm{K_3J_2J_4K_4PJ_3FCH_2}$, *om.* $\mathrm{K_1}$ **4c** °विद्या] °मुद्रा $\alpha_3\mathrm{H_2}$ **4d** तदभ्यासश्च] $\mathrm{S}\alpha_1\beta_1\mathrm{FK_5H_2}$; तदभ्यासं च μ, तदभ्यासंश्च $\mathrm{R_2}$, तदभ्यासो पि *U*T, तदभ्यासाश्च $\mathrm{K_1}$, तद*द्री*वा च $\mathrm{K_3}$, तदभ्यासस्त $\mathrm{K_2}$, तदभ्यासस्य $\mathrm{PC}\gamma_1$, तदभ्यास सुतद $\mathrm{J_3}$ *(unm.)*, तदभासो पि $\mathrm{R_1}$, तदभ्यासस्तु B,तद्भ्यासाश्च $\mathrm{H_2}$ *(unm.)* ◇ दुर्लभः] दुर्लभं $\mu\mathrm{W_2}$, दुर्लभा $\alpha_3\mathrm{J_4H_2}$, दुल्र्लभाः $\mathrm{K_2}$ **5a** अभ्यासो] MFB; अभ्यास $\mu\mathrm{K_3}$, अभ्यासं *cett.* ◇ मेलकं] S; मेलनं *cett.*

अभ्यासमात्रनिरतो न विन्देतेह मेलकम् ॥५॥
अभ्यासाल्लभते देवि जन्मजन्मान्तरे क्व चित् ।
मेलकं जन्मनां तत्तु शतान्तेऽपि न लभ्यते ॥६॥
अभ्यासं बहुजन्मान्ते कृत्वा सद्भावसाधितम् ।
मेलकं लभते देवि योगी जन्मान्तरे क्व चित् ॥७॥
यदा तु मेलकं कामी लभते परमेश्वरि ।
तदा तत्सिद्धिमाप्नोति यदुक्तं शास्त्रसंततौ ॥८॥
ग्रन्थतश्चार्थतश्चैव मेलकं लभते यदा ।
तदा शिवत्वमाप्नोति विमुक्तः संसृतेर्भयात् ॥९॥
[अयं ग्रन्थः]
शास्त्रं विना समाबोद्धुं गुरवोऽपि न शक्नुयुः ।
तस्मात्सुदुर्लभतरं लभ्यं शास्त्रमिदं प्रिये ॥१०॥
यावन्न लभ्यते ग्रन्थस्तावद्गां पर्यटेदिमाम् ।

5c °मात्रनिरतो] $J_6J_7\alpha_3$; °मात्रविरतो A, °मत्रनिरता $R_2J_2K_4$, °निरता देवि S, °माननिरता K_2, °मंत्रनिरता J_4, °मात्रनिरता *cett.* **5d** न] विं° F ◇ विन्देतेह] μ; विंदन्तीह $R_2SMJ_2J_4K_4$-PJ_3B, विंदंते ह *U*T, विंदंति च N, च विंदति W_1, विन्दतीह α_3C *(unm.)*, विंदति स K_2, °दंति न च F, वदंति हि J_1, विदंति ह J_5 ◇ मेलकम्] $\mu\alpha_3J_3$; मेलनं *cett.* **6a** अभ्यासाल्] $\mu\alpha_3H_2$; अभ्यासो B, अभ्यासं *cett.* ◇ लभते] लभ्यते $J_6J_7J_4B$, तत्तु ते R_2 ◇ देवि] ब्रह्मन् *U*, देवीं α_3 **6b** जन्म°] योगी T **6c** मेलकं] *em.*; मेलने A, मेलनं $J_6J_7R_2$*U*T, अभ्यास° $S\alpha_2\beta\gamma$ ◇ जन्मनां तत्तु] *U*; भुजगानां च AJ_7, भुजगा नाम J_6, तत्तु जन्मान्ते R_2, तत्वजन्मीर्गं T, °मात्रनिरता $S\alpha_2\beta\gamma$ **6d** शतान्तेऽपि न लभ्यते] *U*T; जन्मांते तु न लभ्यते μ, लभ्यते मानव प्रिये R_2, न च विंदंति मेलनं $S\alpha_2J_4VK_4J_3$, न च विंदंति मेलकं $J_2PFK_5C\gamma$, न विंदति हि मेलनं K_2 **7a** अभ्यासं] *om.* R_2, अभ्यास° T ◇ बहुजन्मान्ते] तत्तु जन्मांते R_2 **7b** सद्°] A; तद्° $J_6J_7R_2$*U*T ◇ °साधितम्] μ*U*; °साधिते R_2, °साधितः T **7c** मेलकं] मेलके μ, मेलनं R_2*U*TMJ_4 ◇ देवि] कश्चिद् *U* **7d** योगी] जन्म° S, योगे α_3, योगि° V **8a** यदा तु] तदा तन्° μ, तदा तु R_1H_2 ◇ मेलकं] मलकं J_6J_7, मेलनं R_2*U* ◇ कामी] कर्म μ, योगी *U*TR_1, चैव N, देवि M **8b** परमेश्वरि] $\mu R_2SNMJ_4VK_4K_5K_6C\gamma H_2$; गुरुवक्त्रतः *U*, परमेश्वरी $TW_1J_2PJ_3F$, परमेश्वरीम् α_3K_2 **8c** तदा तत्] तदांतः H_2 **8d** उक्तं] उक्ता *U*, उक्तं U^{vl} ◇ °संततौ] °संमतौ J_4, °संमतां J_3, °संततैः J_6, °सत्तमैः γ **9a** ग्रन्थतश्] अभ्यासा° M, ग्रंथादा° K_2 ◇ चार्थतश्] छास्त्रतश् M, चार्यतश् $J_4K_2J_3\gamma$ **9b** मेलकं लभते] *transp.* μ, मे*ल*नं लभ्यते R_2, मेलनं लभते *U*M, मेलकं लभ्यते $J_3\gamma$ ◇ यदा] तदा AJ_7 **9d** विमुक्तः] μ; निर्मुक्तः *cett.* ◇ संसृतेर्] $S\alpha_1\beta_1FK_5$-CB; संसृति° $\mu\alpha_3H_2$ *(unm.)*, संसृतिर् R_2, सर्वसं° *U*, संस्मृति T *(unm.)*, स मृतेर् $K_2PJ_3\gamma_2R_1$, स सृतेर् K_6, संमृतेर् W_2 ◇ भयात्] $S\alpha_1\beta\gamma$; °वृतान् A, °व्र*जा*त् J_6, °वृतात् J_7, व्रजेत् R_2, °सृतेः *U*, प्रजात् $T\alpha_3H_2$ **10a** समाबोद्धुं] $R_2S\alpha_2J_4K_4PJ_3FK_5K_6CH_2$; समावोदुं A, समावोढं J_6J_7, पि संबोद्धुं *U*, पि संभोक्तुं T, बोधयितुं M, सममावोद्धुं K_1 *(unm.)*, मसावोद्धुं K_3, समावोद्धं J_2K_2, समाबोद्धु V, समोबोधं γ_2, समोबोद्धुं W_2B, स[मा]वोद्धं वै R_1 *(unm.)* **10c** सु°] स $AJ_7K_6\gamma_1$, तु α_2, धि M, च K_2 **10d** लभ्यं] $AJ_6U\alpha_3H_2$; लभ्यां J_7, तेभ्यः *cett.* ◇ प्रिये] मुने *U* **11a** लभ्यते] $J_6J_7R_2U\alpha_3J_2J_4K_4J_3H_2$; लभते $A\alpha_1VK_2PFK_5K_6C\gamma$, लभ्[य]ते S ◇ ग्रन्थस्] $\mu S\alpha_2VPFK_6C\gamma H_2$; ग्रंथ R_2, ग्रंथं $M\alpha_3K_5$, ग्रंथ $J_2J_4K_4$, ग्रंथः K_2, शास्त्रं *U*, शास्त्र J_3 **11b** तावद्गां पर्यटेद्] तावन्न पर्यटेद् N, तावत्पर्यटते γ ◇ इमाम्] यतिः *U*, इशां α_3, दिशा γ_2W_2, दिशां R_1, दिशः B

5cd *om.* VK_5W_2 **6ab** *om.* J_3W_2 **6cd** *om.* $M\alpha_3J_3J_1$ **7ab** *om.* $S\alpha\beta\gamma$ **7cd** *om.* K_2J_1 **8a** *start of readings from* K_6 ◇ तदा शिवत्वमाप्नोति विमुक्तः संसृतिवृता*त्* *add.* A **10d – 13a** *om.* T

यदा स लभ्यते देवि तदा सिद्धिः करे स्थिता ॥११॥
न शास्त्रेण विना सिद्धिरटतो ऽपि जगत्त्रये ।
तस्मान्मेलकदातारं शास्त्रदातारमीश्वरि ॥१२॥
तदभ्यासप्रदातारं शिवं मत्वा सदा यजेत् ।
तन्त्राश्च बहवो देवि मया प्रोक्ताः सुरार्चिते ॥१३॥
न तेषु खेचरीसिद्धिराख्याता मृत्युनाशिनी ।
महाकालं च मार्तण्डं विवेकाद्यं च शाबरम् ॥१४॥
विशुद्धेश्वरसंज्ञं च तथा वै जालशंवरम् ।
एतेषु तन्त्रवर्येषु तदभ्यासः प्रकाशितः ॥१५॥
क्व चित्स्पष्टं तथास्पष्टं क्व चित्तन्मेलकादिकम् ।
अस्मिन्तन्त्रवरे दिव्ये मेलकादि प्रकाशितम् ॥१६॥
यद्यज्ज्ञेयं भवेत्किं चिद् दुर्ज्ञेयं खेचरीमते ।
तत्तत्सर्वमिहास्माभिस्तव प्रीत्या प्रकाशितम् ॥१७॥

11c यदा] यावत् K_5 ◇ स लभ्यते] μ; संलभ्यते $R_2 US\alpha_3\beta_1 PJ_3K_5\gamma_1H_2$, संलभते $\alpha_2K_2FK_6$-C, स लभते M, च लभते B ◇ देवि] शास्त्रं $UM\alpha_3$ **11d** सिद्धिः] मुक्तिः M **12b** अटतो ऽपि] दृष्टा चैव *U* ◇ °त्रये] μUMF^{ac}; °त्रयं *cett.* **12c** मेलक°] मेलन° *U* **12d** ईश्वरि] अच्युतम् *U* **13a** °प्रदातारं] °प्रदं देवि M **13b** शिवं] गुरुं S ◇ सदा यजेत्] $\mu R_2S\alpha_1PK_5$-$C\gamma$; समाश्रयेत् *U*, तदाश्रये T, सदा जपेत् $\alpha_3J_2J_4K_4K_2K_6H_2$, सदा जयेत् V, सदा व्रजेत् F **13c** तन्त्राश्] μR_2; मंत्राश् *cett.* **13d** सुरार्चिते] सुरेश्वरी T, सुरेश्वरि S **14a** °सिद्धिर्] विद्यार् R_2 **14b** आख्याता मृत्युनाशिनी] आख्याता पापनाशिनी R_2, विख्यातामृतवासिनी γ **14c** मार्तण्डं] $\mu R_2S\alpha_1K_1\beta_1K_2PK_5K_6CJ_1BH_2$; मार्तांडं T, मार्त्तांडं K_3, मार्तंडो J_3, मार्तांड F, मार्त्तडं $J_5W_2R_1$ *(unm.)* **14d** °आद्यं] $\mu\beta\gamma$; °आहा R_2, °आर्थं T, °आढ्यं S, °आख्यं αH_2 ◇ शाबरम्] *conj.*; शाभरं A, शांवरं J_6J_7, शोभनं α_3, शोभितं H_2, शांभवं *cett.* **15a** विशुद्धेश्वर°] विशुद्धैश्वर्य° R_2, ⌈तंत्रं⌉विशुद्ध° M ◇ °संज्ञं] °तंत्रं T **15b** तथा वै जाल°] तद्भवं जाल° R_2, शास्त्रं वै जाल° M, तथ्य वेताल° T ◇ °शंवरम्] $\mu R_2\alpha_1J_2K_4PK_5C$; °शंबरं T, °शाबरं S, °संज्ञितं M, °मंवरे α_3, °संवरं VK_2, °मेव च J_3, °संभरं F, °शंव*रां* K_6, °शंभवं γ_1, °संभवं B, °संवरे H_2 **15c** तन्त्र°] $\mu R_2\alpha_1\beta_1K_5$; मंत्र° $TS\alpha_3K_2PJ_3FK_6C\gamma H_2$ ◇ °वर्येषु] °चर्येषु α_3K_2 **15d** तदभ्यासः] तदभ्यास $\mu\gamma_2W_2$, तदाभ्यास TK_2R_1, सदाभ्यास H_2 ◇ प्रकाशितः] $S\alpha VK_2J_3K_5K_6CW_2$-$BH_2$; प्रकाशितं $\mu J_2J_4K_4$, प्रभावतः R_2, प्रकाशतः T, प्रकीर्तितः SF, प्रकाशिताः γ_2, प्रकाशित R_1 **16a** स्पष्टं तथास्पष्टं] स्पृष्टं तथास्पृ J_6J_7 *(unm.)*, स्पष्टस्तथास्पष्टः M, स्पृष्टं तथास्पष्टं K_1, स्पृष्टं तथाप्यष्टं K_3 **16b** तन्°] $TS\alpha K_5H_2$; तं $\mu\beta_1K_2PJ_3FK_6C\gamma$ ◇ °दिकम्] °दिक् J_6J_7 *(unm.)*, °धिकं α_3 **16c** अस्मिन्] अस्मिंस् N ◇ तन्त्र°] तंत्रे AJ_7, तंत्रै J_6, मंत्र° α_3H_2 **17a** यद्यज्ज्ञेयं] $STK_2F^{ac}K_5C$; यद्यज्ञेयं $\mu\beta_1BF^{pc}$, यदा ज्ञेय R_2, यदि ज्ञेयं α, यद्यहेयं P, यदज्ञेयं J_3, यद्यद्वेयं K_6, यद्यभयं J_1, यद्यद्ज्ञयं J_5, यद्यद*यं W_2 ◇ किं चिद्] लोके S **17b** दुर्ज्ञेयं खेचरीमते] μTK_2J_3F; दुर्ज्ञेय खेचरीमते R_2, दुर्ज्ञेयं खेचरीमृते $S\alpha_1J_2VK_4PK_5C$, दुर्ज्ञेया खेचरीमता α_3, दुर्गेयं खेचरीं मते J_4, तज्ञेयं खेचरीम् ऋते K_6, गुरुज्ञेयं खेचरीमते γ_1 *(unm.)*, गुरुगम्यं च खेचरी B **17c** तत्तत्सर्वमिहास्माभिस्] ततः सम्यगिहास्माभिस् μ, तत्तत्सर्वं मया देवि MJ_3, तत्तत्सर्वं महात्माभिस् K_2P, मते तत्सर्वमास्माभिस् B **17d** प्रीत्या] देवि μ

12b अभ्यासमात्रनिरता न च विंदंति (विंदति R_1) मेलकं मेलकं लभते देवि योगी जन्मांतरे क्व चित् (*cf.* 5cd, 7cd) *add.* J_1R_1 **13c – 20b** *om.* *U* **16** *om.* R_2

तस्माच्छास्त्रं प्रलभ्येत मयोक्तमिदमद्भुतम् ।
गोपनीयं महेशानि न सर्वत्र प्रकाशितम् ॥१८॥
मन्मुखाम्बुरुहाज्जातं यस्तु शास्त्रामृतं वदेत् ।
स एव हि गुरुः सत्यमर्थतो वेत्ति यः पुनः ॥१९॥
स चाधिकतमः ख्यातो गुरुर्नास्ति ततोऽधिकः ।
लब्ध्वा शास्त्रमिदं गुह्यमन्येषां न प्रकाशयेत् ॥२०॥
सुविचार्य प्रवक्तव्यमेतन्मार्गोपजीविनाम् ।
य इदं परमं शास्त्रं यत्र तत्र प्रकाशयेत् ॥२१॥
स शीघ्रं भक्ष्यते देवि योगिनीभिः शिवाज्ञया ।
ग्रन्थिं नोद्ग्रन्थयेदस्य विना कौलिकतर्पणात् ॥२२॥
पूजितं शुभवस्त्रस्थं दिव्यधूपसुधूपितम् ।
श्रावयेद्द्विजनस्थाने योगिने योगशालिने ॥२३॥

18a प्रलभ्येत] $\mu\alpha_3$FR_1; प्रलीभ्यते T, प्रयुक्तैतन् R_2, प्रलभ्यैतन् *cett.* **18b** मयोक्तम्] यथोक्तम् α_3 **18c** गोपनीयं] सुगृह्यत्वान् R_2, गुह्याद् गुह्यं T, सुगुह्यत्वान् VK_5 ◇ महेशानि] सुगुप्तत्वा A, सुगुह्यत्वान्महेशानि J_6K_4 *(unm.)*, सुगुप्तत्वान्महेशानि J_7 *(unm.)* **18d** न सर्वत्र] μ; सम्यक्सर्वं $R_2\beta_1K_5$, सम्यक्सत्यं T, यतः सर्वं *cett.* **19b** वदेत्] $\mu\alpha_3$; पिवेत् R_2, ददेत् S$\alpha_2K_5\gamma$, च तत् T, ददत् M$J_2K_4K_2$PK_6C, ददात् J_4, ददत् V, महत् J_3, धधत् F **19d** अर्थतो वेत्ति यः] वेदयेद्यः पुनः α_2, यो वेत्ति च पुनः M **20a** स] μSF; न *cett.* ◇ चाधिकतमः] S; चाधिक समा° A, चाधिकः समा° J_6J_7, वाधिकस्तमा R_2K_3, चाधिकस् स*मा° T, चाधिकतमा W_1J_2PK_6Cγ, वाधिक*त*मा K_1, वाधिकतमया J_4 *(unm.)*, वाधिकतमा VK_4J_3, चाधिकमया K_2, हित्यधिकमा F, चाधिकतया K_5, बाधिकस्तमा H_2 ◇ ख्यातो] खातो J_2VK_4 **20b** गुरुर्नास्ति ततोऽधिकः] न गुरुस्तेन चाधिकः μ **20c** गुह्यम्] मह्यम् *U*T, गुह्यम् U^{vl} **20d** न] म AJ_7, त R_2, तत् J_2K_4, नत् J_4 **21a** सुविचार्य] μR_2MS$\alpha_3\beta H_2$; विचार्येव T, सुविचार्या α_2, सविचार्य γ_2W_2, सर्व*व*[र्य] R_1, सम्यग्विचा° B ◇ प्रवक्तव्यम्] μTS$W_1\alpha_3\beta_1$FK_5; श्ववक्तव्यम् R_2, प्रवक्तव्य NM, प्रकर्त्तव्यम् K_2PC$K_6\gamma_1H_2$, प्रकर्त्तव्यः J_3, °र्य कर्तव्यम् B **21b** एतन्मार्गोपजीविनां] SPFK_6C; एकमार्गोपजीविना μ, एष मार्गो य जीवतु R_2, एतदात्मोपजीविनं T, एष मार्गो पजीविनाम् NMβ_1K_5, एष मार्गोऽपि जीवनं W_1, एकं मार्गोपजीविनं K_1, एकं मार्गोपजीवितं K_3, एतत्मार्गोप्रजीवनां K_2, तेन मार्गोपजीविना J_3, एतन्मार्गो पि जीवनं J_1R_1, एतन्मार्गे पि जीवनं J_5W_2, एतन्मार्गे च जीवनं B, एकमार्गोपजीवितं H_2 **21c** य इदं परमं शास्त्रं] षत्पदं परमं शास्त्रं μ, प्रकाशितं यदि पुनर् G, जपदं परमं शास्त्रं K_2 **21d** यत्र तत्र प्रकाशयेत्] यथा तथा प्रकाशयेत् μ *(unm.)*, म्मूढेनात्माभियातिना G, साधकैश्च प्रका*श्*येत् R_2, यत्र कुत्र प्रकाशयेत् TSα_1^{ac} **22a** भक्ष्यते] वद्यते G **22c** ग्रन्थिं] *em.*; ग्रंथि μ, श्रजं T, ग्रंथं *cett.* ◇ नोद्ग्रन्थयेदस्य] μ; समर्पयेत्तस्य G, तु नार्पयेद्देवी R_2, सदाच्चयेकृस्य T, तु नार्पयेद्देवि SJ_2VK_4K_2PK_5K_6C, सम्अर्पयेदस्य α_1, समार्पयेद्यस्य α_3, तु नार्चयेद्देवि J_4F, तु नाये देवि J_3 *(unm.)*, तु चार्चयेद्देवि γ, समर्पयेद्यस्य H_2 **22d** विना कौलिकतर्पणात्] विना च गुरुतर्पणात् G, विना कौषकदर्पणम् T, विना कौलिकतर्पणं αH_2, नास्तिके कौलतर्प्पणात् K_2, विना शंकरपूजनात् K_5 **23a** पूजितं] पूजिते T ◇ शुभवस्त्रस्थं] शुभ्रवस्त्रेण G, तु भवेत्स्वस्थं T, शुभवस्त्रेण Sα_1, शुभवस्तुस्थं γ_1 **23b** °धूपसु°] °धूपैस्तु $R_2J_2K_4$, °धूपैश्च TS **23c** विजनस्थाने] विजने स्थाने μ, द्विजसंस्थाने Sα_2 **23d** योगिने] योगिनी M ◇ °शालिने] μGR_2TM$\alpha_3J_3K_5\gamma H_2$; °शीलिने SNJ_2K_4PFC, °शीलने W_1J_4VK_2K_6

18cd *om.* NMα_3 **20ab** *om.* NM **20b** कः : *start of readings from* G **21ab** *om.* G**21a – 25b** *om.* *U*

यस्मिन्नपूजितं शास्त्रमिदं तिष्ठति वै गृहे ।
तत्राग्निरुग्ग्रहारातिपीडा भवति निश्चितम् ॥२४॥
यत्रेदं पूजितं ग्रन्थं गृहे तिष्ठति पार्वति ।
तत्र सर्वार्थदायिन्यो वसन्ति कुलदेवताः ॥२५॥
तस्मात्सर्वप्रयत्नेन गोपनीयं विजानता ।
यस्तु योगी मया प्रोक्ता इमाः सिद्धीः समीहते ॥२६॥
स योगी सर्वभावेन गोपयेत्पुस्तकं त्विदम् ।
अहं तस्य गुरुर्देवि यत्रास्ते पुस्तकं स्वयम् ॥२७॥
गुणागुणं महेशानि पुस्तकस्य च रक्षणात् ।
प्रकटं च मया प्रोक्तमिदानीं खेचरीं शृणु ॥२८॥
यत्रास्ते च गुरुर्देवि दिव्ययोगप्रसाधकः ।
तत्र गत्वा च तेनोक्तां विद्यां संगृह्य खेचरीम् ॥२९॥
तेनोक्तं सम्यगभ्यासं कुर्यादादावतन्द्रितः ।
विद्यां च खेचरीं देवि प्रवक्ष्ये योगसिद्धिदाम् ॥३०॥

30c – 33b *cit.* "खेचरीविद्या" (O) f.1v

24a ऋपूजितं] पूजितं नु G, वै पूजितं γ 24b तिष्ठति] तिष्ठंति $\mu TJ_4J_3J_5W_2$ ◇ वै गृहे] विग्रहे A, वै ग्रहे TJ_3, चैव हि α_2, सुन्दरि M, य∗हे B 24c °रुग्ग्रहाराति°] SK_5; °रुद्रहारात्रि° AJ_6, °रुद्रहारात्रि° J_7, °रुग्रहाराति° $R_2\alpha_2J_2K_4FB$, °चोरजा पीडा T, °ररातीरणां M^{ac} *(unm.)*, °वार्रारातीरणां M^{pc}, °रुग्नहारात्रि° α_3, °रुग्राहाराति J_4, °रुग्महाराति° V, °रुग्रग्राहार्त्ति° K_2, °रुग्ग्रहारार्ति° P, °रुग्ग्रहारार्ति° J_3, °स्तग्रहारार्त्ति° K_6, °रुग्रहारार्ति° C, °रुग्णाहाराति° γ_2W_2, °∗ग्णाहारात्ति° R_1, °रूपहाराभि° H_2 24d °पीडा भवति निश्चितम्] भवत्येव हि निश्चयम् T 25a यत्रेदं] यत्रेमं μ, यत्रायं TB, यत्रेयं γ_1 ◇ पूजितं] पूजिते γ ◇ ग्रन्थं] शास्त्रं $R_2W_1MC^{pc}$, ग्रंथे γ 25b गृहे] ग्रहे AVK_2 25d वसन्ति कुल°] वसंत्यखिल° R_2 26b विजानता] प्रयत्नतः G, विजानतः α_3, विजानताः K_4K_6 26c यस्तु] $G\alpha_1$; यो ऽस्मिन् μ, यस्मि∗ R_2, यश्च T, यस्मिन् $S\beta\gamma$, तस्मिन् α_3H_2 ◇ योगी] योगि A, योगे $S\gamma$, योगो J_2, योग∗ P, योगा J_3 ◇ मया प्रोक्ता] α_2; मयोक्तानि $\mu GTS\alpha_3\beta_1PJ_3FK_5C\gamma H_2$, [....] R_2, इमां प्रोक्तां M, मया प्रोक्तान् K_2, ⌈म⌉यो भक्ता K_6 26d इमाः सिद्धीः] W_1; संसिद्धीनि μ, संसिद्धानि G, सिद्धिवाव्या° R_2, संसिद्धिर्न $T\alpha_3H_2$, सिद्धवाक्या° $S\beta\gamma$, इमाः सिद्धि N, मया सिद्धिं M ◇ समीहते] $\mu GT\alpha H_2$; °नि संवते R_2, °नि संवदेत् $S\beta\gamma$ 27c तस्य गुरुर्] तस्तु गुरुं μ 27d स्वयम्] त्विदं GMK_5B 28a °गुणं] °शुणं AJ_7, °गुणा G, °गुणां R_2, °गुणौ T, °गुण $K_2K_6\gamma$ 28b रक्षणात्] रक्षणे $\mu R_2T\alpha H_2$ 28c प्रकटं च मया प्रोक्तम्] प्रकटां च मया प्रोक्ताम् G, प्रकटत्वमिति प्रोक्तं S, प्रकटं च मया प्रोक्तां W_1F, तत्प्रकटं मया प्रोक्तम् H_2 29a च] μGR_2*U*TMF; स $S^{pc}\beta_1K_2PJ_3FK_5C\gamma$, सद् $S^{ac}J_3$, त्व N, त्वद् W_1, चा α_3, सन् K_6 ◇ गुरुर्] गुरु ATM^{ac}, गुरुं J_6J_7, गुरोर् K_2 ◇ देवि] ब्रह्मन् *U* 29b °प्रसाधकः] °प्रभावतः G, °प्रदायकः *U*, °स्य साधकः S 29c तेनोक्तां] तेनोक्त° *U*, तेनोक्तं $R_2U^{vl}S\alpha J_4J_3FJ_1R_1H_2$ 29d विद्यां संगृह्य खेचरीम्] दिव्यां संगृह्य खेचरीं G, संप्रधार्य प्रयत्नतः α_1, संप्रदायत्नयत्नतः α_3H_2 30a तेनोक्तं] $GR_2S\beta J_1R_1$; तेनोक्ते μ, तेनोक्तः *U*, तेनोक्त U^{vl}T, सम्यग° α, तेनोक्तां J_5W_2B, सम्यक् भ्या° H_2 ◇ सम्यगभ्यासं] °भ्यासं यत्नेन MK_3, °भ्यासयत्नेन α_2K_1, °सं प्रयत्नेन H_2 30b ऋादावतन्द्रितः] ऋाहावत्लंद्रितः A, ऋाहावलंद्रितः J_7, वेत्ता ऋतंद्रितः α_3, ऋादौ च तं ततः γ, *धि*त्वा ऋतन्द्रितः H_2 30c विद्यां च] तां विद्यां G ◇ देवि] देवीं GW_1 30d योग°] गण° $\alpha_2\alpha_3$, सर्व° M

24b वै – 25b तिष्ठति *om.* G (*eye-skip* तिष्ठति – तिष्ठति) 26c – 28d *om.* *U* 30cd *om.* *U*

न तया रहितो योगी खेचरीसिद्धिभाग् भवेत् ।
खेचर्या खेचरीं युञ्जन्खेचरीबीजपूर्वया ॥३१॥
खेचराधिपतिर्भूत्वा खेचरेषु सदा वसेत् ।
[मन्त्रोद्धारः]
खेचरावसथं वह्निमम्बामण्डलभूषितम् ॥३२॥
व्याख्यातं खेचरीबीजं तेन योगः प्रसिध्यति ।
मस्तकाख्या महाचण्डा शिखिवह्निकवज्रभृत् ॥३३॥
पूर्वबीजयुता विद्या व्याख्याता ह्यतिदुर्लभा ।
षडङ्गविद्यां वक्ष्यामि तया षट्स्वरभिन्नया ॥३४॥
कुर्याद्देवि यथान्यायं सर्वसिद्ध्याप्तिहेतवे ।

31a न तया रहितो] $\mu R_2\alpha_3\beta O$; *आदौ हि कशितो* G, अनया विद्यया *U*, अनया सहितो T, नैतया रहितो $S\alpha_2$, नैतया खेचरी M, न खेचर्या हितो $\gamma_2 W_2 B$, न खेचर्या विना R_1 **31b** खेचरी°] रहितो M ◇ °भाग्] °वान् R_2 **31c** खेचर्या] खेचर्यो A, खेचर्यां $G\alpha_3$ ◇ खेचरीं] $\mu R_2 US\alpha_2\alpha_3 J_3 K_5 COH_2$; खेचरी $GTM\beta_1 K_2 PF\gamma$, *om.* K_6 ◇ युञ्जन्] $\mu R_2 UTSJ_2 VK_4 PFK_5$; युजन् GC, युंज्यात् α_2, पूज्या M, योज्या K_1, योज्यात् K_3, पुंजन् J_4O, जंपन् K_2, च्युबन् J_3, *om.* K_6, युंजान् $\gamma_2 R_1$, पुंजान् W_2B, युज्यात् H_2 **31d** °पूर्वया] °पूर्वकं G, °पूरया $U\alpha_3$, °पूर्वयाः $J_2J_4K_4$ **32b** खेचरेषु] खेचरीषु K_2 **32c** खेचरा°] खेचरी° $GJ_3\gamma$, खेचरे R_2 ◇ °वसथं] $AJ_7 UTS\alpha_1\beta_1 PJ_3 FK_5 CO$; °वसंथं J_6 *(unm.)*, °वसतं G, वसथो R_2, °वसथ α_3, °हस्त्रवं K_2, °वस*थं* K_6, °वसतां J_1R_1, °वसथां J_5W_2B, वसथों H_2 ◇ वह्निम्] वह्निर् μ, वह्नीम् R_2, वह्नि MK_6, वह्निं α_3, वह्निर्म J_2K_4, वव्रज्विम् V *(unm.)* **32d** अम्बा°] $R_2SJ_4VK_4K_2PK_5C\gamma O$; अह्नी° μ, अंभो° G, अम्बु° *U*, अभ्र° T, अंडवा° N *(unm.)*, आया° W_1, वडवा° M *(unm.)*, सर्वा α_3, अवा° J_2, अथा° J_3, आबा° F, वाम K_6, अम्वा° H_2 ◇ °भूषितम्] °भूषितां FW_2B **33a** व्याख्यातं] आख्यातं *U*T, व्याख्याता K_2, व्याख्यानं γ **33b** योगः] योगी α_3H_2 **33c** मस्तकाख्या] *em.*; मस्तकाख्यो μ_a, शनैः शनैश् G, शनैः शनैर् *cett.* ◇ महाचराडा] μ_a; शिरोव्योम° G, मस्तकाश्च α_3, मस्तकार्ध V, मस्तकस्थ° H_3, मस्तकाच्च *cett.* **33d** शिखि°] J_7; शिवि° A^a, शिंखि° J_6^a, सह° α_3, महा° *cett.* ◇ °वह्नि°] μ_a; °वस्त्रं μ_b, °वज्र° $GR_2 UTS\alpha J_3H_2H_3$, °वस्त्र° $\beta_1 PK_5K_6C\gamma$, वस्त्रा° F ◇ °कवज्र°] μ_a; °कपाट° $A^bJ_7^bR_2S\alpha\beta_1PJ_3FK_5K_6C\gamma H_2H_3$, °कयाट° J_6^b, °कवाट° G*UT* ◇ °भृत्] μ_a; °धृक् $\mu_b\beta\gamma$, °वित् G, °हृत् R_2, °भित् $UTS\alpha H_2H_3$ **34a** पूर्व°] पूर्वं *U*, पूंर्व° K_1 ◇ °बीजयुता°] बीजयुतां GW_1H_2, °वीजोजिता° α_3 ◇ विद्या] विद्यां GW_1H_2 **34b** व्याख्याता] $\mu_aR_2TSM\beta_1F$; °प्याख्याता A^b, ख्याता $J_6^bJ_7^b$ *(unm.)*, व्याख्याताम् GH_2, ह्याख्याता *U*, विख्याता $N\alpha_3\gamma$, विख्यातां W_1, व्याख्याताद् K_2PK_5C, विख्याताद् J_3 ◇ ह्यतिदुर्लभा] μ_aS; यातिदुर्लभा $\mu_b\beta_1K_2PJ_3K_5C\gamma$; अतिदुर्लभा* G, ह्यतिदुर्लभ R_2, याति दुर्लभां *U*T, चान्यदुर्लभां α_2, चान्यदुर्लभा M, तिसुर्दुर्लभा K_1, निसुदुर्लभा K_3, °प्यतिदुर्लभा F, यातादू*र्ल्ल*भा K_6, अतिदुर्लभाम् H_2 **34c** षडङ्गविद्यां वक्ष्यामि] μ_a; तस्याः षडंगं कुर्वंत $J_2J_4K_4J_3F$, तस्याः षडंगं कुर्वंति K_2K_6, तस्य स्वंडं प्रकुर्वीत K_1, तस्य षंडं प्रकुर्वीत K_3, अस्याः षडङ्गं कुर्वीत H_2, तस्याः षडङ्गं कुर्वीत *cett.* **34d** तया] तथा $\mu_a\mu_b$ ◇ षट्स्वर°] $\mu_a GUT\alpha$; षट्द्वार° μ_b, षड्स R_2 *(unm.)*, षड्दीर्घ° $S\beta\gamma$, षट्चक्र° H_2 **35a** देवि] देवी GK_3, एवं *U*T, देवीं K_1, दिवि J_3 ◇ यथान्यायं] यथा न्यासं $A^aJ_7GK_5K_6$, करन्यासं *U*T, यथात्यास्त्रं J_2, यथाशास्त्रं J_4, यथात्यांस्त्रं K_4 **35b** °सिद्ध्याप्ति°] $\mu_bS\beta$; °विद्याप्ति° μ_a, सिध्यंति G, °सिद्ध्यादि° *U*T, °सिद्धिप्र° α_1, °विद्याप्र° α_3, °सिद्धार्थ° γ ◇ °हेतवे] °हेतवः G

32c – 33b *and* **35c – 36b** *transp.* R_1 **33c – 35b** *is found after* 53d *in all the witnesses that report it* $(\mu UTS\alpha\beta\gamma)$; *μ has the passage twice, at both* 33c–35b ($\mu_a=A^aJ_6^aJ_7$) *and after* 53d ($\mu_b=A^bJ_6^bJ_7^b$) **35ab** *om.* R_2

सोमेशान् नवमं वर्णं प्रतिलोमेन चोद्धरेत् ॥३५॥
तस्मात् त्रिंशकमाख्यातमक्षरं चन्द्ररूपकम् ।
तस्मादप्यष्टमं वर्णं विलोमेनापरं प्रिये ॥३६॥
तथा तत्पञ्चमं देवि तदादिरपि पञ्चमः ।
इन्द्रो ऽपि बिन्दुसंभिन्नः कूटो ऽयं परिकीर्तितः ॥३७॥
गुरूपदेशलभ्यं च सर्वलोकप्रसिद्धिदम् ।
यतस्य देहजा माया विरूपा करणाश्रया ॥३८॥
स्वप्ने ऽपि न भवेत्तस्य नित्यं द्वादशजाप्यतः ।
य इमां पञ्च लक्षाणि जपेदतिसुयन्त्रितः ॥३९॥
तस्य श्रीखेचरीसिद्धिः स्वयमेव प्रवर्तते ।
नश्यन्ति सर्वविघ्नानि प्रसीदन्ति च देवताः ॥४०॥
वलीपलितनाशश्च भविष्यति न संशयः ।

35c – 44d *cit.* “खेचरीविद्या” (O) f.2r

35c सोमेशान्] सोमेशा GO, सोमांश *U*T, सोमेशन् γ_1, सोमेशं B, शोमेशान् H_2 ◇ नवमं] नवमे G, नवकं *U*, नवमा F, नंवमं O ◇ वर्णं] वर्णा AK_3, वर्णो G^{ac} **36a** तस्मात्] तस्यास् μ, तस्माद् TM, तस्या J_4, ततस् K_2, तस्मीस् P ◇ त्रिंशकम्] $\mu GSJ_2VK_4PFK_5K_6C\gamma O$; त्रिंशकाम् R_2, त्र्यंशकम् *U*, त्र्यम्बकम् U^{vl}, अंशम् T *(unm.)*, त्रिंशाद्य° $\alpha_2\alpha_3H_2$, वि⌈शंति⌉ M, त्रि*शिं*क*म् J_4, मान्त्रिंशम् K_2, त्रिशकम् J_3 ◇ आख्यातम्] °रं शास्त्रम् α_2, ⌈मं⌉ शास्त्रम् M, °रशास्त्रम् α_3, °रं शस्त्रं H_2, आख्यातं O **36b** अक्षरं] मकारं O ◇ °रूपकम्] °भूषितं G, °सूर्यकं M **36c** अप्यष्टमं] G*U*T; अप्यष्टकं μ, अप्यष्*मं R_2, अथाष्टमं $S\alpha_1\beta\gamma$, अधाम व° α_3, अधाष्टमं H_2 ◇ वर्णं] वर्णो μ, °र्णं च α_3 **36d** विलोमेनापरं] $GR_2USα_2\beta_1PFK_5C\gamma O$; विलोमेन्य वरं A, विलोमेनावरं J_6J_7, विलोमेनापुरं TK_6, विलोमेन परं MK_2, विलोमं परमं α_3, विलोमेनाप्रियं J_3, विलो*मेनापरं* H_2 ◇ प्रिये] मुने *U* **37a** तथा] तदा U^{vl}, तस्मात् αH_2 ◇ तत्पञ्चमं] $S\beta_1PJ_3FK_5K_6C\gamma_1O$; तत्वंचमे A, तत्वंचमं J_6J_7, तत्वंचमां G, तत्पचमं R_2, तत्परमं *U*, तत्पुरमन् T, पंचममित्य् α_1H_2, परममित्य् α_3, तां पंचमं K_2, °न्यत्पंचमं B ◇ देवि] विद्धि *U*, उक्तं αH_2 **37b** तदादिर्] वेदादिर् H_2 ◇ पञ्चमः] पंचमं $\mu TK_2J_3R_1$, पंचमा *U* **37c** इन्द्रो ऽपि] इंदोश्च *U*T, चंद्रो यं M, इदापि K_2, इन्द्रापि γ_1 ◇ बिन्दुसंभिन्नः] $S\alpha_1K_2FK_5$; बिंदुसंभिन्नं $\mu\alpha_3\beta_1$-$J_3PK_6C\gamma H_2$, बिंदुसंभिंनां G, विंदुसभिंन R_2, बहुभिन्नं च *U*, बहुभिश्चल T, भिन्नसंभिन्नं O **37d** कूटो] मोच्चो G ◇ °कीर्तितः] °कीर्तितं AJ_7T **38a** गुरूपदेश°] $\mu GR_2UTK_3H_2$; गुरूपदेशाल् *cett.* **38b** सर्वलोक°] $GR_2S\beta\gamma$; सर्वयोग° μU, स वै योग° T, सर्वलोके αH_2 ◇ °सिद्धिदम्] °सिद्धि*द*: G, °सिद्धिदः F **38c** यतस्य] $K_2\gamma O$; यत्तस्य $\mu GR_2UJ_2J_4K_4C$, युक्तस्य T, न स्पृशेद् $S\alpha_1$, या तस्य $\alpha_3VK_5H_2$, यत्रस्य PF, प्रत*च्च्य* J_3, यात्रस्या K_6 ◇ देहजा] *U*T; देवजा μ-$GR_2\alpha_2J_2VK_4K_5K_6$, देवता $SMK_2PJ_3FC\gamma O$, देवया $\alpha_3J_4H_2$ ◇ माया] मायां MK_2 **38d** विरूपा] μCO; विरूप° $GR_2S\alpha_1\beta_1K_2PJ_3FK_5K_6\gamma H_2$, निरुद्ध° *U*, निरूढ° T, तद्रूप° α_3 ◇ करणाश्रया] कारणाश्रया μ, करणाश्रयां M, करणाश्रयः α_3H_2 **39a** स्वप्ने] स्वप्नो $\mu GNM\alpha_3$-$K_2K_6H_2$ ◇ न] ना $K_2PK_6J_1W_2R_1B$ ◇ भवेत्तस्य] लभेत्तस्य *U*, भवेतस्य $J_4\gamma O$ **39b** °जाप्यतः] °जप्यतः *U*T, °भावतः J_3, °जापतः K_5, °जाप्यतेः K_6 **39d** अतिसु°] μ; आसंनि° G, अपि सु° $R_2UTS\alpha_1\beta\gamma H_2O$, अपि स्व° α_3 ◇ °यन्त्रितः] °यंत्रितं J_6J_7, °यत्नतः α_1, °यांत्रितः K_6 **40a** तस्य श्री] $R_2UTS\beta\gamma O$; तस्मात् श्री μ, तस्यास्ति $\alpha_2\alpha_3$, तस्यापि M, तस्यास्त्रि H_2 **40d** प्रसीदन्ति] प्रसीदति AJ_7, प्रसीदंते α_3 ◇ च] थ AJ_7, ⌈*⌉ J_6, न K_2 ◇ देवताः] देवता $AJ_6R_2K_2J_3$ **41a** °नाशश्च] $\mu U\alpha_1K_5BO$; °नाशं च $GR_2S\alpha_3\beta_1K_2PJ_3FK_6C\gamma_1H_2$, सर्वं च T, नाश्यंति J_4

एवं लब्ध्वा महाविद्यामभ्यासं कारयेत्ततः ॥४१॥
अन्यथा क्लिश्यते देवि न सिद्धिः खेचरीपदे ।
यद्यभ्यासविधौ विद्यां न लभेत सुधामयीम् ॥४२॥
ततः संमेलकादौ च लब्ध्वा विद्यां समुज्जपेत् ।
अनया रहितो देवि न क्व चित्सिद्धिभाग् भवेत् ॥४३॥
यदेदं लभ्यते शास्त्रं तदा विद्यां समाश्रयेत् ।
ततस्तत्रोदितां सिद्धिमाशु संलभते प्रिये ॥४४॥
[खेचर्यभ्यासक्रमः]
तालुमूलं समुद्घृष्य सप्तवासरमात्मवित् ।
स्वगुरूक्तप्रकारेण मलं सर्वं विशोधयेत् ॥४५॥
स्नुहीपत्रनिभं शस्त्रं सुतीक्ष्णं स्निग्धनिर्मलम् ।
समादाय ततस्तेन रोममात्रं समुच्छिनेत् ॥४६॥

---

45 – 49 *cit.* नारायणदीपिका *(D) ad* क्षुरिकोपनिषद् 11, ĀSS 29, p.151
46 = हठरत्नावली 2.136
46 – 48 = हठप्रदीपिका *(H$_1$)* 3.33–35

41d अभ्यासं कारयेत्ततः] अभ्यासं कारयेत् बुधः G, अभ्यासात्कोऽपि साधयेत् K$_2$ **42a** क्लिश्यते] क्लिश्यतो μ, क्लेशतो G ◇ देवि] देवी GTW$_1$, ब्रह्मन् *U*, ब्रह्म *U*^{vl} **42b** सिद्धिः] सिद्धिं A, क्व चित् R$_2$ ◇ खेचरीपदे] सिद्धिवान्भवेत् R$_2$, खेचरीपथे *U*, खेचरीं विना α, खेचरी विना H$_2$ **42c** यद्यभ्यास॰] μ; यथाभ्यास॰ GSαJ$_2$J$_4$K$_2$PJ$_3$FK$_6$CH$_2$O, यदभ्यास॰ *U*, यदाभ्यास॰ T, यश्चाभ्यास॰ VK$_5$, यथाभ्यस॰ K$_4$, यथाभास॰ γ ◇ विद्यां] देवि A, वि J$_7$ *(unm.)*, विद्याम् α_1 **42d** न लभेत] K$_5$; लभेद्यश्च μ, न लभेद्यः G*U*TS$\beta\gamma$, आलभ्येमां α_1, नालभेये K$_1$, नालभेयं K$_3$, नालभ्येयं H$_2$, न लभेव्यः O ◇ ॰मयीम्] ॰मयं A, ॰मयां J$_6$J$_7$K$_4$, ॰मयी VJ$_3\gamma$ **43a** ततः] μG*U*TSαH$_2$; नातः J$_2$J$_4$K$_4$PFCγ_2W$_2$BO, जातः VK$_5$K$_6$, नात J$_3$R$_1$ ◇ सं॰] μG*U*TH$_2$; सा γ_2, शा R$_1$, स *cett.* ◇ ॰मेलका॰] ॰मेऴना॰ G, मेलेका॰ R$_1$ **43b** लब्ध्वा] लव्धां α_3, लध्वां H$_2$ ◇ विद्यां] विद्या GW$_1$V, विद्याम् M ◇ समुज्जपेत्] SJ$_2$VK$_4$K$_5$J$_5$W$_2$B; समुज्जयेत् $\mu\alpha_2\alpha_3$J$_1$, समजिते G, सदा जपेत् *U*T, अमुं जपेत् M, समुच्चयेत् J$_4$, समुजुयेत् P, समुंजयेत् J$_3$, समुद्धरेत् F, समं जपेत् K$_6$, समुजुपेत् C, समाज्जयेत् R$_1$, समुंजपेत् H$_2$, समुजपेत् O **43c** अनया] SαVK$_5$H$_2$; नानया μGJ$_2$J$_4$K$_4$PJ$_3$FCγ_2W$_2$BO, नान्यथा *U*T, न तया K$_6$, नातया R$_1$ ◇ रहितो] सहितो AJ$_7$ ◇ देवि] ब्रह्मन् *U*, देवी TV, विद्या N **43d** न क्व चित्] कुत्र चित् G, न किं चित् *U*TJ$_3$ ◇ सिद्धिभाग् भवेत्] सिद्धिमेष्यति α_1J$_3$ **44a** यदेदं] J$_6$J$_7$Sβ_1PK$_5$CO; यदिदं AG*U*TK$_6\gamma$, यदीदं R$_2$, यदि तं *U*^{vl}, यदैव αH$_2$, यदेतल् F ◇ लभ्यते] लभते $\alpha_2\alpha_3$FK$_6$H$_2$ **44c** तत्रो॰] R$_2\alpha$VPK$_5$Cγ; तंत्रो॰ μSJ$_2$F, त्वत्रो॰ G, तदो॰ *U*TJ$_4$, *त्रचे*॰ K$_2$, ततो॰ K$_4$J$_3$ **44d** आशु] [आश्रि]॰ T, अयु॰ α_3 ◇ संलभते] J$_6$; शंलनते A, तां लभ्यते R$_2\gamma$, तां लभते *cett.* ◇ प्रिये] मुनिः *U* **45a** तालुमूलं] स्वतालुमू॰ H$_2$*H$_3$* ◇ ॰उद्घृष्य] GSJ$_2$VJ$_3$K$_5$K$_6$Cγ; ॰उत्कृष्य AJ$_7$T, ॰उ*ष्य J$_6$, ॰उधृ R$_2$ *(unm.)*, ॰उत्कृप्य *U*, ॰उद्धर्ष्य N, ॰उद्धर्ष्य W$_1$, ॰उद्*त्य M, ॰उद्धृत्यै α_3, ॰उद्धृत्य J$_4$, ॰उद्घष्य K$_4$, ॰उघृष्य K$_2$, ॰उद्घष्य P, ॰उद्धृत्य F, ॰उत्कृत्य *D*, ॰लं संघृष्य H$_2$*H$_3$* **45b** आत्मवित्] आत्मनि H$_2$*H$_3$* **45c** ॰ऊक्तप्रकारेण] ॰ऊक्तेन मार्गेण G **45d** विशोधयेत्] विशोषयेत् R$_2$*D* **46a** स्नुही॰] स्नुहि॰ G*U*MJ$_4$K$_4$W$_2$, सहि॰ T, सुहि J$_2$, पप्नी J$_3$, स्नुहा F, स्नुह γ_2R$_1$ ◇ ॰पत्र॰] पत्रं AJ$_6$K$_6$, यंत्रं J$_7$, पर्व K$_3$ **46b** सुतीक्ष्णं स्निग्ध॰] सुक्ष्मं स्निग्धं च V ◇ ॰निर्मलम्] निर्मलः A **46c** ॰आदाय] ॰आधाय AW$_2$B, ॰आदाया॰ G ◇ ततस्तेन] ॰थ जिह्वाधो G, यतस्तेन *D* **46d** रोममात्रं] लोममात्रं *U*, संछिद्याद्रो॰ *H$_3$* ◇ समुच्छिनेत्] समुच्छिदेत् SK$_2$*D*, ॰ममात्रकम् *H$_3$*

42c – 43d *om.* R$_2$ **42c – 44b** *om.* K$_2$ **44ab** *om.* J$_3$ **45ab** *found after* 45d *in* α_2

छित्त्वा सैन्धवपथ्याभ्यां चूर्णिताभ्यां प्रघर्षयेत् ।
पुनः सप्तदिने प्राप्ते रोममात्रं समुच्छिनेत् ॥४७॥
एवं क्रमेण षण्मासं नित्योद्युक्तः समाचरेत् ।
षण्मासाद्रसनामूलशिराबन्धः प्रणश्यति ॥४८॥
अथ वागीश्वरीधामशिरो वस्त्रेण वेष्टितम् ।
शनैरुत्कर्षयेद्योगी कालवेलाविधानवित् ॥४९॥
पुनः षण्मासमात्रेण नित्यसंकर्षणात्प्रिये ।
भ्रूमध्यावधि साभ्येति तिर्यक्कर्णबिलावधि ॥५०॥
अधश्च चिबुकं मूलं प्रयाति क्रमकारिता ।
पुनः संवत्सराणां तु त्रितयादेव लीलया ॥५१॥
केशान्तमूर्ध्वं क्रमति तिर्यक्शङ्खावधि प्रिये ।

47a छित्त्वा] कृत्वा R_2H_2, हित्वा $UT\alpha_3$, ततः H_1, आदौ H_1^{vl} ◇ सैन्धव°] सजव° T ◇ °आभ्यां] °आदि° H_2 47b चूर्णिताभ्यां] प्रणीताभ्यां T, चूर्णं तेन *D* ◇ प्रघर्षयेत्] प्रकर्षयेत् R_2UT, च घर्षयेत् α_2, च चर्षयेत् M, प्रदर्शयेत् α_3 47d समुच्छिनेत्] समुच्छिदेत् SH_2D 48b नित्योद्युक्तः] $UTSW_1VK_2PJ_3FK_5C$, नित्यो युक्तः $\mu J_2J_4K_4K_6$, इत्युद्युक्तस् G, नित्ययुक्तः $R_2MDH_1H_3$, नित्योद्वक्त्व N, नित्यं संदर्श α_3, नित्याप्युक्तः γ_1, नित्यं युक्तः BH_1^{vl}, नित्यमुक्तं H_2, नित्ययुक्तं H_1^{vl} ◇ समाचरेत्] °अनात्प्रिये α_3 48c °मूल°] °मूलं $R_2UTK_2\gamma$, °मूले VH_3 48d शिरा°] शरा H_2, शिला° H_1^{vl}, नाडी° H_3 ◇ °बन्धः] °बंधं UH_2, °बजं T, °मूलं K_5, °बंधात् γ 49a वागीश्वरी°] वागीश्वरि N, वागीश्वरीं MJ_2K_4D, वागेश्वरी° H_3, प्रिये च वाग् H_3^{vl} ◇ °धाम°] देवि α_1H_3, °धस्ता° α_3, °मध्य° J_3, नाम *D* 49b °शिरो] सिक्त° G, शिवे J_1 ◇ वेष्टितम्] μ; वेष्टयेत् *cett.* 49c उत्कर्षयेद्] उत्घर्षयेद् G, अद्वर्तयेद् R_2, उद्धार्षयेद् α_3 49d °वेला°] °देश° M 50b नित्य°] $\mu R_2C\gamma_2$; नित्यं $GUTS\alpha\beta_1K_5K_6R_1H_2$, योनि° K_2F, नि P *(unm.)*, योनी° J_3, निस W_2, निःशे° B, पुनः H_3 ◇ °संकर्षणात्] $R_2\alpha_1\beta_1K_2PJ_3FK_5CH_2H_3$; °संघर्षणात् μTSK_6, संघर्षयेत् G, संघर्षनान् *U*, °संदर्शनात् α_3, संकर्षयेत् J_1R_1, शकर्षत् J_5 *(unm.)*, शकर्षणात् W_2, °षं कर्षणात् B ◇ प्रिये] मुने *U* 50c साभ्येति] G; चाभेति AJ_4, चाभ्येति $J_6J_7\alpha_2\alpha_3K_5$, चाप्येति $R_2UTJ_2VPJ_3FK_6C\gamma$, वर्धेत SH_2H_3, लभ्येत M, चापोप्येति K_4 *(unm.)*, चाप्नोति K_2 51a अधश्च] *UT*; अध स्वा AJ_7, अधः स्वा J_6, अथ स्व° $GF^{pc}J_1R_1$, अधस्ताच् $R_2S\alpha_1\alpha_3H_2H_3$, अध स्व° $J_2J_4K_4J_5W_2$, अधः स्व° $VPJ_3F^{ac}K_5K_6CB$, अधः शस्व K_2 *(unm.)* ◇ चिबुकं] $\mu R_2W_1\beta H_3$; चुबुके G, चुबुकं *U*NB, अब्रकर् T, चिबुक° SMH_2 *(unm.)*, चिवुके α_3, चुबकं γ_1 51b प्रयाति] प्रजाति K_1, पूजाति K_3, प्रवाति γ ◇ क्रम°] $\mu GR_2UTSNM\alpha_3H_2H_3$; भ्रम° βJ_1W_2, श्रम° W_1J_5B, रस° H_3 ◇ °कारिता] $\mu R_2S\alpha\beta H_2$; °कारिका $G\gamma_2W_2BH_3$, °चारिता *U*, °चारितः U^{vl}, °चारिताम् U^{vl} T, °कारका R_1, °नाक्रमात् H_3 51c संवत्सराणां तु] संवत्सराद्देवि H_2H_3 51d त्रितयाद्] μT; तृतीये GB, तृतीयाद् $R_2U\alpha\beta$, द्वितीयाद् S, तृतीया γ, द्वितीया H_2H_3 ◇ एव] देव G, देवि γ, चैव H_2H_3 52a केशान्तम्] केशांते α_2, केशामू° B, क्रोशादू° H_2, केशादू° H_3 ◇ ऊर्ध्वं] $\mu UTSVFK_5$; ऊर्ध्व GK_3C, ऊर्धं R_2, ऊर्ध्वम् M, मूर्धम् N, मूर्द्धम् W_1, ऊर्द्ध $K_1J_4K_4J_3K_6$, उर्द्ध J_2P, उर्द्धं K_2, ऊर्ध γ_1, °र्ध क्र° B, °र्द्धं च° H_2, °ध्वं क्र° H_3 ◇ क्रमति] $\mu R_2UTSJ_2J_4K_4J_3F^{ac}K_5K_6C$; क्रमणा G, आक्रम्य α_1, क्राम्पंति α_3, क्रममिति V *(unm.)*, क्रमते K_2, क्रमाति $P\gamma_2W_2$, क्रमत्*: F^{pc}, क्रमा ती° R_1, °मा तिर्यक् B, °क्रमिति H_2, °माति च H_3 52b तिर्यक्] र्यक् μJ_1R_1 *(unm.)*, तिर्यक GP *(unm.)*, तिर्यग् α_3J_4, °र्यक् मि J_5, °र्यच्चि W_2, शिखा B ◇ शङ्खावधि] $R_2S\alpha_1VPJ_3FK_5CJ_5W_2R_1B$; सखावधि μ, कर्णावधेः G, शाखावधिर् *U*, शंकापति T, वत्सरवा° α_3, आख्यवधि J_2J_4, यांखावधि K_4, संख्यावधि $K_2K_6H_2H_3^{vl}$, श्रोत्रावधि H_3 ◇ प्रिये] मुने *U*, °वधि K_1, °विधि K_3

---

47 *om.* K_6

अधस्तात्कण्ठकूपान्तं पुनर्वर्षत्रयेण तु ॥५२॥
ब्रह्मरन्ध्रान्तमावृत्य तिष्ठत्यमरवन्दिते ।
तिर्यक्चूलितलं याति अधः कण्ठबिलावधि ॥५३॥
शनैरेव प्रकर्तव्यमभ्यासं युगपन्न हि ।
युगपद्यश्चरेत्तस्य शरीरं विलयं व्रजेत् ॥५४॥
तस्माच्छनैः शनैः कार्यमभ्यासं वरवर्णिनि ।
यदा च बाह्यमार्गेण जिह्वा ब्रह्मबिलं व्रजेत् ॥५५॥
तदा ब्रह्मार्गलं देवि दुर्भेद्यं त्रिदशैरपि ।
अङ्गुल्यग्रेण संघृष्य जिह्वां तत्र निवेशयेत् ॥५६॥
एवं वर्षत्रयं कृत्वा ब्रह्मद्वारं प्रविश्यति ।
[मथनम्]
ब्रह्मद्वारे प्रविष्टे तु सम्यङ्मथनमारभेत् ॥५७॥
मथनेन विना के चित्साधयन्ति विपश्चितः ।

55c – 56d *cit.* नारायणदीपिका *(D) ad* क्षुरिकोपनिषद् 11 (ĀSS 29, p.151)

52c कण्ठ°] कंठं A, क* G, कर्ण° M, कंव° J_2, कूट° K_2 53a °रन्ध्रान्तमावृत्य] °रंध्रं समावृत्य *U*, °रज्जुं समाप्रत्य T, °रंध्रांतमावृत्या R_1 53b तिष्ठत्यमरवन्दिते] तिष्ठेदेव न संशयः *U*, तिष्ठ परमवन्दिते J_3, तिष्ठेत्परमवन्दिते H_2, तिष्ठेदमरवन्दिते H_3 53c तिर्यक्चूलितलं] तिर्यक्चूलीतले A, तिर्यक्चूलीतलै J_6J_7, तिर्यक्तूलीतलं R_2, तस्मादाषतलं T 53d अधः कण्ठ°] $\mu U F^{pc}$; अधः कर्ण° R_2, अधः कणा° T, अथ कर्ण° $S\alpha\beta_1K_2PJ_3K_5K_6C\gamma$, अध कठ° F^{ac} ◇ °बिलावधि] °बिलावधिः *U*, बिलादधः S^{pc} 54a शनैरेव] $S\beta\gamma$; शनैः शनैः μ, अनेनैव G, क्रमेणैव R_2H_3, शनैरेवं *U*, शनैरिमं α_1, शनैरियं α_3 ◇ °कर्तव्यम्] °कर्तव्यो GSH_3, °कुर्वीत α_1, °कर्तव्याम् γ_1 54b अभ्यासं] ह्यभ्यासो G, *यासो न R_2, भ्यासश्च S, अभ्यासो B, ऽभ्यासो वै H_3 ◇ युगपन्न हि] युगपत्प्रिये R_2, वरवर्णिनि H_3 54c युगपद्] युगपन् T ◇ यश्चरेत्] *em.*; यश्वरेद् A, यश्चरेद् J_6J_7, य[..]स् G, यतते $R_2SH_2H_3$, वर्तते *U*, मुच्यते T, यश्च तत् NW_1^{ac}, यस्य तत् W_1^{pc}, कुर्वतस् M, यस्वते α_3, यत J_2K_4 *(unm.)*, कृपत J_4, यततस् $VK_2PJ_3FK_5K_6C\gamma_1$, यततः B ◇ तस्य] अस्य μ, यस्य *U*T, पुंसः B 54d विलयं] विमलं H_2 55a छनैः शनैः] छनैरियं α_2, छनैरिदं M, छनै रसं α_3 ◇ कार्यम्] कुर्याद् G, कार्यो $R_2H_2H_3$, कार्या α_2, कार्य B 55b अभ्यासं] अभ्यासो GB, भ्यासो न R_2, अभ्यासाद् α_2, भ्यासेन H_2, ऽभ्यासो च H_3 ◇ वरवर्णिनि] वरवर्णि* R_2, मुनिपुंगव *U*, युगपन्न हि M, युगपत्प्रिये H_2H_3 55c बाह्य°] वायु° α_3 55d ब्रह्म°] मूल° G ◇ °बिलं] °किलं α_3 56a देवि] ब्रह्मन् *U* 56c अङ्गुल्यग्रेण संघृष्य] अंगुल्यग्रे समुत्घृष्य G, अंगुष्ठाग्रेण संघृष्य S^{ac} 56d जिह्वां तत्र] DH_2H_3; जिह्वामंत्रं A, जिह्वामत्र $J_6J_7SK_3K_2PFK_5K_6$-CH_2^{vl}, जिह्वामं* G, जिह्वामात्रं *U*TB, जिह्वामंत्रे° N, जिह्वामंत्र W_1J_3, जिह्वां मत्रे° M, जिह्वामत्रं K_1, जिह्वामात्र $\beta_1\gamma_1$ ◇ निवेशयेत्] °ण वेशयेत् NM, प्रवेशयेत् W_1K_6D 57b प्रविश्यति] प्रविशति A *(unm.)*, विशेद्ध्रुवं $R_2H_2H_3$, प्रपश्यति U^{vl}, प्रवेशते α_2, प्रवेशति M, ⌈प्रविश्यति⌉ J_2, प्रवेश्यति VK_6, प्रविश्यंति K_4, प्र⌈वेश्य⌉ति C 57c °द्वारे] °द्वारं AJ_4K_2 ◇ प्रविष्टे] प्रशुद्धे $\alpha_2\alpha_3H_2$ 57d सम्यङ] सदा G ◇ मथनम्] मंथनम् R_2S ◇ आरभेत्] आचरेत् $GUT\alpha J_4$-$J_3\gamma H_2$ 58a मथनेन] मंथनेन R_2S ◇ विना] विशु° H_2 ◇ के चित्] देवि $\beta_1K_2PJ_3FC\gamma$, नैव K_5, देवी K_6, °द्धासु H_2 58b विपश्चितः] विचक्षणाः α_1, विचक्षणैः α_3H_2

53cd *om.* G 55 *om.* K_5 55b प्रकर्तव्यं तमभ्यासं कारयेद्वर*णि*नि *add.* G

खेचरीमन्त्रसिद्धस्य सिध्यते मथनं विना ॥५८॥
जपं च मथनं चैव कृत्वा शीघ्रं फलं लभेत् ।
स्वर्णजां रौप्यजां वापि लोहजां वा शलाकिकां ॥५९॥
नियोज्य नासिकारन्ध्रे दृढस्निग्धेन तन्तुना ।
प्राणान्निरुध्य हृदये दृढमासनमास्थितः ॥६०॥
शनैश्च मथनं कुर्याद् भ्रूमध्ये न्यस्य चक्षुषी ।
षण्मासान्मथनावस्था तावतैव प्रजायते ॥६१॥
सम्यक्संरुद्धजीवस्य योगिनस्तन्मयात्मनः ।
यथा सुषुप्तिर्बालानां तथा भावस्तदा भवेत् ॥६२॥
न सदा मथनं शस्तं मासे मासे समाचरेत् ।
सदा रसनया देवि मार्गं तु परिसंक्रमेत् ॥६३॥
एवं द्वादशवर्षान्ते संसिद्धिः परमेश्वरि ।
शरीरे सकलं विश्वं पश्यत्यात्माविभेदतः ॥६४॥

---

64 *cit.* नारायणदीपिका *(D) ad* क्षुरिकोपनिषद् 11 (ĀSS 29, p.151)

58c खेचरी°] खेचरो J_2K_4 ◇ °सिद्धस्य] सिध्यंते α_2, °सिद्धास्ते M, °सिद्धिः स्यात् α_3, °सिध्यर्थं B **58d** सिध्यते] संसिद्धेन् R_2, सिध्यंते $T\alpha_2J_4$, कुर्वते M, सिद्धा ते K_6 ◇ मथनं] मंथनं μR_2S **59a** मथनं] मंथनं μR_2S **59b** लभेत्] व्रजेत् G, भवेत् α **59c** स्वर्णजां रौप्यजां] μGR_2-$UTW_1\alpha_3$; स्वर्णजा रौप्यजा $SNM\beta\gamma$ **59d** लोहजां वा शलाकिकां] $\mu GR_2UTW_1\alpha_3$; लोहजा वा शलाकिका $SNM\beta\gamma$ **60a** नियोज्य] नियोज्या μNMC, नियोज्यं V ◇ °रन्ध्रे] °रन्ध्रं *U* **60b** दृढस्निग्धेन] दुग्धसिक्तेन *U* **60c** प्राणान्] प्राणं GU^{vl} **60d** दृढम्] सुखम् *U*T ◇ आसनमास्थितः] आसनमात्मनः *U*, आसनसंस्थितः α_2, आसनसंस्थिते α_3 **61a** च] $S\beta\gamma$; स AJ_6R_2, सं° $J_7\alpha H_2$, तु G, सु° *U*, सृ T ◇ मथनं] मंथनं AS ◇ कुर्याद्] कार्यं αH_2 **61b** न्यस्य] न्यस्त° $GUS\gamma$ ◇ चक्षुषी] $J_6J_7T\alpha_1\beta_1PK_5C\gamma$; चक्षूषी A, चक्षुषि GUK_6, चक्षुषीं R_2, लोचनः S, चक्षुषां α_3, वक्षषी K_2, चक्षुषा J_3F, चक्षुषम् H_2 **61c** षण्मासान्] षण्मासं U^{vl} **61d** तावतैव] $J_7GR_2S\alpha_2K_4PK_5K_6CR_1$; तावनैव A, तावन्नैव J_6, भावेनैव *U*T, तद्विनैव M, तावन्नैव α_3, तावैतैव $J_2J_4V\gamma_2W_2B$, भावनैव K_2, तावतैतैव P *(unm.)*, स्यतंवैव J_3, तावदैव F **62a** सम्यक्°] संज्ञा° G ◇ °संरुद्ध°] $\mu R_2TS\alpha$; °निरुद्ध° G, °संरुध° J_2K_4, संरुध्य $J_4K_2PFC\gamma_1$-, संरूध्य V, संद्रध्य J_3, °संरूध° K_5, संरुद्ध्य K_6, संरुह्य B **62b** तन्मयात्मनः] स्यान्मनोन्मनी S, स्यान्मनो यथा α_1, तन्मनो यथा α_3 **62c** यथा सुषुप्तिर्बालानां] $R_2UTS\beta\gamma$; यथा सुषुप्ति वलिनां μ, यथा सुषुप्तिर्बहुळा G, सुषुप्तिर्बालकानां च α **62d** तथा भावस्] $VK_2PFK_5K_6C\gamma$; यथा भावस् μR_2GUT, तथा वै सा S, यथा वै सा α_2, यथा सैव M, बालकानां α_3, तथा भवेस् J_2, तथा भावेत् J_4, तथा भवस् K_4, तदा भावस् J_3 ◇ तदा भवेत्] $GK_2PFK_6C\gamma$; तथा भवेत् $\mu R_2UT\alpha_3\beta_1J_3K_5$, प्रजायते $S\alpha_1$ **63a** न सदा] स तथा G, रसना R_2 ◇ शस्तं] शक्तिं G, सह्यं S, कार्यं α_1, सक्तः J_4 **63b** मासे मासे] मासि मासि A, मासि मासे J_6J_7, शस्तमासे R_2 **63c** सदा] यदा $GMJ_2J_4K_4$ ◇ देवि] योगी G*U*T, मार्गम् M **63d** मार्गं] मार्ग° R_2, मार्गम् α_2, उपर्य M, मार्गे α_3H_2 ◇ तु परि°] °तः परि° R_2, न परि° *U*T, चोपरि SW_1, उपरि NM **64a** °वर्षान्ते] μGR_2UTD; °वर्षेण $SVK_2PJ_3FK_5K_6CJ_1R_1$, °वर्षं च $\alpha_2\alpha_3H_2$, °वर्षे च M, °वर्षाणि $J_2J_4K_4B$, °वर्षण J_5W_2 **64b** °सिद्धिः] °सिद्धि $A\alpha_3\gamma_1$, °सिद्धे M, °सिद्धः J_3F, °सिद्धिं BH_2 ◇ परमेश्वरि] भवति ध्रुवा *U*, भवति ध्रुवम् U^{vl}, परमेश्वरी $T\alpha_3K_2J_3K_6H_2$ **64d** पश्यत्य्] पश्यंन् G ◇ आत्मावि°] $J_6J_7UTJ_3$; आत्मादि° R_2, आत्मवि° *cett.*

58cd *om.* K_2 **62ab** *om.* *U* **41a – 43b** *repeated after* 62d G

[अमृतपानम्]
ब्रह्माण्डे यन्महामार्गं राजदन्तोर्ध्वमण्डले ।
भ्रूमध्ये तद्विजानीयात् त्रिकूटं सिद्धसेवितम् ॥६५॥
चणकाङ्कुरसंकाशं तत्र संयोजयेन्मनः ।
लिहन्रसनया तत्र स्रवन्तं परमामृतम् ॥६६॥
शनैरभ्यासमार्गस्थश्चतुर्वर्षं पिबेत्प्रिये ।
वलीपलितनाशश्च संसिद्धिः परमा भवेत् ॥६७॥
सर्वशास्त्रार्थवेत्ता च जीवेद्वर्षसहस्रकम् ।
खन्याबिलमहीवादरसवादादिसिद्धयः ॥६८॥
योगिनः संप्रवर्तन्ते पञ्चवर्षेण पार्वति ।
सम्यग्रसनया योगी स्रवन्तममृतोदकम् ॥६९॥
संपीत्वोपवसेत्स्वस्थो व्रतस्थो द्वादशाब्दकम् ।
अनेनाभ्यासयोगेन वलीपलितवर्जितः ॥७०॥
वज्रकायो महायोगी वर्षलक्षं स जीवति ।
दशनागसहस्राणां बलेन सहितः प्रिये ॥७१॥

68c – 69b ≃ हठरत्नावली 2.153

65a ब्रह्माण्डे] ब्रह्माण्डो *UT* ◇ यन्] मन् A, यो R_2, ऽयं *UT* ◇ °मार्गं] °मार्गे $AK_2\gamma$, °मार्गो GR_2U, °मार्ग α_2 **65b** °मण्डले] °कुण्दली *UT*, °मंडलं $J_4\gamma$ **65c** °मध्ये] °मध्यं M ◇ तद्] F; तं *cett.* **65d** त्रिकूटं] भ्रूकुटं A, भ्रूकूटं J_6J_7 ◇ सिद्ध°] सिद्धि° $\mu K_3K_2\gamma_1$ **66b** °योजयेन्] °कोचयेन् G, °योज्य यन् α_3, °योजयन् γ **66c** तत्र] तंतु μ, तंत्र R_2 **66d** स्रवन्तं] स्रवंत° μGNM, संवर्त्तं K_1, संवर्त्त K_3, संश्रवत् R_2 **67a** °मार्गस्थश्] °मार्गस्य μJ_4, °मार्गेण K_2F **67b** पिबेत्] पिबन् $J_2VK_4PK_5C$ **67c** °नाशश्] °नाशं $S\beta\gamma$ **67d** संसिद्धिः परमा] μ; संसिद्धिश्च परा $GJ_2J_4J_3K_5K_6$, यं सिद्धिश्च परा R_2, सिद्धिश्च परमा $S\alpha_2\gamma$, परमा⌈मृततो⌉ M, संसिद्धिर्निश्चला α_3, संसिद्धश्च परो VPC, संसिद्धिश्च परो K_4, स सिद्धश्चापरो K_2, संसिद्धस्य परो F **68c** खन्याबिलमहीवाद] *em.* Sanderson; कन्याविलं महीपाद° A, कन्याविलमहीपाद J_6J_7, कन्याबलमहावाद° G, खनीविलमहानाद° R_2, खन्याद्विलं महावादे S, खन्याबिल NM, खन्याविलं W_1, खनित्याविमहावादे α_3, खन्याविलमहावादे $\beta_1K_5K_6C$, स्वर्णादिधातुवादानि K_2, खन्याविलं महावादे $PJ_3J_1W_2B$, खन्यानिलमहावादे F, स्वन्याविलं महावाटे J_5R_1, खनित्या*क्ति*महारन्ध्रे H_2 **68d** °रसवादादि°] °रसवादाश्च G, °रसनादादि S, °रसनादीनि α_3H_2 ◇ °सिद्धयः] $\mu GR_2\alpha_3$-H_2; °सिद्धये *cett.* **69d** स्रवन्तममृतोदकम्] μ; स्रवन्तं तं परामृतं G, संश्रवच्चामृतोदकं R_2 **70a** संपीत्वोपवसेत्] G; पीत्वा रस विशे R_2, पीत्वा पीत्वा विशेत् *cett.* ◇ स्वस्थो] स्वस्थं $\mu\alpha_3H_2$, षस्यं R_2 **70b** व्रतस्थो] $\mu GR_2SJ_2VK_4K_5K_6C$; व्रतस्यो α_3H_2, ⌈वस्थो⌉ J_4 *(unm.)*, यतस्थे K_2, यतस्थो $P\gamma$, यातस्यो J_3, यतस्था F^{ac}, यत्नस्** F^{pc} ◇ °आब्दकम्] °आत्मकम् $\alpha_3K_2H_2$, °आब्दके $J_2J_4K_4K_6$, °आष्टकं J_3, °आब्दकः γ **71b** स जीवति] प्रजीवति $\mu\alpha_3$, संजीवति B **71d** बलेन] बलवान् $J_2J_4K_2PJ_3C\gamma$, वलं वा K_6

65b *end of witnesses UT* **68c** °मही – **71a** °कायो *om.* α_1 *(eye-skip from* °मही *to* महा) **69** *om.* $S\alpha\beta\gamma$ **70b** पीत्वा पीत्वा विशेषेण द्वौ प्रस्थौ द्वादशाब्दकं *add.* G **70cd** *om.* K_2 **71ab** *found after* 72b *in* γ

स दूरदर्शनश्चैव दूरश्रवण एव च ।
निग्रहानुग्रहे शक्तः सर्वत्र बलवान् भवेत् ॥७२॥
एता हि सिद्धयो देवि भ्रूमध्ये संभवन्ति हि ।
आकाशे रसनां कृत्वा दन्तपङ्क्तिं निपीडयेत् ॥७३॥
काकचञ्चुपुटं वक्त्रं कृत्वा तदमृतं पिबेत् ।
पानाद्वत्सरतः सत्यं जरामरणवर्जितः ॥७४॥
खेचरत्वमवाप्नोति जीवत्याचन्द्रतारकम् ।
पादुकाखड्गवेतालसिद्धिद्रव्यमनःशिलाः ॥७५॥
अञ्जनं विवरं चैव चेटकं यक्षिणी तथा ।
यत्किं चित्सिद्धिसमयं विद्यते भुवनत्रये ॥७६॥
तत्सर्वमेव सहसा साधयेत्साधकोत्तमः ।

इति श्रीमदादिनाथप्रोक्ते महाकालयोगशास्त्रे
उमामहेश्वरसंवादे खेचरीविद्यायां प्रथमः पटलः

72a स] सु° $J_6J_7R_2\alpha_1$, सं° G ◇ °दर्शनश्] $S\alpha_2\alpha_3K_2P$; °दर्शनं $\mu GR_2\beta_1FK_5K_6C\gamma$, °श्रवणश् M, °श्रवणा J_3 ◇ चैव] लब्ध्वा J_3, वेद F **72b** दूर°] दूरा° $\alpha_3\gamma_2B$ ◇ °श्रवण] $S\alpha_2$; °श्रवणम् $\mu GR_2\beta_1K_2PFK_5K_6C\gamma_1$, °दर्शनम् MJ_3, °छ्रवणम् α_3B **72c** शक्तः] शक्तिः μR_2 **73a** एता हि] एताद्य μ, एताश्च α_3 **73b** भ्रू°] भू° J_6J_7 **73d** °पङ्क्तिं] °पंक्तिर् A, °पंक्तीर् J_6J_7, °पक्ति R_2K_3, °पंक्ति NPJ_3J_5, पंक्ता K_2, पं*क्ति*: F ◇ निपीडयेत्] न पीडयेत् AR_2K_3, निपीज्येत् J_6 *(unm.)* **74a** °पुटं] पदं α_3 ◇ वक्त्रं] कृत्वा α_1, चक्रं α_3 **74b** कृत्वा] चक्रं α_2, वक्त्रं M, दत्वा VK_5 **74c** पानाद्वत्सरतः] $G\alpha H_2$; भानुवत्सरतः μ, पानाद्वत्सतर R_2-, तेनाब्दशतसा° SF, तेनाव्दा[नी]शतं J_2, तेन चावृषतं J_4, तेना*षु*सं*श*तं V, तेनाव्दशतं K_4 *(unm.)*, तेनाष्टशतसा° K_2J_3, तेनाव्दशतः PW_2 *(unm.)*, तेनाव्दानां शतं K_5, तेन नादात्स्मृत K_6, तेनाव्दात्स्मृतः C *(unm.)*, तेनावृशतः γ_2 *(unm.)*, तेनावृतः R_1 *(unm.)*, तेनैवाब्दशतं B ◇ सत्यं] °हस्त्रं SJ_3F, °हस्रयं K_2 **75a** खेचर°] खेचरी° R_1 **75b** जीवत्याचन्द्रतारकम्] जीवेच्चंद्रार्कतारकं G, जीवेदाचंद्रतारकं S, जीवेद्वर्षसहस्रकं α_1 **75c** पादुका°] पादुके S ◇ °खड्ग°] °खड्गर् A, °खड्गु° R_2J_3, °षड° α_3, खड्गः V *(unm.)*, °खर्ड्ग° K_4, °खेच[री]° R_1 *(unm.)* ◇ °वेताल°] J_7R_2-$SMFK_6\gamma$; °वेतोलः AJ_6, °वेतालं α_2K_3, °वेता*ल*° K_1, °वेताला° $J_2J_4K_4PK_5C$, °वैताला° VJ_3, °वेतालाः K_2 **75d** °सिद्धि°] °सिद्ध° $\mu R_2VK_5K_6$, °सिद्धिं α_3 ◇ °द्रव्यमनःशिलाः] AK_6; °द्रव्यमनःशिला $J_6J_7R_2\beta_1K_2PJ_3FK_5C$, °द्रव्यमभीप्सितं $S\alpha$, °द्रव्यमनेकशः γ **76b** चेटकं] खेटकं μ, चेटको R_2, चेटका N ◇ यक्षिणी] चाक्षिणी α_1, यक्षणी $K_1\beta_1K_5\gamma_1$ **76c** यत्किं चित्] ये के चित् α_3, पंक्तिवित् β_1K_6C ◇ सिद्धिसमयं] $\alpha_1K_2FW_2$; सिद्धमयं A *(unm.)*, सिधमयं J_6J_7 *(unm.)*, स तु यं ज्ञात्व G^{ac}, सफलं ज्ञात्व G^{pc}, सिद्धसमयं $S\alpha_3\beta_1J_3PK_5K_6C$, सिद्धिसमये γ_2R_1B **76d** विद्यते] विद्याने A, विद्या ते J_6J_7, भिद्यते G **77a** तत्] त्वत् A **77b** साधयेत्] सेवयस् γ_1, सेवयेत् B ◇ साधकोत्तमः] तारकोत्तमः γ

75cd *om.* G **76cd** *om.* R_2 **77ab** *om.* V

द्वितीयः पटलः

[ब्रह्मद्वारार्गलकलाः]

यत्र ब्रह्मार्गलद्वारं दुर्विज्ञेयं महेश्वरि ।
कलाचतुष्कं तत्रस्थं चतुर्वर्गात्मकं परम् ॥१॥
पूर्वभागे कृता नाम गुप्ता दक्षिणगोचरा ।
शिवा पश्चिमदिग्भागे परापरशिवोत्तरे ॥२॥
तद्द्वारं रसनाग्रेण भित्त्वा पूर्वकलामृतम् ।
यदा पिबति वै योगी मासाद्धर्माधिपो भवेत् ॥३॥
यदा गुप्तामृतं दक्षे योगी रसनया लिहेत् ।
मासादेव न संदेहः साक्षादर्थेश्वरो भवेत् ॥४॥
तत्पश्चिमकलाजातममृतं जिह्वया पिबेत् ।
यदा तदा महायोगी मासात्कामेश्वरो भवेत् ॥५॥
उत्तरस्थकलाजातममृतं प्रपिबेद्यदा ।
तदासौ परमेष्ठीनामाधिपत्यमवाप्नुयात् ॥६॥
तदूर्ध्वमण्डले लीनं ब्रह्मरन्ध्रे परामृतम् ।

Witnesses for the second paṭala:
$AJ_6J_7GR_2SNW_1MK_1K_3J_2J_4VK_4K_2PJ_3FK_5K_6J_1J_5W_2R_1B$;
C (*up to* 14d); H_2 (78c-81b, 93c–94b, 95cd, 96cd, 105); *D* (72–73b).
μ=AJ_6J_7 ◇ α=$NW_1MK_1K_3$ α_1=NW_1M α_2=NW_1 α_3=K_1K_3 ◇
β=$J_2J_4VK_4K_2PJ_3FK_5K_6C$ β_1=$J_2J_4VK_4$ ◇ γ=$J_1J_5W_2R_1B$ γ_1=$J_1J_5W_2R_1$ γ_2=J_1J_5

1a यत्र] μ; तच्च G, यत्तद् $R_2S\beta_1PJ_3FK_5CJ_5W_2B$, एतद् $\alpha_1J_1R_1$, यत्तज् α_3, यत्तु K_2, तत्र K_6 ◇ ब्रह्मार्गल°] $J_6J_7GR_2\beta_1K_2PF\gamma_1$; ब्रह्मार्गलं $ASJ_3K_5K_6CB$, गुह्यार्गल° α_1, जिह्वार्गल° α_3 ◇ °द्वारं] देवि S, देवी J_3 **1b** दुर्विज्ञेयं] दुर्जेयं वै F ◇ महेश्वरि] महेश्वरी $AJ_6J_4VK_2K_6CW_2B$, सुरेश्वरि G, कुलेश्वरी J_3 **1c** °चतुष्कं] °चतुर्क्क A, °चतुष्कं J_6J_7, °चतुष्ट R_2 ◇ तत्र°] तंत्र° $J_3\gamma$ **1d** °वर्गात्मकं परम्] °वक्त्रात्मकं परं AJ_7, °वर्गफलप्रदं G, वर्षात्परंयरं R_2 **2b** °गोचरा] °गोचरं G, °गोचरः R_2, °गोचरे α_3 **2c** शिवा] $\mu GR_2SMVK_5K_6$; शिवः α_2PJ_3FC, दिवा α_3, शिव $J_2J_4K_4\gamma$, शिवाय K_2 *(unm.)* **2d** परा°] परात् G ◇ °शिवोत्तरे] °शिवोत्तरा $R_2\beta\gamma$ **3c** यदा] यदि γ_1 **3d** मासाद्धर्माधिपो] G; मासार्द्धे माधिपो A, मासा धर्माधिपो J_6J_7, मासार्धमधिपो $R_2S\alpha\beta_1PK_6C\gamma_2W_2$, मासार्द्धमधि यो $K_2J_3R_1$, मासार्धेमधिपो F, मासार्द्धादधिपो K_5, मासार्द्धमपि यो B **4a** यदा] तदा W_1K_1, यदि J_3W_2B ◇ दक्षे] दत्ते γ **4b** लिहेत्] पिबेत् $GS\alpha_1$ **4c** मासादेव] मासार्धेन α **4d** अर्थेश्वरो भवेत्] स खेचरो भवेत् G, दीर्घश्चिरो भवेत् R_2, अर्थो भवेन्नरः α_2, अर्थे भवेन्नरः M **5a** तत्पश्चिम°] पश्चिमन्तु α_3, यत्पश्चिम° $J_5W_2R_1$, यत्पश्चिमं J_1 ◇ °कलाजातम्] °कलाजालं μ, °कलायातम् α_2, °कलायांतम् α_3 **5b** अमृतं जिह्वया पिबेत्] शुद्धं पिवति जिह्वया μ, सुधां पिबति जि[.]या G **6a** उत्तरस्थ°] उत्तस्था A *(unm.)*, उत्तरस्य α_3J_4, उत्तरस्था γ **6b** यदा] μ; यदि *cett.* **6c** परमेष्ठीनाम्] पारमेष्ठीनाम् μG **7a** °ऊर्ध्व°] $J_6J_7R_2S\alpha_2J_2VK_4K_5K_6\gamma$; °ऊर्ध्वं $AGMJ_4K_2PJ_3FC$, °ओर्ध्वं α_3 ◇ लीनं] लीने AJ_7

---

4 *added in margin by later hand* K_6 5 *om.* K_5B *and found after* 7 *in* J_1R_1 **5b – 6a** *om.* α_1K_2 **6ab** *om.* K_6

यदा पिबति योगीन्द्रो जीवन्मुक्तः शिवो भवेत् ॥७॥
मासमासावधि यदा द्वादशाब्दं समाचरेत् ।
सर्वरोगविनिर्मुक्तः सर्वज्ञो मुनिपूजितः ॥८॥
जायते शिववद्योगी लोके ऽस्मिन्नजरामरः ।
चतुष्कलामृतं वारि पीत्वा पीत्वा महेश्वरि ॥९॥
ब्रह्मस्थाने तथा जिह्वां संनियोज्यामृतं पिबेत् ।
सुस्वादु शीतलं हृद्यं क्षीरवर्णमफेनिलम् ॥१०॥
मासमात्रप्रयोगेन जायते देववत्स्वयम् ।
द्विमासे सर्वशास्त्रार्थं सम्यग्जानाति पार्वति ॥११॥
स्वतन्त्रः शिववन्मासत्रयाद्भवति वै शिवे ।
चतुर्मासान्महेशानि सर्वज्ञत्वं प्रवर्तते ॥१२॥
पञ्चमासे महासिद्धस्त्रैलोक्यमपि पश्यति ।
षण्मासे परमानन्दगुणसद्भावपूरितः ॥१३॥
जायते नात्र संदेहो जीवन्मुक्तः परापरे ।
सप्तमासे महाभूतपिशाचोरगराक्षसैः ॥१४॥
सह संवर्तते नित्यं स्वेच्छया हृष्टमानसः ।
अष्टमे मासपर्यायि देवैः संमेलनं भवेत् ॥१५॥

7c यदा पिबति योगीन्द्रो] M; यदा तदासौ पिबति $\mu GR_2SW_1\beta B$, यदासौ संपिबति N, यदासौ पिवते योगे α_3, यदा तदासो पिबति γ_1 **8a** मासमासावधि] मासे मासे विधि A, मासमासविधि J_6J_7, मासान्मासावधिर् G, मासमासावधौ R_2, मासमासावपि α_2, मासं मासं पिबेद् M ◇ यदा] याव G, देवी R_2, एवं M, यद्वा γ **8d** सर्वज्ञो मुनिपूजितः] सर्वज्ञगुणपूरितः μ, सर्वज्ञस् सर्वपूजितः G, सर्वज्ञगुणपूजितः R_2, सर्वलक्षणसंयुतः α_1, सर्वसंपूर्णलक्षणः α_3, सर्वतो मुनिपूजितः $J_4\gamma$ **9c** वारि] द्वापि μ **9d** महेश्वरि] महेश्वरी $AK_3J_4J_3K_6\gamma_1$, °मरेश्वरी B **10a** तथा] तदा GF, निजां M, स्थिता α_3 ◇ जिह्वां] जिह्वा $\alpha_3J_4K_4PJ_3K_5K_6\gamma_2W_2$ **10d** श्रफेनिलम्] मनोहरं G **11b** जायते] ज्ञायते β_1PJ_3C ◇ देववत्] शिववत् μ, देवता S **12a** स्वतन्त्रः] $\mu S^{vl}\alpha_1$; स्वतंत्र° G, स्वयं च S, स्वतंत्रं α_3, स्वतत्वं $J_2VK_4K_5C$, स्वतत्रं J_4, स्वतुल्मं K_2, स्वतलं $P\gamma$, स्वतुल्यं J_3, स्वस्तलं F, स्वत*त्व* K_6 ◇ शिववन्] °वद्वसन् G **12b** °त्रयाद्] °त्रये μG, यावद् R_2 ◇ भवति वै शिवे] भवति पार्वति G, ऊर्ध्वं भवेछिवे M, भव∗ वै शिवो K_6 **12c** चतुर्मासान्] $G\alpha VK_2F$; चतुर्मासे $\mu SJ_2J_4K_4J_3K_5K_6C$, चतुमासान् R_2, चतुर्मास P, धातुमांस γ_2, धातुभास W_2, धातुभासा B **13a** °मासे] °मासान् F ◇ °सिद्धस्] $R_2S\alpha_2VK_4J_3K_5K_6$; °सिद्धिस् $\mu GM\alpha_3$-$J_2J_4K_2\gamma$, °सिद्धश् PC, °सिद्धिं F **13c** परमानन्द°] परमानंदं μR_2, शिवसत्भाव° G, परमानंदो $S\alpha$, परमानंदः K_2 **13d** °गुणसद्भाव°] °परमानंद° G, °गुणः सद्भाव° α_1 ◇ °पूरितः] *em.* Sanderson; °पूजितः *codd.* **14b** परापरे] परावरेः A, परावरे $J_6J_7R_2S\alpha_2$, परात्परे GK_2 **14c** सप्तमासे] μ; सप्तमे च GK_5, सप्तमेन *cett.* ◇ महाभूत°] μG; महाकायः $R_2SM\alpha_3\beta$, महाकाया α_2, महाकायो γ **15a** सह संवर्तते] सदा संवेष्टितो G **15b** हृष्ट°] μGR_2SK_1VF; तुष्ट° α_1, दृष्ट° K_3PJ_3, दृष° J_2K_4, दृष्य° J_4, दृढ° $K_5^{pc}\gamma$, दृश° K_5^{ac}, दृष्ट्र° K_6 **15c** मास°] मासि $\alpha_2J_2VK_4PK_6B$, °मासे J_4 ◇ °पर्यायि] °पर्याप्ते R_2K_5, °पर्यायैर् $K_2J_5W_2$, °प्रजाये J_4, °पर्यायै PJ_3K_6B **15d** देवैः संमेलनं] वैष्णवं मेलनं N, सहसा मेलनं W_1, देवसंमीलनं α_3

13cd *om.* J_3 **14d** शाचोरग° – **17a** त्रिकालज्ञः *om.* R_1 (f.17v *missing*) ◇ °राक्ष *end of* C

नवमे मास्यदृश्यत्वं सूक्ष्मत्वं चैव जायते ।
दशमे कामरूपत्वं सर्वलोकप्रकाशकम् ॥१६॥
एकादशे त्रिकालज्ञः सर्वलोकेश्वरः प्रभुः ।
जायते शिववद्देवि सत्यमेतन्मयोदितम् ॥१७॥

[केदारकलाः]

यत्र चूलितलं प्रोक्तं केदारं प्राहुरीश्वरि ।
तत्र सोमकलाश्चाष्टौ विख्याता वीरवन्दिते ॥१८॥
अमृता प्रथमा देवि द्वितीया मानदाह्वया ।
पूषा तुष्टिश्च पुष्टिश्च रतिश्चैव धृतिस्तथा ॥१९॥
शशिनी चाष्टमी सर्वाः परामृतमहार्णवाः ।
तद्धामाभिमुखीं जिह्वां यदा योगी करोति च ॥२०॥
अष्टधा स्रवते तत्र तदा तुहिनसंततिः ।
तदाप्लावनसंयोगात्कलेवरगदक्षयः ॥२१॥
अष्टभिर्मासपर्यायैः खेचरत्वं प्रजायते ।

[सोममण्डलकलाः]

16a नवमे मास्य्] μR_2MB; नवमासेषु G, नवमे स्याद् K_5, नवमासे ह्य् *cett.* **16c** दशमे] दशाभिः N, दशभिः W_1 **16d** ◦लोक◦] ◦लोम◦ A, ◦ज्ञत्व◦ M ◇ ◦प्रकाशकं] ◦प्रकाशना AK_6, प्रकाशता J_7, ◦प्रकाशितं GR_2, प्रकाशनं K_6 **17b** ◦लोकेश्वरः] ◦लोकेश्वर◦ AJ_7K_3 **17c** देवि] देवी R_2K_6, योगी $MFK_5^{ac}\gamma$, विद्धि α_3 **17d** सत्यम्] तत्वम् α_3 **18a** चूलितलं] $S\alpha K_4PK_5$-K_6W_2B; तूलीतलां AJ_7, तूलीतलं J_6, चोळुतं G *(unm.)*, चु*ीतलम् R_2, वूलितलं J_2V, चूलतलं J_4, *हिलिनलं K_2, चूलितरं J_3, चूलीतलं F, चुलित्तरं J_1, चुलित्तलं J_5, चुलितरं R_1 **18b** ईश्वरि] ईश्वरी $\alpha_3K_2J_3K_6J_1W_2R_1$ **18c** सोम◦] सौम◦ μ ◇ ◦कलाश्] $\mu GNMJ_2VK_4$; ◦कला *cett.* ◇ चाष्टौ] चाष्ट GF^{pc}, अ्रष्टौ R_2, *शा*ष्ट F^{ac} **18d** विख्याता] विख्यातास् G, विख्यातौ R_2 ◇ वीरवन्दिते] $\mu\alpha_3$; सुरवंदिते G, वीरवन्दितौ R_2, [ऽ]मरवंदिते S, अ्रमरार्चिते α_2, भ्रमरार्चिते M, ◦मरवन्दिते $\beta\gamma$ **19a** देवि] देवी $R_2J_3K_6F^{pc}$ **19b** मानदाह्वया] मानदातुया M, मानवाह्वया α_3 **19c** पूषा तुष्टिश्च पुष्टिश्च] $GSVK_4K_2PJ_3K_5K_6B$; पूषा तुष्टिश्च μ *(unm.)*, पूषा पुष्टिश्च तुष्टिश्च R_2, सुपुष्टिश्चाथ तुष्टिश्च α_2, ⌈पू⌉षा पुष्टिश्चाथ तुष्टी M, पुष्टिश्चाथ तुष्टिश्च α_3 *(unm.)*, पुषा तुष्टिश्च पुष्टिश्च $J_2\gamma_1$, पूषा तुष्टश्च पुष्टिश्च J_4, पूषा तुष्टिश्च युष्टिश्च J_3F^{ac}, पूषा तुष्टिश्च मष्टिश्च F^{pc} **19d** रतिश्] शांतिश् SJ_3, शक्तिश् K_2, स्मतिश् F **20a** शशिनी] $GS\alpha_1\beta_1FK_5B$; शंखिनी μR_2K_6, सात्मीनि α_3, अ्रशिनी K_2, शशिना PJ_3, रासिनी J_1W_2, रासिनि J_5, शसिनी R_1 ◇ चाष्टमी] शंखिनी R_2 ◇ सर्वाः] $\mu GR_2SM\alpha_3F$; सर्व N, सर्वा $W_1\beta\gamma$ **20b** परामृत◦] $GR_2S\alpha\beta B$; परमामृ◦ μ, परामृता◦ γ_1 ◇ ◦महार्णवाः] GR_2SF; ◦तहार्णवाः A, ◦तमहार्णवाः J_6J_7 *(unm.)*, ◦रसार्णवा N, ◦रसार्णव W_1, ◦रसार्णवाः $M\alpha_3$, ◦महार्णवा $J_2PJ_3K_5K_6$, ◦महाररणवा J_4 *(unm.)*, ◦महार्णवी $V\gamma$, ◦मर्हर्णवा K_4 *(unm.)*, ◦महार्णदा K_2 **20c** ◦मुखीं] J_6J_7GSVPB; ◦मुखी $AR_2K_2K_6\gamma_1$, ◦मुखं $\alpha_2\alpha_3J_2J_4K_4$, ◦मुखां MFK_5, ◦मुखिं J_3 ◇ जिह्वां] जिह्वा $\alpha_3J_4K_4K_6\gamma_1$ **21a** स्रवते] च्यवते β, द्रवते γ **21c** ◦प्लावन◦] ◦प्लुवन◦ $\mu\alpha_2\alpha_3$, ◦प्[...] G, ◦श्र⌈व⌉ण◦ M ◇ ◦संयोगात्] ◦संयोगः α_1, ◦संयोगे α_3 **21d** ◦गद◦] ◦वद◦ G, ◦मत◦ K_2 **22b** प्रजायते] प्रपेदिरे $\beta\gamma$

16b – 17a *om.* K_2

भ्रूमध्यं नाम यद्धाम तत्प्रोक्तं सोममण्डलम् ॥२२॥
कलाचतुष्कं तत्रोक्तं परामृतनिकेतनम् ।
चन्द्रिकाख्या च कान्तिश्च ज्योत्स्ना श्रीश्चेति नामतः ॥२३॥
तत्र जिह्वां समावेश्य पीत्वा पीत्वा समापिबेत् ।
योगी मासचतुष्केण जायते निरुपद्रवः ॥२४॥
वज्रकायो भवेत्सत्यं तदाप्लावनपानतः ।
[खेचरमण्डलकलाः]
तदूर्ध्वं वज्रकन्दाख्यं शिला खेचरमण्डलम् ॥२५॥
ललाटान्ते विजानीयात्तत्र देवि कलात्रयम् ।
प्रीतिस्तथाङ्गदा पूर्णा तत्र जिह्वां प्रवेशयेत् ॥२६॥
क्षीरधारामृतं शीतं स्रवन्तं जिह्वया पिबेत् ।
मासत्रयेण देवेशि सर्वव्याधिविवर्जितः ॥२७॥
अच्छेद्यः सर्वशस्त्रैश्च अभेद्यः सर्वसाधनैः ।
अचिन्त्यः सर्वविज्ञानैर्विरूपविषयान्वितैः ॥२८॥

22c भ्रूमध्यं] μG; भ्रूमध्ये $R_2S\alpha_1\beta\gamma$, भ्रूमध्यो° α_3 ◇ नाम यद्धाम] G; नाम युद्वाम A, नाम युद्धाम J_6J_7, वाम यत्प्रोक्त R_2, धाम यत्प्रोक्तं $S\alpha_1\beta\gamma$, °र्ध्वं मया प्रोक्तं α_3 **22d** प्रोक्तं] प्रभो α_3 ◇ °मण्डलम्] °मंडले S **23a** तत्रोक्तं] तंत्रोक्तं AB **23b** परामृत°] परमामृत° $\mu\gamma$ *(unm.)* **23c** चन्द्रिका°] चंडिका° μK_4, चंदिका α_3, चंद्रका° $J_4\gamma$ ◇ °ख्या च कान्तिश्च] °ख्याथ कांतिश्च G, °ख्याश्च कांतिश्च R_2K_2, नवकांतिश्च α, °ख्यं चंद्रकांति B **23d** श्रीश्चेति] श्री प्रीति F, सुश्रेति γ **24a** जिह्वां] जिह्वा $N\alpha_3J_4K_2\gamma_1$ ◇ समावेश्य] समावेश्या $S\alpha$ **24b** पीत्वा पीत्वा] °मृतं पीत्वा $S\alpha_1$ ◇ समापिबेत्] *conj.* Sanderson; समालिहेत् G, समं विशेत् W_1, समाविश्येत् J_4, संविशेत् R_1 *(unm.)*, समाविशेत् *cett.* **24c** योगी] *conj.*; देव μ, देवी J_3K_6, देवि *cett.* ◇ मास°] भास° μ **25b** तद्°] μGMJ_4; सद्° *cett.* ◇ °आप्लावन°] °आपवन° J_6F, °आस्रवन° J_7, °आपावन° $NM\alpha_3J_1R_1$ ◇ °पानतः] $AGSJ_2VK_4PFK_5K_6J_5W_2B$; °पाततः J_6, °यावन R_2, °पावनः α, °मानतः J_4, °पातनः K_2, °याततः J_3, °प्लावनतः J_1 *(unm.)*, °प्लानतः R_1 **25c** °ऊर्ध्वं] $J_6J_7SM\alpha_3$-$K_2J_3FK_6J_1B$; °ऊर्ध्व° $A\alpha_2PJ_5W_2$, °ऊर्ध्व G *(unm.)*, °ऊर्ध्वैं R_2, °ऊर्ध्वे $J_2VK_4K_5$, °ऊर्द्धे J_4, °उर्द्धे R_1 ◇ वज्र°] वज्रे G ◇ °कन्दाख्यं] $\mu R_2S\alpha_1\beta_1K_2J_3K_5$; नंदाख्यं G, °कंदाख्य° α_3PF, °कदाख्यं K_6, °कन्दाख्या γ **25d** शिला] शिरा K_5 ◇ खेचर°] रसे च α_3, खेचरी R_1 ◇ °मण्डलं] °मध्यगं μG, °मंडलः F **26a** ललाटान्ते] $R_2SW_1\beta$; ललाटं तं μGNM, ललाटान्तं α_3, ललाटांतो γ **26b** कलात्रयम्] कलान्वितं G, कलात्रये $J_2J_4K_4$ **26c** तथाङ्गदा] GF; तथांगजा μ, तथांग[दा] M, तथा गजा *cett.* ◇ पूर्णा] पुण्या α_3 **27a** क्षीर°] एतत्सुधामयं क्षीर° G *(unm.)* ◇ शीतं] शितं J_6J_7 *(unm.)*, शांतं J_3 **27b** स्रवन्तं] संश्रवज् R_2 **27c** °त्रयेण] $\mu\alpha FJ_1R_1$; °मात्रेण $GR_2S\beta J_5W_2B$ **28a** अच्छेद्यः] अभेद्यः α_3, अवेद्यः J_3 ◇ °शस्त्रैश्च] J_6J_7G, °शस्त्रेश्च A, °शस्त्रैस्त R_2, °शास्त्रौघैर् J_3K_6, °शस्त्रौघ R_1, °शस्त्रौघैर् *cett.* **28b** अभेद्यः] $\mu G\alpha K_4$; ख्य R_2 *(unm.)*, अलक्ष्यः SJ_2PFK_5, अलक्षः J_4K_2, अलभ्यः V, अलक्ष J_3, अलख्यः K_6, उल्लिख्य J_1, उल्लक्ष्यः J_5W_2B, नल्लिख्य R_1 ◇ °साधनैः] G; °लोकशै A, °लेखकैः $J_6S\alpha_3VK_4PJ_3FK_5\gamma$, °लेशकैः J_7, °लेखनै R_2, °भेदकैः α_1, °लौकिकैः J_2, °लोककैः J_4K_6, °लक्ष्यकैः K_2 **28d** विरूप°] $\mu GR_2M\alpha_3$; निरूपो S, विरूपं N, निरूपं W_1, निरूप° $\beta_1PJ_3FK_6\gamma$, अरूप° K_2, निरूप्यो K_5 ◇ °विषयान्वितैः] °विषमान्वितैः μ, विषयान्वितः K_6

22d – 23a *om.* J_4 **24 – 30** *found in margin of* f.29v J_6 (*eye-skip* तत्र–तत्र) **25c** शिवश् शिखरी मण्डलं तदूर्ध्वं वज्रकेशाख्यं *add.* G

भैरवाभो भवेत्सत्यं वज्रकन्दप्रभावतः ।

[राजदन्तकलाः]

नासिकाधो ɔधरोष्ठोर्ध्वं राजदन्तं महापदम् ॥२९॥

तत्र पूर्णामृता देवि शीतला च कलाद्वयम् ।

संप्राप्य कुम्भकावस्थां रसनाग्रेण संस्पृशेत् ॥३०॥

तत्र संजायते देवि सुस्वादु शीतलं जलम् ।

स्वमनस्तत्र संयोज्य पिबेन्मासत्रयं व्रती ॥३१॥

अजरामरतामेति सर्वव्याधिविवर्जितः ।

[आधारकलाः कुण्डलिनीशक्तिश्च]

गुदबीजान्तरस्थानमाधारं परिकीर्तितम् ॥३२॥

तत्र पञ्च कलाः प्रोक्ताः प्रगलत्परमामृताः ।

सुधा सुधामयी प्रज्ञा कालघ्नी ज्ञानदायिनी ॥३३॥

कलाः पञ्च सुधाधाराः कीर्तिताः सर्वसिद्धिदाः ।

तत्रस्था परमा शक्तिराद्या कुण्डलिनी शिवे ॥३४॥

तत्राकुञ्चनयोगेन कुम्भकेन सुरार्चिते ।

29a °आभो] °आंगो M, °आंभो α_3 **29b** °कन्दप्र°] °कन्दर्प° γ **29c** नासिकाधो] $GR_2SJ_2J_4$-$VK_2FK_5K_6$; नासिकोर्धो AJ_7, नासिकोर्द्धो J_6, नासिकाधों° α_1, नासिकाधा° α_3, नासिका*° K_4, नासिकाद्यो° $P\gamma$, शशिंकाद्यो° J_3 ◇ ɔधरोष्ठोर्ध्वं] *em.*; °धरोष्ट्राई A *(unm.)*, °धरौष्ठार्द्ध° J_6, धरौष्ट्रार्द्र J_7, धरोष्ठोर्ध्वे G, धरोष्ठौध R_2, °त्तरोष्ठोर्ध्वे S, °तरोष्ठोधो N, °तष्टोरोधो W_1^{pc}, °तष्टोराधो W_1^{ac}, °तरोष्ठाधो M, °तरोष्टोर्ध्वो α_3, °त्तरोष्ठोर्ध्वं β, °तरोष्टाधः γ **29d** °दन्तं] °दंत° $R_2MJ_4\gamma$ ◇ °पदम्] $R_2\beta\gamma$; °पथां AJ_7, °पथं $J_6G\alpha_1K_5^{ac}$, °पदः α_3 **30a** पूर्णामृता] GR_2SVK_6; पूर्णामृतं $AJ_7\alpha_1$, पूर्णामृते J_6, पूर्णामहं α_3, पुर्णामृतो $J_2J_4K_4K_2PF$, पारिणामृता J_3, पूर्णानिना K_5, पूर्णा ततो γ ◇ देवि] देवी $R_2J_3K_6$ **30b** शीतला] $GS\beta\gamma$; शीतता AJ_7, शीलता J_6, शीत*ल*ा R_2, शीतलं α ◇ कलाद्वयम्] कलाह्वयां μ, कलाह्वया G **30c** संप्राप्य] पूर्णापि α ◇ कुम्भका°] कुलका° J_3 ◇ °वस्थां] °वस्था $R_2M\alpha_3K_2PFK_6\gamma$ **30d** रसनाग्रेण संस्पृशेत्] रसनाग्रं प्रवेशयेत् B **31a** देवि] *om.* μ, सत्वं α_1, सत्यं $GR_2\alpha_3$ **31b** सुस्वादु शीतलं जलम्] μ; जलं सुस्वादु शीतलं G, सुखदं शीतलं जलं $R_2S\alpha\beta\gamma$ **31c** स्वमनस्] सुमनस् α_3, स्वं मनस् B **31d** पिबेन्] पिबन् $SJ_4PF\gamma_1$ ◇ मासत्रयं व्रती] μ; मासद्वयं प्रये G, मासत्रयं ज इति R_2 *(unm.)*, मासद्वयं व्रती $S\beta\gamma$, मासचतुष्टयं α **32c** °बीजान्तर°] °बीजांतरं S, °बीजांकुर° α **33a** पञ्च] सोम° G ◇ कलाः] कला $J_6J_7G\alpha_2\alpha_3K_2J_3K_5^{ac}K_6\gamma_1$ ◇ प्रोक्ताः] [पूर्णाः] G, प्रोक्ता NM-$\alpha_3K_2J_3$, सक्ताः J_4, प्रोक्तः PJ_5, प्रोक्त J_1R_1 **33b** प्रगलत्] प्रस्रवत् G, विगलत् M ◇ °मृताः] $\mu GS\alpha_1\beta_1PFK_5K_6$; °मृ*ता* R_2, °मृतः K_1, °मृतः K_3, °मृतां $K_2J_5W_2$, °मृता J_3, °मृतं J_1R_1B **33c** सुधा°] रस° R_2 ◇ प्रज्ञा] प्राज्ञा $G\beta_1J_3K_5K_6J_5W_2B$, धारा J_1R_1 **33d** कालघ्नी] कलघ्नी α_2J_4VB ◇ ज्ञानदायिनी] ज्ञानदायका μ, कामदायिनी GF **34a** कलाः पञ्च] $S\alpha_1$; कला पंच $\mu\alpha_3J_3$, कला*:* पंच G, ककता पंच R_2 *(unm.)*, कल्पं पंच J_2J_4, कल्प पंच VK_4PFK_6, कलाः च J_3 *(unm.)*, कस्य पंच K_5, कल्पय च γ_1, कल्पयेच्च B ◇ सुधाधाराः] सुधाराश्च α_1, सधारा च α_3 **34b** कीर्तिताः] कीर्तिता $AJ_7\alpha_3\gamma_1$ ◇ °सिद्धिदाः] °सिद्धिदा $\alpha_3J_3K_5^{ac}\gamma_1$ **34c** तत्र°] मंत्र° J_4 ◇ शक्तिर्] शक्ति μM, शक्तिः α_2, शक्तिःर् J_3B **34d** आद्या] माया μG, आह्री R_2, ख्याता α_1, अद्या α_3, आधा VK_2 ◇ शिवे] परा S, शिवा α_2, सिता α_3, प्रिये B **35a** तत्रा°] तत्र MK_2PJ_3, तत्रां γ_1

33c – 34b *om.* K_2

मूलशक्त्या समासाद्य तत्रस्थं शीतलामृतम् ॥३५॥
सुषुम्णया समानीय स्वाधिष्ठानादिपङ्कजात् ।
तत्सुधावृष्टिसंसिक्तं स्मरेद् ब्रह्माण्डकावधि ॥३६॥
तत्रस्थममृतं गृह्य शक्तिः श्रीकुण्डली परा ।
सुषुम्णामार्गमासाद्य ब्रह्मधामान्तमीयुषी ॥३७॥
मूलपञ्चकलाजातसुधातृप्तिपरिप्लुता ।
आपादमस्तपर्यन्तं व्यापयन्तीं तनुं स्मरेत् ॥३८॥
पञ्चमासप्रयोगेन पञ्चभूतलयो भवेत् ।
शिवसाम्यं भवेत्सत्यं त्रिकालाभ्यासयोगतः ॥३९॥
[स्वाधिष्ठानकलाः]
लिङ्गस्थानं हि यद्देवि स्वाधिष्ठानं तदुच्यते ।
तत्र दिव्यामृतमयं कलात्रयमुदीरितम् ॥४०॥
सुसूक्ष्मा परमाह्लादा विद्या चेति प्रकीर्तिताः ।
पूर्ववत्कुम्भकावस्थां प्राप्य शक्तिं प्रबोध्य च ॥४१॥

35c °शक्त्या] °शक्तिं G   35d तत्रस्थं] तत्रगं μG   36a सुषुम्णया] $AJ_6^{pc}J_7VK_5$; सुषुम्नया $J_6^{ac}GJ_2K_4J_3PFB$, सुषुम्णयां R_2, सुषुम्नायां $SW_1\alpha_3$, सुषुम्नयां N, सुषुम्णायां M, सुषुम्नाया J_4-J_1, सुषुम्णाया K_6R_1, सुषुमृणाया J_5W_2 ◇ समानीय] $GS\beta\gamma$; समुन्नय्य A, समुन्नध्य J_6J_7, समीनीय R_2, समासीना α_2, समासीनः M, समासीन α_3 36b °ष्ठानादि°] °ष्ठानाद्य° α_2 ◇ °पङ्कजात्] °पंकजान् VJ_3, °पंचकात् K_2B 36c तत्सुधावृष्टि°] G; वसुधावृष्टि° μ, तं सुधारस° K_5, तत्सुधारस° *cett.* ◇ °संसिक्तं] °ससिक्ता R_2, °संसिक्तां $S\alpha_2$ 36d स्मरेद्] स्मरद् $R_2\gamma_1$, स्रवद् B ◇ °कावधि] °वत्*सु*धीः G, °कार्यधीः α_3 37a तत्रस्थममृतं] μGR_2; तत्र स्थाने मृतं $S\alpha$, तत्र संस्थामृतं $\beta\gamma$ ◇ गृह्य] μ; गुह्यं $GR_2S\alpha_2\alpha_3\beta$, [मयी] M, गुह्य γ 37b श्रीकुण्डली] $\mu K_3\beta_1K_5K_6$; कुंडलिनी $GR_2S\alpha_1$, कुंडली K_1J_3 *(unm.)*, कुडलनीं K_2, थी कुंडली P, सा कुंडली F, यत्कुंडलिका J_1R_1 *(unm.)*, यत्कुंडलि J_5W_2, य कुंडलिनी B *(unm.)* ◇ परा] पराः A, परां K_2P, पुरा B   37c सुषुम्णा°] सुषुम्ना° $J_6^{ac}\alpha_3J_2J_4K_4PJ_3FB$ 37d °धामान्तम्] $J_6GR_2S\alpha_2K_5B$; °धामं तम् $AJ_7\alpha_3$, °धामातम् $J_2J_4K_4$, °धामांत $VJ_3F\gamma_1$, °धायांन K_2, °धामात P, °धामांत्तर् K_6 ◇ ईयुषी] $\mu SW_1J_2J_4K_4K_5K_6B$; श्रायुषी $GN\alpha_3$, उन्मुखीं R_2, पीयुषी $VP\gamma_1$, पीयुषा K_2, यायुषा J_3, पीयुषि F   38a °पञ्च°] °पर्व° α_3 ◇ °कला°] °कसा° A ◇ °जात°] $GR_2SJ_2VK_4K_2$-PFK_5; °जाता $\mu\alpha_2K_6\gamma$, °जाताः M, °याता α_3, °जातं J_4J_3 38b °तृप्ति°] °वप्ति° J_2, °तप्ति° γ_2R_1 ◇ °प्लुता] *प्ल*तां R_2, °प्लुताः MK_5 38c °मस्त°] μ; °तल° *cett.*   38d व्यापयन्तीं] $\mu R_2SMK_1J_2K_4PK_5$; [वि]ख्यायंती N, व्यापयंती $W_1K_3J_4VK_2FB$, व्यापयंतिं J_3, व्यापती[त] K_6, व्यापयंति γ_1 ◇ तनुं] $J_6J_7R_2SMK_1$; तनु $A\alpha_2K_3$, तु तां $\beta_1PJ_3FK_5K_6\gamma$, तु सं° K_2 39b °लयो भवेत्] °जयं लभेत् μ 39c °साम्यं] GR_2; °तुल्यो K_2B, °सम γ_1, °साम्यो *cett.*   39d त्रिकाला°] त्रिविधा° G   40a लिङ्गस्थानं हि यद्] G; नाभिस्थानं हि यद् μ, नाभिस्थानादधो *cett.*   40c °मयं] °मयी γ 41a सुसूक्ष्मा] सुषुम्णा $S\alpha\gamma$ ◇ परमाह्लादा] GSJ_4K_6; परमा हृद्या α_1, परमाह्लाद *cett.*   41b विद्या चेति] कला विद्या G, दिव्या चेति R_2, नाम्ना देवि M ◇ प्रकीर्तिताः] $J_6GR_2MK_5$; प्रकीर्तिता *cett.*   41d प्राप्य] प्राण° α_1 ◇ प्रबोध्य] प्रयोध्य AJ_7

35d – 36a *om.* K_2 37cd *om.* M   38cd *om.* G39a – 40d *om.* α_3

नीत्वा ब्रह्माण्डपर्यन्तं प्लावयेच्च स्वकां तनुम् ।
योगी त्रिमासपर्याये पूर्वोक्तं लभते फलं ॥४२॥
[वेणुदण्डकलाः]
गुदमेढ्रान्तरं यद्वै वेणुदण्डं तदुच्यते ।
कलाचतुष्कं तत्रोक्तं परामृतरसात्मकम् ॥४३॥
सुशीता च महातृप्तिः पलितघ्नी वलिक्षया ।
तत्र शक्तिं समुद्बोध्य पूर्ववत्प्लावयेत्तनुम् ॥४४॥
चतुर्मासप्रयोगेन पूर्वोदितफलं लभेत् ।
पिङ्गला रविवाह्या स्यादिडा स्याच्चन्द्रवाहिनी ॥४५॥
विषवाहो रविः प्रोक्तः सुधावाहो निशाकरः ।
अभ्यासः सूर्यवाहाख्ये चन्द्रवाहे च शस्यते ॥४६॥
†धारणा चन्द्रवाहे च† योगी कुम्भकमाचरेत् ।
शशिवाहेन पवनं पूरयेदात्मनस्तनुम् ॥४७॥
रविवाहेन चोत्सर्गः शस्यते देहवृद्धये ।
एतत्ते व्याहृतं देवि कलास्थानं चतुर्गुणम् ॥४८॥

42a नीत्वा ब्रह्माण्डपर्यन्तं] पीत्वा ब्रह्मांडपर्यंतं μ, कलां प्राप्य पीत्वा ब्रह्मादिपर्यंतं G *(unm.)* **42b** प्लावयेच्च स्वकां] प्लावयेद्यः स्वकां μ, प्लावयित्वा स्वकां G, प्लावयेच्च स्वकीं $R_2J_4K_4$, प्लावयेदात्मनस् M **42c** °पर्याये] °पर्यायैः $S\alpha_1K_2J_3$, °पर्याय γ_1, °पर्यायात् B **43a** गुद°] गुह्य° α_3 ◇ °मेढ्रान्तरं यद्] °मेढ्रांततंतुर् G, °मेढ्रांतरे यद् R_2F **43b** वेणु°] वीणा° G **44a** सुशीता च] सुगतं च G, सुशांता च J_3, सुशीतला B ◇ महातृप्तिः] परा तृप्तिः $R_2\alpha$, महातृप्ति $J_2VK_4PJ_3\gamma$ **44b** पलितघ्नी] वलिघ्नी च G, तदंघ्रीव N ◇ वलिक्षया] परिक्षया G, वलीजय R_2 **44d** प्लावयेत्] भावयेत् $SPJ_3F\gamma$ **45c** रवि°] विष° G ◇ °वाह्या] $AJ_6SJ_2J_4K_4PK_6\gamma$; °वाज्या° J_7, °वाहा $GR_2W_1MK_5$, °वाह $N\alpha_3F$, °वाह्य VK_2J_3 ◇ स्याद्] °ख्या μG, °स्थाद् α_2 **45d** इडा स्याच्] इडाख्या μ, चेडाख्या G ◇ चन्द्र°] छशि° M **46a** विषवाहो] $\mu R_2\alpha_1\gamma$; विषवाहा G, विषवाही S, विषवाहस् α_3, विषमहो β_1PJ_3, विषमंहो K_2, विषवाह F, विषमहा K_5, विषमाहो K_6 ◇ रविः प्रोक्तः] B; रवेर्बाहुः A, रवेर्वाहुः $J_6J_7K_6$, रवेर्वाहा G, रविर्वार्वाहो R_2 *(unm.)*, रवेर्वाहः SMJ_2K_4PF, रवेर्वाह α_2, तु खे वाहः K_1, तु रवे वाहः K_3 *(unm.)*, रवे वहिः J_4, रारवेर्वाहः V *(unm.)*, रचे वहिः K_2, रवे वह्निः J_3, रविवाहः K_5 *(unm.)*, रवेर्काहः γ_1 **46b** सुधावाहो] सुधावाहा GK_2, क्षुधावाहो α_3, सुधावा*हे* F ◇ निशाकरः] निशाकरे $\mu GR_2\alpha_2\alpha_3$, निशाकरं V **46c** अभ्यासः] अभ्यासं μ, अभ्यास $W_1K_2FJ_1R_1$ ◇ सूर्य°] पूर्व° R_2 ◇ °वाहाख्ये] μ-α_3; °वाहस्य G, °वादौ स्या R_2, °वाहाच्च $SK_4K_2J_3FK_6$, °वाहाख्य N, °वाहाख्यश् W_1, वाहाख्यः M, °वाहच्च J_2V, °वावा च J_4, °वाह च P, °वाहाद्ये K_5, °वाहे च γ **46d** चन्द्र] शिशि M ◇ °वाहे] °वाह° G, °वाहश् NM, वाहः W_1, °वाहो $V^{ac}J_3$ ◇ च शस्यते] $J_6J_7R_2NM\alpha_3$; च शम्यते A, °स्य शस्यते G, प्रशस्यते $W_1\beta_1PJ_3FK_5\gamma$, प्रकाश्यते K_2, प्रशास्यते K_6 **47a** †धारणा†] $S\alpha_2VK_4\gamma$; धारणं μJ_2, धारणां GJ_3K_5, धारणाच् R_2K_2PF, धीरः स्याच् M, न रक्षा α_3, धारःणा J_4, धारनाच् K_6 ◇ †°वाहे च†] °वाहेन μ **47c** °वाहेन] °वाहे च $\beta\gamma$ ◇ पवनं] पवनैः K_5 **47d** पूरयेदात्मनस्] पूरयित्वात्मनस् G ◇ तनुम्] पदं K_2 **48a** रविवाहेन] विषवाहेन G, रविवाहे च γ_1, रविवाहे त° B ◇ चोत्सर्गः] त्वोत्सर्गः α_2, वोत्सर्गः VK_4, °थोत्सर्गः B **48b** °वृद्धये] °सिद्धये G **48c** एतत्] एवं AB ◇ व्याहृतं] कथितं S, व्याकृतं α_3 **48d** चतुर्गुणम्] च तद्गुणः AJ_7, च ⌈त⌉द्गुणं J_6

42d लभते तनु संगम् *add.* G ◇ **42d** लभते – **43c** तत्रोक्तं *om.* V

[परामृतमहापदम्]

अतः परं प्रवक्ष्यामि परामृतमहापदम् ।
वज्रकन्दं ललाटे तु प्रज्वलच्चन्द्रसंनिभम् ॥४९॥
लंगर्भं चतुरस्रं च तत्र देवः परः शिवः ।
देवताः समुपासन्ते योगिनः शक्तिसंयुतम् ॥५०॥
चूलितले महादेवि लक्षसूर्यसमप्रभम् ।
त्रिकोणमण्डलं मध्ये देवं लिङ्गात्मकं शिवम् ॥५१॥
रंगर्भमध्यमं देवि स्वशक्त्यालिङ्गितं परम् ।
देवतागणसंजुष्टं भावयेत्परमेश्वरि ॥५२॥
दक्षशङ्खे महाभागे षड्बिन्दुवलयान्वितम् ।
यंगर्भं धूम्रवर्णं च तत्र देवं महेश्वरम् ॥५३॥
लिङ्गाकारं स्मरेद्देवि शक्तियुक्तं गणावृतम् ।
वामशङ्खे ऽर्धचन्द्राभं सपद्मं मण्डलं शिवे ॥५४॥
वंगर्भं च दृढं मध्ये तत्र लिङ्गं सुधामयम् ।
गोक्षीरधवलाकारं शरच्चन्द्रायुतप्रभम् ॥५५॥

49b °महापदम्] μ; महापथं GSM$\alpha_3\beta_1$PF$K_5K_6\gamma$, महापथां R_2, महामृतं α_2, महामथं K_2, महीपथं J_3 49c °कन्दं] °कंदे μ, °कंद α_2, °कुंद J_1R_1 ◇ ललाटे तु] ललाटोक्तं S, ललाठं च R_2, ललाटे च αJ_3 49d प्रज्वलच्°] प्रस्फुरच्° R_2 50a लंगर्भं] μG; लंभग° R_2, लंगर्भे S$\beta\gamma$, लं[बीजं] N, लंबितं W_1, लंबीजं M, लीगलं K_1, लांगलं K_3 ◇ चतुरस्रं] °र्भचतुस्रं R_2, चतुरस्रे VK_5 50b तत्र देवः परः शिवः] तत्र देवं पर ग्रावरं G *(unm.)*, तावदेव परः शिवः α_3 50c देवताः] $R_2S^{pc}\alpha_3J_2VK_4K_5$; देवतास् μ, देवता GJ_4P$J_3\gamma_1$, तद्देवाः S^{ac}, ते देवाः N, तं देवाः W_1, त देवाः M, देवतां K_2FK_6B ◇ समुपासन्ते] तमुपासंते J_6, तुमुपासंते AJ_7, समुपासते J_2, समुपासत्ते VK_4, शक्तिसंयुक्ता M 50d योगिनः] Sα_1B; योगिन्यः μGR_2, योगिन्याः α_3, योगीभ्यः β_1K_2PK_5K_6, योगीन्यः J_3, योगिभ्यश् F, योगिभ्यां γ_1 ◇ शक्तिसंयुतम्] $\mu R_2\beta\gamma_1$; शक्तिसंयुताः S$\alpha_2\alpha_3$, समुपासते M, शक्तिसंयुतां B 51a चूलितले] चुलितले A, चूलीतले J_6J_7-$R_2K_1K_2$F$K_5\gamma$, चूळीतले G, चूलिताले α_2 ◇ °देवि] °भागे G 51b °प्रभम्] °प्रभां γ 51c °मराडलं] °मराडल° W_2, °मरादले B 51d देवं] देव $\alpha_2J_2J_4$PFK_6, देवि $K_2\gamma$ ◇ शिवम्] μR_2SαV; शिवे G$J_2J_4K_4K_2$PJ_3F$K_5K_6\gamma$ 52a °गर्भ°] °गर्भं GSαVF ◇ °मध्यमं] °मध्यगं μG, °परमं α_3, °मध्यम° γ_1 52b °लिङ्गितं] °लिंगितां γ ◇ परम्] परे G 52c °संजुष्टं] °संवीतं G, °संयुक्तं αJ_4, °संतुष्टं K_2, °जुष्तं च γ 52d भावयेत्] प्लावयेत् J_2, सावयेत् J_4, लावयेत् K_4 ◇ परमेश्वरि] परमेश्वरी $K_3J_4K_2K_6$, परमेश्वरं J_3B 53a दत्त°] लत्त° R_2 ◇ °शङ्खे] °संख्ये R_2K_6, °शाखे α_3 53b °ग्रान्वितम्] °ग्रांकितं M, °ग्रान्विते $\alpha_3\gamma_2R_1$ 53c °गर्भं] °गर्भ° R_2NJ_2J_4VPγ_1, °गर्भे B 53d देवं महेश्वरम्] देवो महेश्वरः SαK_6 54b शक्तियुक्तं] शिवयुक्त α_3, शक्तियुक्ति K_2 ◇ गरणावृतम्] गुरणीवृत R_2, गुरणावृतं K_2, गुरणान्वितं J_3 54c °शङ्खे] °शंखो $\mu J_2J_4\gamma_1$, °शाखे α_3, °संखो K_2, °[स]खे P, °सेखे J_3 54d सपद्मं] स्वपद्मं μ, सपद्म° $K_2\gamma_1$, पापद्मं J_3 55a वं°] व° μ, य° K_3, तं° J_3 ◇ च दृढं] टढं पत्त्य° A *(unm.)*, दृढं पत्त° J_6J_7 *(unm.)*, च कूरितं G *(unm.)*, च टृटं M, चन्द्राद्य° K_6 55b लिङ्गं] लिंग° γ_1

स्वशक्तिसहितं सर्वदेवतागणसेवितम् ।
एवं देवि चतुर्दिक्षु स्थानान्युक्तानि वै मया ॥५६॥
तेषां मध्ये महावृत्तं हंगर्भं तत्र पार्वति ।
परमेशः परः शम्भुः स्वशक्तिसहितः स्थितः ॥५७॥
लिङ्गाकारो गणयुतः सूर्यकोटिसमप्रभः ।
पृथिव्यधिपतिर्भाले पश्चिमे सूर्यनायकः ॥५८॥
दक्षशङ्खे ऽनिलपतिर्वामे जलपतिः शिवे ।
मध्ये व्योमाधिपः शम्भुस्थानाः पञ्च मयोदिताः ॥५९॥
व्योमाधिपस्य देवस्य शिरोर्ध्वे चतुरङ्गुलम् ।
ज्योतिर्मण्डलमध्यस्थं कोटिचन्द्रसमप्रभम् ॥६०॥
दिव्यामृतमयं भाण्डं मूलबन्धकपाटकम् ।
ऊर्ध्वचन्द्रं महाशैलमभेद्यममृतास्पदम् ॥६१॥
शीतलामृतमध्ये तु विलीनं लिङ्गमीश्वरि ।
त्रसरेणुप्रतीकाशं कोटिचन्द्रसमप्रभम् ॥६२॥

56a स्वशक्ति॰] संशक्ति॰ N, सशक्ति॰ W_1, सुशक्ति॰ γ ◇ सर्व॰] $\mu G\alpha_1 K_1 K_2 K_6 B$; [..] R_2, सर्वं $SK_3 J_2 VK_4 FK_5 \gamma_1$, सर्वे J_4, संर्व P, तत्र J_3 **57a** ॰वृत्तं] $\mu GS\alpha_2\alpha_3 VK_5$; ॰वृत्यं R_2, ॰वृत्ते M, ॰वृत्तं $J_2 PJ_3 FK_6\gamma$, ॰वृतं $J_4 K_4$, ॰वृत्तां K_2 **57b** ॰गर्भं] ॰गर्भे $M\gamma_1$ ◇ तत्र] तव M, तत्त्व α_3 **57c** परमेशः] μFK_5; परेश्वर॰ G, परमेश्व॰ R_2, परमेश्वरः $SNJ_2 VK_4 K_2 PK_6\gamma$ *(unm.)*, परेश्वरः $W_1 M\alpha_3 J_4$, परमे J_3 *(unm.)* ◇ परः] ॰रश्च R_2 **57d** स्वशक्ति॰] स्वशक्त्या μG, स्वसिन॰ K_1, खसित॰ K_3, स्वशक्तिः $J_3 K_6$ ◇ ॰सहितः स्थितः] $J_6 SNMJ_2 J_4 K_4 PJ_3 F$; ॰सहितस्थितः $AJ_7 GR_2 W_1 VK_2 K_6$, ॰शक्तिसंस्थितः α_3, ॰सहितः शिवः K_5, ॰परतः स्थितः γ_1, ॰परिसेवितः B **58a** ॰आकारो] ॰आकारा R_2, ॰आकारे $NK_3 J_2 K_6$, ॰आकारैर् W_1, ॰आकार M, ॰आकारै K_1 ◇ गण॰] $J_6 J_7 GK_6 B$; गुण॰ $AR_2 S\beta_1 K_2 PFK_5\gamma_1$, गुणैर् α, गुणी॰ J_3 ◇ ॰युतः] ॰युक्तः α **58b** सूर्यकोटि॰] कोटिसूर्य॰ G **58c** पृथिव्य॰] पृथिव्या॰ $AR_2 M\alpha_3\beta W_2 B$ ◇ ॰पतिर्] $J_6 J_7 GR_2\alpha_1 K_2$; ॰पति $A\beta_1$, ॰पतिः $SPJ_3 FK_5 K_6\gamma$, ॰पतेर् α_3 ◇ भाले] $\mu\alpha_2\alpha_3$; जाले G, वामे $R_2 K_4$, लाभे M, पूर्वे $SVK_5 K_6\gamma$, पुर्वे J_2, पूर्व $J_4 K_2 F$, पुर्वैर् P, पूर्वैः J_3 **59a** दक्ष॰] तथा G, दक्षि॰ γ_1 ◇ ॰शङ्खे] ॰शाखे α_3 ◇ निल॰] नील॰ μ **59b** शिवे] शिवः μGM **59c** मध्ये] *om.* G ◇ व्योमाधिपः] μ; व्योमाधिप॰ G, व्योमपति॰ $R_2 W_1 M\alpha_3\beta_1 K_2 PFR_1$, व्योमपतिः $SNK_5\gamma_2 W_2 B$, सोमपति॰ J_3, यामपतिः K_6 ◇ शम्भु॰] μ; स्थानान्य् $GR_2\beta\gamma$, स्थाने $S\alpha$ **59d** ॰स्थानाः] μ; एताः G, एषां $R_2 J_2 J_4 K_4 PJ_3 FK_5 K_6\gamma$, एते $S\alpha$, एषा VK_2 ◇ मयोदिताः] $J_6 GSW_1 MK_1$; मयोदिता $AJ_7 NK_3 R_1$, मयोदितं $R_2\beta_1 PK_5 K_6 B$, मयोदित K_2, मयोदितः $J_3 F$, मयोदितां $\gamma_2 W_2$ **60b** शिरोर्ध्वे] $J_6 J_7 R_2 SFK_5$; शिरोर्द्धे $A\alpha_1\beta_1 K_2 PJ_3 FK_6$, शिरोर्ध्वश् G, शिरोर्धे α_3, सिद्धं च γ ◇ ॰अंगुलम्] $SJ_2 PJ_1 R_1 B$; ॰अंगुले $\mu GR_2\alpha J_4 VK_4 K_2 K_5 K_6$, ॰अंगुलां $J_5 W_2$ **61a** ॰मयं] $\mu GR_2 S\alpha K_5$; ॰मये $\beta_1 K_2 PK_6\gamma$, ॰मयो F ◇ भाण्डं] $\mu GR_2 S\alpha K_5$; भांडे $J_2 J_4 K_2 PK_6\gamma$, भांड V **61b** कपाटकम्] कवाटकं AGK_4, कवाठकं $J_6 J_7$ **61c** ऊर्ध्वचन्द्रं] $K_5 B$; ऊर्ध्वेरुर्ध्व॰ A, ऊर्ध्वेरूद्र्ध्व॰ J_6, ऊर्ध्वेरूर्ध्व॰ J_7, ऊर्ध्वरंध्र॰ G, ऊर्ध्वे चंद्र R_2, ऊर्ध्वचंद्र $S\alpha J_2 J_4 K_4 K_2 PJ_3 F\gamma_2 W_2$, ऊर्ध्वशैलं V, ऊर्द्धच*न्द्र K_6, उर्द्धं चंद्रं R_1 ◇ महाशैलम्] तथा चंद्र॰ V **61d** अभेद्यम्] $\mu GR_2\alpha K_5$; अभेदम् $SJ_2 J_4 K_4 K_2 PF$, भवेदम् V, अभेदाम् J_3, अहाभेद् K_6, अमेदम् γ ◇ अमृतास्पदम्] अमृतं परं α_3, अमृतात्मकं J_4 **62a** शीतलामृत॰] शीतरमृत G **62b** ईश्वरि] ऐश्वरं R_2, ईश्वरं $\beta\gamma$ **62d** ॰चन्द्र॰] ॰सूर्य॰ S

58c – 62d *found after 2.66d in* R_2 *(probably as a correction of an eye-skip to 2.63a)* **60c – 61a** *om.* J_3
62a ॰मध्ये तु – **64a** परामृत॰ *om.* G *(eye-skip)*

हेयोपादेयरहितमज्ञानतिमिरापहम् ।
अतीत्य पञ्च स्थानानि परतत्त्वोपलब्धये ॥६३॥
परामृतघटाधारकपाटं कुम्भकान्वितम् ।
मनसा सह वागीशामूर्ध्ववक्त्रां प्रसारयेत् ॥६४॥
निरुद्धप्राणसंचारो योगी रसनयार्गलम् ।
लीलयोद्घाटयेत्सत्यं संप्राप्य मनसा सह ॥६५॥
शीतलेक्षुरसस्वादु तत्र क्षीरामृतं हिमम् ।
योगपानं पिबेद्योगी दुर्लभं विबुधैरपि ॥६६॥
तत्सुधातृप्तिसंतृप्तः परावस्थामुपेत्य च ।
उन्मन्या तत्र संयोगं लब्ध्वा ब्रह्माण्डकान्तरे ॥६७॥
नादबिन्दुमयं मांसं योगी योगेन भक्षयेत् ।
एतद्रहस्यं देवेशि दुर्लभं परिकीर्तितम् ॥६८॥
सर्वज्ञेन शिवेनोक्तं यत्फलं शास्त्रसंततौ ।
तत्फलं लभते सत्यं षण्मासान्नात्र संशयः ॥६९॥
संप्राप्य सिद्धिसंतानं यो योगमिममीश्वरि ।
न वेत्ति तस्य वक्तव्यं न किं चित्सिद्धिमिच्छता ॥७०॥

63c अतीत्य] अभीष्ट α ◇ पञ्च] ॰तत्व॰ M ◇ स्थानानि] शून्यानि α **63d** परतत्त्वोपलब्धये] परं तत्वे पि लभ्यते $\alpha_2\alpha_3$, परतत्वे च लभ्यते M, परतत्त्वोपलभ्यते J_3, परं तत्वे *पि* लब्धये K_5 **64a** ॰घटाधार॰] J_6J_7; ॰चटाधार॰ A, ॰घडाधार॰ G, ॰षडाधार॰ $R_2SK_3J_4VK_4PJ_3FK_5K_6\gamma$, ॰षडाधारं $\alpha_1K_1J_2$, ॰षडाधारा॰ K_2 **64b** ॰कपाटं] ॰कवाटं μG; कपालं α_1, कपाल α_3 **64c** वागीशाम्] $S\alpha_1J_3$; वागीशीम् $\mu G\alpha_3FK_5$, वागीशी* R_2, वागीशिम् $J_2J_4K_4PK_6\gamma_1$, वागीशम् V, वागीश K_2, वागीशी B **64d** ऊर्ध्व॰] ऊर्ध्वं $G\alpha_3R_1B$ ◇ ॰वक्त्रां] वक्त्रे G **65a** निरुद्ध॰] संरुद्धा॰ A, संरुद्ध॰ J_6J_7G, निरुद्धा॰ J_2P ◇ ॰संचारो] ॰संस्थानो R_2 **66a** शीतलेक्षु॰] शीतलक्षण॰ A, शीतेक्षुर॰ α ◇ ॰रसस्वादु] ॰रसस्वादं S, ॰ससुस्वादं α, रसः स्वादु γ_1 **66b** तत्र क्षीरामृतं] μ; हृद्यं क्षीरोपमं G, ****मृतं R_2, तत्क्षीरममृतं $S\alpha_2\alpha_3\beta_1K_2PFK_5\gamma$, तत्क्षरममृतं M, तत्क्षारममृतं J_3, *तत्*क्षिरममृतं K_6 ◇ हिमम्] हितं μK_2, परं α **66c** योगपानं] परामृतं G ◇ पिबेद्योगी] $GS\alpha$; पिबेन्मध्यं μ, पिबेत्क्षीरं $R_2\beta_1K_2PFK_6\gamma$, पिबेत्क्षारं J_3, भवेत्क्षीरं K_5 **66d** विबुधैर्] विविधैर् μK_2, त्रिदशैर् S **67a** ॰तृप्ति॰] ॰पान॰ G, ॰रस॰ M ◇ ॰तृप्तः] GSK_5; ॰तप्तः μ, ॰तृप्त्यै α_2, ॰तृप्त्य M, ॰तृप्तो *cett.* **67c** उन्मन्या तत्र] उन्मन्यंते त्र॰ α_2, तन्मयं नेत्र॰ α_3, उन्मना तत्र K_5 **67d** लब्ध्वा] बध्वा γ ◇ ॰कान्तरे] ॰काननं G **68a** मांसं] मासं $AJ_6W_1J_4J_3B$, मास W_2R_1 **68d** परिकीर्तितम्] त्रिदशैरपि M **69a** सर्वज्ञेन] सर्वज्ञानं G, सर्वं तेन γ **69b** यत्फलं] μ; सकलं R_2, सफलं *cett.* ◇ ॰संततौ] ॰संमतौ J_4, ॰संसृतौ P, ॰संमतं B **69c** फलं] μ; सर्वं *cett.* ◇ लभते] लभ्यते $\alpha_2\alpha_3\gamma$ ◇ सत्यं] नित्यं GR_2, सिद्ध N, सिद्धं W_1 **69d** ॰मासान्] ॰मासां G, ॰मासे α_2 **70a** सिद्धि॰] सिद्धिं AJ_2VK_2 ◇ ॰संतानं] $\mu GR_2J_2VK_4FK_5K_6\gamma$; ॰सोपानं $S\alpha_1$, ॰संपानं α_3, ॰संज्ञानं J_4, ॰संतानां K_2, ॰सतांनां P, ॰संतानो J_3 **70b** यो योगमिममीश्वरि] योगगम्यमपीश्वरि A, योगयोगममीश्वरि J_6J_7, यो योगमिममीश्वरम् K_5, *य*ोगगम्यं महेश्वरि B **70d** किं] क्व μ, च α ◇ चित्सिद्धिम्] सिद्धिं प्र॰ α_1, सिद्धिं नि॰ α_3 ◇ इच्छता] $\mu SK_2PJ_3FK_6$; इच्छतां $G\gamma$, इच्छतः $R_2S^{vl}J_2J_4K_4K_5$, ॰यछति α_1, ॰यच्छसि K_1, ॰यक्कसि K_3, इच्छति V

---

67 found after 68 J_3

न जानन्ति गुरुं देवं शास्त्रोक्तान्समयांस्तथा ।
दम्भकौटिल्यनिरतास्तेषां शास्त्रं न दापयेत् ॥७१॥

[अमृतेनाङ्गमर्दनम्]
जिह्वामूले स्थितो देवि सर्वतेजोमयो ऽनलः ।
तदग्रे भास्करश्चन्द्रो भालमध्ये प्रतिष्ठितः ॥७२॥
एवं यो वेत्ति तत्त्वेन तस्य सिद्धिः प्रजायते ।
मथित्वा मण्डलं वह्नेः समुद्बोध्य प्रयत्नतः ॥७३॥
तदुष्णसारद्रवितं भालजं चन्द्रमण्डलम् ।
भास्कराधिष्ठिताग्रेण रसनेन समाश्रयेत् ॥७४॥
तच्चन्द्रगलितं देवि शीतलं परमामृतम् ।
नासिकारन्ध्रनिर्यातं पात्रेण परिसंग्रहेत् ॥७५॥
तेनाङ्गमर्दनात्सत्यं नाडीशुद्धिः प्रजायते ।
गुदलिङ्गोद्गतं पात्रे निर्गतं चामरीरसम् ॥७६॥
कक्षामृतं च संलोड्य संस्कृतं चाधरारसैः ।

72a – 73b *cit.* नारायणदीपिका *(D) ad* ब्रह्मविद्योपनिषद् 8, ĀSS 29, p.341

71a गुरुं] गुरून् F **71b** °श्रोक्तान्] °श्रोक्त° $G\gamma_2$, °श्रोक्तं K_1W_2, °श्रोक्तः K_3 ◇ समयांस्तथा] समयं तथा G, समयान् पुनः K_5 **71c** दम्भकौटिल्यनिरतास्] ये दंभ्यकुटिलास्तेभ्यश् G **71d** तेषां शास्त्रं] शस्त्रमेतं G **72a** °मूले] °मूल° G ◇ स्थितो] स्थिति A, स्थिते J_6, स्थिता $G\alpha_3$ ◇ देवि] देवी $R_2\alpha_3J_4J_3K_6$, देवः D_1 **72b** ऽनलः] निलः J_4B, जलः J_3 ◇ **72c** चन्द्रो] μ; चंद्रस् $GSNM\alpha_3J_4VK_4FK_5BD$, चंद्र $R_2W_1K_2J_3J_1R_1$, चंद्रः J_2PJ_5, चेंद्र K_6, चद्रः W_2- **72d** भालमध्ये] μ; तालुमूले GM, तालुमध्य° K_5, तालुमध्ये *cett.* ◇ प्रतिष्ठितः] व्यवस्थितः G **73a** तत्त्वेन] देवेशि μ, तत्वज्ञस् G, तत्वे च R_2 **73b** प्रजायते] प्रयुज्यते γ **73c** वह्नेः] वन्हिं G **74a** तदुष्णसारद्रवितं] GR_2B; उष्णसारद्रवितं A *(unm.)*, दुष्णसारद्रवितं J_6J_7 *(unm.)*, तदुष्णत्वद्रवीभूतं $S\alpha_1$, तदुष्णं चंद्रवीभूतं α_3, तद्विष्णुसारद्रवितं K_5 ($\beta_1K_2PJ_3F\gamma_1$ *have corruptions of* तदुष्णसारद्रवितं) **74b** भालजं] μ; तज्जलं α_3, वह्निजं K_5, तालुजं *cett.* ◇ °मण्डलम्] °मंडले α_3 **75a** तच्] μR_2K_6B; त्वं γ_1, तं *cett.* ◇ चन्द्र°] चंद्रा° A **75b** शीतलं] शीतं[*] G, शितला γ_1 ◇ परमामृतं] तत्पयोमृतं AJ_7, यत्पयोमृतं J_6, *यंप*योगी तं G **75d** पात्रेण] पात्रे च α_3 **76a** तेनाङ्ग°] तदंग° G, तेभ्यांग° γ ◇ °मर्दनात्सत्यं] °मर्द्दनां नित्यं G, °मर्दनं कृत्वा R_2 **76b** नाडी°] नाडि° AGJ_3, नदा° R_1 ◇ °शुद्धिः] °सिद्धिः μ **76c** गुद°] गुह्य° J_3, गुड° K_6, गूढ° γ ◇ °लिङ्गोद्गतं] $GR_2SJ_2VPJ_3FK_5\gamma$; °लिङ्गोहतं μK_6, °लिंगद्रुतं α_2, °लिंगं द्रुतं M, °लिंगाद्रुतं α_3, °लिंगाहृतं J_4, °लिंगोहृतं K_4, °लिंगागतं K_2 ◇ पात्रे] देवि μ **76d** निर्गतं] निर्गमं μ, निर्मथ्यम् α_1, निर्मथ्या α_3, निर्गत° K_2FK_6 ◇ चामरी°] μG; यपुरी R_2, यो मरी° SJ_4J_3, अमरी° α_1, सशरी° α_3, व्योमरी° $J_2VK_4PFK_5\gamma$, °त्त्योमरी° K_2, °स्यामरी° K_6 ◇ °रसम्] °रयं R_2, °रकं α_3 **77a** कक्षामृतं] कलामृतं μ, काक्षामलं R_2, कद्यामृतं α_3, कक्षामतं J_2V, कंक्षामृतं P, संख्यामृतं J_3, कथामृतं γ ◇ °लोड्य] °योज्य M, °लेप K_2, °लोद्य P, °लेद्य J_3, °लेप्य γ **77b** संस्कृतं] $R_2S\alpha_1J_2VK_2FK_5K_6B$; संस्कृत्यं μ, संस्कृत्य G, स सत्यं α_3, सस्कृतं J_4K_4, संस्कृजं P, संस्कार्यं J_3, संस्कृतां γ_1 ◇ चाधरा°] स्वामरी° G, वाधरा° B ◇ °रसैः] °रसं G, °रसः α_3, °रसौ $J_2J_4K_4$

72b *all witnesses except* μGD *insert corrupt versions of* 75ab **72b – 73a** *om.* V **75** *om.* J_3

तेनाङ्गमर्दनं कृत्वा योगी लोके निरामयः ॥७७॥
बलवान् जायते सत्यं वलीपलितवर्जितः ।
जिह्वामूलं समुद्घृष्य तत्र जातं महाद्रवम् ॥७८॥
स्वदेहं मर्दयेत्पूर्वं रसना वत्सरार्धतः ।
चतुरङ्गुलवृद्धा च जायते नात्र संशयः ॥७९॥

[खेचरीमुद्रा]
उत्कृष्य रसनामूर्ध्वं दक्षिणाङ्गुलिभिः शिवे ।
वामहस्ताङ्गुलीभिश्च घण्टिकां स्फोटयेच्छिवे ॥८०॥
मथित्वा पावकस्थानमूर्ध्ववक्त्रं शनैः शनैः ।
त्रिकूटोर्ध्वे च चन्द्रांशे शिवस्थानं समाश्रयेत् ॥८१॥
एषा ते खेचरीमुद्रा कथिता मृत्युनाशिनी।
[भटनटदोषाः]
एवमभ्यासशीलस्य तद्विघ्नार्थं भवन्ति हि ॥८२॥
भटभेदाश्च चत्वारो नटभेदास्तथैव च ।
अङ्गशोषः क्षुधालस्यं कण्डूर्देहविवर्णता ॥८३॥
भटस्य प्रत्यया एते तेषां शृणु च भेषजम् ।

77d योगी लोके] योगी स्यात्तु G, *transp.* $S\beta\gamma$ 78c समुद्घृष्य] GW_2; समूद्घृष्य A, समुद्धृष्य J_6J_7, च संघृष्य $S\alpha_1H_2$, च संमर्द्य α_3, संमुद्*घृ*ख्य J_2, समुद्धृत्य J_4VK_5, समुद्धृत्य K_4, समुत्कृष्य K_2PB, समुद्धष्य J_3, समुघृ*ष्य*K_6, समुद्*ुष्य γ_2, समुष्टाष्य R_1 78d जातं] जात° GK_2 ◇ महाद्रवम्] मदद्रवं μ 79a स्वदेहं] स्वदेहे $AJ_2J_4K_4K_2$ ◇ पूर्वं] पूर्वाद् μ, पूर्व° α_2 79b रसना] रसेन $M\alpha_3H_2$ 79c °वृद्धा] μJ_3; °वृद्ध्या *cett.* 80a उत्कृष्य] आकृष्य G ◇ ऊर्ध्वं] ऊर्ध्वे J_6J_7, ऊर्ध्व° $R_2\alpha_2\beta_1K_2PJ_3FK_6$ 80d घण्टिकां] $GR_2SNJ_2K_5$; रसनां M, घटिका H_2, घंटिका *cett.* 81a पावकस्थानं] वामकं स्थानं μ, पावकास्थाने G, पावकं स्थानं F 81b °वक्त्रं] $\mu SJ_2J_3FR_1$; °वक्त्रः $G\alpha_1K_5$, °वक्त्र $R_2K_1J_4K_4$, °चक्र K_3K_6, °चक्रः V, °चक्रं $K_2P\gamma_2W_2B$, °चक्त्र H_2 81c °ध्वें च] GNM; °ध्वं च μ, °द्धें च R_2W_1, °ध्वें र्ध° SF, °ध्वोंर्चे K_1, °ध्वोंर्ध च K_3 *(unm.)*, °द्धैंद्व J_2, °द्धैंद्वं J_4, °द्धें द्य V, °द्धें द्यं K_4, °द्धं K_2 *(unm.)*, °द्वें P *(unm.)*, °द्धें द्धं° J_3K_6, °ध्वें थ K_5, °द्धाट° $J_1J_5R_1$, °द्धात्य W_2B ◇ चन्द्रांशे] $SM\beta_1FK_5K_6$; वज्रांत्यो μ, वज्रांते G, वज्रांशे R_2, चांद्रांशे α_2, चक्रांशे α_3, चंद्रांसो K_2, चंद्राशे P, चंद्रातं J_3, °यच्चंद्रो J_1, चंद्रोंशे J_5, चंद्रोशे W_2, °यच्चंद्रा R_1, चंद्रांशं B 81d समाश्रयेत्] समाचरेत् G 82a एषा] एषां $AJ_4V\gamma_1$ 82d °विघ्नार्थं] विज्ञानं G, °विद्यार्थं α_3, °विद्याश्च J_2J_4, °विज्ञार्थं J_3, °विघ्नाश्च K_6 ◇ भवन्ति हि] भवति हि A, भवत्यथ G, भवेंति हि J_2, भवेति हि J_4, भवन्न हि K_2 83a भट°] μB; हट° $GR_2\alpha_2J_2K_5$, हठ° $SMK_1J_4K_4K_2FK_6$, ह° K_3 *(unm.)*, हर° V, हव° P, देह° J_3, म° J_1R_1 *(unm.)*, भ° J_5W_2 *(unm.)* 83b नट°] नर° V, नट° P *(unm.)* 83c °शोषः] $\mu S\alpha_1K_5$; °दोषः G, °शोष° $R_2\alpha_3J_2^{pc}$, °सोक° $J_4\gamma_1$, °शोष्क° V, °शोक° $J_2^{ac}K_4K_2PJ_3K_6$, °शोकः F, °सेक° B ◇ °आलस्यं] °आलस्य° $GK_2PFK_6\gamma$ 83d कण्डूर्] $GSNMVK_4F$; कंड $AR_2\alpha_3$, कंडू $J_6J_7J_4K_6$, कडूर् W_1, कंडुर् $J_2K_2PK_5$, कुंडर् J_3, कदु J_1W_2B, कडु J_5, कदु R_1 84a भटस्य] $J_6J_7VPK_5^{ac}\gamma$; भटःस्य A, हटस्य $GR_2NK_4FK_5^{pc}$, हठस्य SW_1MJ_4, नटस्य $\alpha_3K_2J_3K_6$, भ्दतस्य J_2 ◇ प्रत्यया] प्रत्ययाश् μG ◇ एते] चेते A, चैते J_6J_7, चैव G, °प्येते α_3 84b शृणु च] $\mu G\alpha$; स शृणु R_2, *transp.* $S\beta\gamma$

78c – 79b *om.* R_2 80ab *om.* J_4K_2F 82b सर्वसिद्धिप्रदा देवि जीवन्मुक्तिप्रदायिनी ॥ इति श्रीमत्स्येन्द्रसंहितायां पंचदशः पटलः *add.* μ

मनो निर्विषयं कृत्वा त्रिमासममरीरसम् ॥८४॥
देहमुद्वर्तयेत्तेन देहवृद्धिः प्रजायते ।
त्रिस्त्रिरुद्वर्तनं कुर्याद्दिवा रात्रौ तथैव च ॥८५॥
रसनामूर्ध्वमायोज्य वज्रकन्दपदोन्मुखीम् ।
तत्सुधां लिहतः सत्यं क्षुधालस्यं च नश्यति ॥८६॥
तत्सुधाममरीं देवि गृहीत्वा चाङ्गमर्दनात् ।
स्वशरीरविवर्णत्वं कण्डूश्चापि प्रणश्यति ॥८७॥
नटभेदाश्च चत्वारो बहुधा संस्थिताः प्रिये ।
नेत्ररोगो ऽङ्गवेपश्च दाहो भ्रान्तिस्तथैव च ॥८८॥
भेदमेकं मया प्रोक्तं द्वितीयमधुना शृणु ।
दन्तरुक्चाल्पसत्त्वं च देहलाघवनाशनम् ॥८९॥
तृतीयभेदं च तथा शृणु देवि महाज्वरः ।
शिरोरुक्श्लेष्मदोषश्च चतुर्थः संप्रधार्यताम् ॥९०॥
वमनं श्वासदोषश्च नेत्रान्धत्वं तथैव च ।

84c कृत्वा] पुडका A *(unm.)*, पुड्का J_6, पुदका J_7 **84d** °मासम्] °मासाद् G, °वारम् B ◇ अमरीरसम्] μG; अमृतारसैः B, अमरीरसैः *cett.* **85a** तेन] α_3B; तस्य *cett.* **85c** त्रिस्त्रिरुद्वर्तनं] त्रिरुद्वर्त्तनकं μ, त्रिस्त्रि कुर्यादह्नि R_2, निरुद्वर्त्तनकं α_3 ◇ कुर्याद्] रात्रौ R_2 **85d** दिवा] μM; सप्त° G, अह्नि *cett.* ◇ रात्रौ] °रात्रं G, कुर्या R_2 **86b** °पदोन्°] °परोन्° AJ_6, °वदुन्° G ◇ °मुखीं] °मुखी $\alpha_3J_2K_4K_2K_6\gamma$ **86c** °सुधां] °सुधा $R_2\alpha_3K_2\gamma$ ◇ लिहतः] लिहितः K_5, लिहितं γ **87a** अमरीं देवि] G; अमरी देवी A, अमरी देवि J_6J_7, अमरीं चापि R_2M, अमृतं चापि $SFK_5\gamma$, अमरी चाथ α_3, अमृतश्चापि $J_2VK_4K_2PK_6$, अमृतं J_4 *(unm.)*, अमृतं त्रापि J_3 **87b** गृहीत्वा] कषित्वा G **87c** स्वशरीरविवर्णत्वं] $\mu GR_2M\alpha_3$; सर्वं शरीरवैवर्ण्यं *cett.* **87d** कण्डूश्चापि प्र°] $SM\alpha_3J_4K_4$F; कंडूत्वं च प्र° μ, कंडुश्चापि प्र° R_2, कंडूकत्वं च G, कंदुश्चापि प्र° $J_2PJ_3K_5\gamma_1$, कडूस्यापि प्र° V, कुण्डश्चां प्र° K_2 *(unm.)*, कन्तुश्चापि प्र° K_6, कंडूश्चापि वि° B **88a** नटभेदाश्] नभटेदाश् A, नवभेदाश् J_4 **88b** बहुधा] हि मुदा G ◇ संस्थिताः] J_6GSMF; संस्थिता $AJ_7R_2W_1J_2J_4K_4K_2PJ_3\gamma_1$, संस्थितां NK_6, शंसिना K_1, शंसिता K_3, संस्थिते VK_5, संस्थिताश् B ◇ प्रिये] च ये B **88c** नेत्ररोगो] नेत्ररोगा° $GR_2N\alpha_3$, नेत्ररोगश् K_2, नेत्रे रोगं J_3, नेत्रस्य रो° B ◇ ऽङ्गवेपश्] G; ङ्गशेषश् A, ङ्गशोषश् $J_6J_7R_2S\alpha J_2VK_5$, ङ्गशोकश् $J_4K_4K_6$, च शोकश् K_2, शोकश् PJ_5W_2 *(unm.)*, च शोकं J_3, पि शोकश् FJ_1R_1, °गो शोकश् B **88d** दाहो भ्रान्तिस्तथैव च] भ्रांतिदाहोपशोषकाः G **89a** भेदमेकं] $\mu\alpha$; इदमेकं G, एको दवो R_2, एको भेदो S, एको दोषो $\beta\gamma$ ◇ मया] तथा α ◇ प्रोक्तं] $\mu G\alpha$; प्रोक्तो $R_2S\beta\gamma$ **89c** °रुक्] $\mu GR_2M\alpha_3VPJ_3K_6$; °रुग् SFK_5, °कं N, °क° W_1, °क् J_2 *(unm.)*, °*तुक*J_4 *(unm.)*, तुक्रु K_4 *(unm.)*, °हः K_2, °रुक्* J_1, °रुक्र $J_5W_2R_1$ *(unm.)*, °रुक B *(unm.)* ◇ चाल्पसत्त्वं] J_6J_7G; वाल्पसत्वं A, चालसत्वं R_2, अलसत्वं S, कायसत्वं N, °षायसत्वं W_1, कायशोषश् M, वलसत्वं $K_1\beta_1PJ_3FK_6\gamma$, कलशत्वं K_3, खलसत्त्वं K_2, गलसत्त्वं K_5 **89d** देहलाघव°] देहरोमवि° G **90a** तृतीयभेदं च तथा] तथा त्रितीयं भेदं च G, तृतीयभेदमधुना B **90b** देवि महाज्वरः] $\mu S\alpha_3J_2J_4VK_2PJ_3K_5$; देवि महाज्वरं G, *छे*को महेश्वर R_2, देवि महेश्वरि α_2, वक्ष्यामि सुंदरि M, देवि महा*घ*रः K_4, देवि भयज्वरः F, देवी महाज्वरः K_6, देवि महज्ज्वरः γ **90c** °दोषश्] °शोषश् M, °दोषाश् F **90d** चतुर्थः] $S\alpha_2$; चतुर्थं $\mu G\alpha_3J_2J_4K_4K_5$, चतुर्थश् M ◇ संप्रधार्यताम्] चावधार्यतां M **91a** वमनं श्वासदोषश्] वमनश्वासदोषं A, वमनं श्वासदोषं J_6J_7, पंचम*श्*वासदोषश् G **91b** तथैव च] प्रजायते S

86cd *om.* J_4 (*eye-skip from* तत् *to* तत्) 87 *om.* α_2 **89bc** *om.* J_4 **90d – 91a** *om.* $R_2VK_2PJ_3F\gamma$

दुर्जया च तथा निद्रा तेषां शृणु च भेषजम् ॥९१॥
मूलाधारात्सुषुम्नायामूर्ध्वं कुण्डलिनीं नयेत् ।
निश्चलामूर्ध्वगां जिह्वां कृत्वा कुंभकमाश्रयेत् ॥९२॥
शक्तिक्षोभान्महेशानि महानादः प्रवर्तते ।
यदा शृणोति तं नादं तदा मुक्तः स उच्यते ॥९३॥
चिन्तयेदमृतासिक्तं स्वदेहं परमेश्वरि ।
अनेन देवि मासेन पूर्वदोषैः प्रमुच्यते ॥९४॥
अनेनैव विधानेन द्विमासं तु यदाचरेत् ।
तदा शृणोति कर्णाभ्यां महागजरवध्वनिम् ॥९५॥
पूर्ववच्चिन्तयेद्देहं द्वितीयैर्मुच्यते गदैः ।
त्रिमासाद् ब्रह्मनादं च शृणुत्वा पूर्ववत्स्मरेत् ॥९६॥
तृतीयभेददोषैश्च मुच्यते नात्र संशयः ।
मेघनादमघोराख्यं चतुर्थे मासपर्यये ॥९७॥
श्रुत्वा पूर्ववदभ्यस्य भ्रान्तिदोषैः प्रमुच्यते ।

91d तेषां शृणु च] $J_6J_7R_2W_1M\alpha_3K_6$; तिषां शृणु च A, तदा शृणुत G, तेषां च शृणु $S\beta_1$-$K_2PJ_3FK_5\gamma$, शृणु देवि च N **92a** मूलाधा°] G; संमूला A, समूला $J_6J_7\gamma_1$, स्वमला R_2, स्वमूलो $SW_1M\alpha_3$, समूलो $NVK_4K_2J_3FK_5$, समूलात् J_2J_4, समूलाच् PK_6, समूलां B ◇ °रात्सु°] G; छास° A, छ्वास° $J_6J_7\alpha_2K_1VPFK_5K_6$, °श्वास° R_2, च्छ्वास° S, °द्वान° M, क्वास° K_3, स्वास° J_2, स्वाश° J_4, ष्वास° K_4, °त्थास° K_2, साव° J_3, चशि° γ ◇ °षुम्नायाम्] G; °संयुक्तां S^{ac}, °रांभिन्नाम् B, °सम्भिन्नाम् *cett.* **92b** ऊर्ध्वं] $\mu R_2MK_2K_6B$; ऊर्ध्वां F, ऊर्ध्व° *cett.* ◇ कुण्डलिनीं] कुंडलिनी $W_1M\alpha_3K_2PJ_3K_6\gamma_1$ **92d** आश्रयेत्] आचरेत् F **93b** महानादः] जलनादः μ, महानांदः γ_2R_1 **93d** स उच्यते] स मुच्यते $J_2K_4PJ_3$, प्रमुच्यते VK_5 **94a** चिन्तयेद्] सेचयेद् G ◇ अमृतासिक्तं] अमृतांत्राभि G, अमृताशक्तिं α_3H_2, अमृताशक्तं J_3 **94b** स्वदेहं परमेश्वरि] सांगोपांगकलेवरे H_2 **94c** अनेन देवि] क्रमेण देवि R_2, तेन देवेशि F **94d** पूर्व°] सर्व° μV ◇ प्रमुच्यते] विमुच्यते G **95b** द्विमासं तु] द्विमासांत A, द्विमासांतं J_6J_7G, द्विमासं च $K_2J_1R_1$ ◇ यदाचरेत्] सदा चरेत् R_2, समाश्रयेत् M, यदा*ध*रेत् J_2, यदा धरेत् J_4K_4, समाचरेत् K_2K_6 **95d** °गज°] °राज° α_2 ◇ °रव°] GMF; °वर° $\mu R_2S\alpha_2\alpha_3K_2J_3H_2$, °वरं $J_2VK_4PK_5\gamma$, र J_4 *(unm.)*, °रवं K_6 **96a** चिन्तयेद्] कुंभयेद् M ◇ देहं] देवि $G\alpha_1J_4$, देह $R_2\gamma$, देहे J_2 **96b** द्वितीयैर्] μM; द्वितीयो α_3, द्वितीयै K_4, द्वितीय K_2K_5, द्वितीयं F, द्वितीये *cett.* ◇ गदैः] भ्रमैः G **96c** त्रिमासाद्ब्रह्मनादं च] त्रिमासात्सिंहनादं च μ, त्रिमासाज्जिह्वया नादं G, त्रिमास ब्रह्मवन्नादं H_2 **96d** श्रणुत्वा] μ; शृणुयात् *cett.* **97a** तृतीय°] तृतीये $GR_2\gamma$, तृतीयैर् M **97d** चतुर्थे] चतुर्थं γ ◇ मासपर्यये] $K_4K_2FK_5K_6$; मासि पर्ययेत् μ, मासि पर्याये GJ_3, मास पर्ययेत् R_2, मासि श्रूयते $S\alpha_2\alpha_3$, श्रूयते प्रिये M, मासे ** J_2, मास श्रूयते J_4, मासपर्ययत् V, मासपर्य्यये P, मासपर्यते γ_1, मासपर्यतः B **98a** श्रुत्वा] स्मृत्वा $\alpha_2J_2J_4$, शृण γ_1, शृणु B ◇ अभ्यस्य] $\mu G\alpha_2$; अभ्यासे $R_2\alpha_3$, अभ्यस्येद् M, अभ्यासाद् *cett.* **98b** भ्रान्ति°] भ्रांत्या R_2 ◇ °दोषैः] $GS\alpha FB$; °दोषैश् μ, °शेषैः $\beta_1K_2PJ_3K_5K_6W_2$ ◇ प्रमुच्यते] च मुद्यते A, च मुच्यते $J_6J_7R_2$

94ab *om.* K_2 **98bcd** *om.* γ_2R_1

एवं स्थिरमतिर्ध्यानमभ्यासं च त्रिकालतः ॥९८॥
साधयेत् त्र्यब्दतः सत्यं जायते ह्यजरामरः ।
भटदोषचतुष्कस्य नटदोषस्य चैव हि ॥९९॥
निवारणं मया प्रोक्तं भूयः शृणु सुराधिपे ।
यो ऽस्मिन् शान्ते परे तत्त्वे योगे योगी सुखात्मके ॥१००॥
प्रविष्टः सर्वतत्त्वज्ञस्तस्य पादौ नमाम्यहम् ।

[अभ्यासक्रमः]

प्रथमं चालनं देवि द्वितीयं भेदनं भवेत् ॥१०१॥
तृतीयं मथनं शस्तं चतुर्थं च प्रवेशनम् ।
तालुमूलं समुद्घृष्य जिह्वामुत्कर्षयेत्प्रिये ॥१०२॥
चालनं तद्विजानीयाद् ब्रह्मार्गलविभेदनम् ।
भेदनं तद्वदन्ति स्म मथनं तन्तुना प्रिये ॥१०३॥
लोहकीलप्रवेशेन यदा मथनमाचरेत् ।

98c एवं] ब्रह्म॰ G ◇ स्थिरमतिर्ध्यानम्] $\mu R_2 SNM\alpha_3$; स्थिरमतिध्यानम् GW_1, सर्वस्थिरमतिध्यानम् J_2 *(unm.)*, सर्वस्थिरमतिर् $J_4K_4J_3B$, सर्वं स्थिरमतिर् $VPFK_5$, स्थिरसर्वमतिर् K_2, सर्वस्थिरसरमतिर् K_6 *(unm.)*, सर्वास्थिरमतिर् W_2 98d अभ्यासं च] अभ्यसेच्च μ, अभ्यासेन K_2 ◇ त्रिकालतः] द्विकालकं μ, त्रिकालकं G, त्रिकालिकाः α_2, त्रिकालिकः α_3, त्रिकालसः $J_2J_4K_4$ 99a साधयेत्] μMK_1VK_2; कृत्वाथ G, साधयेद् $R_2SJ_2J_4K_4PJ_3FK_5K_6$, [धारयत्] N, धारयेत् W_1, साधयत् K_3, साधू यद् γ_2, साधयद् W_2, साध्यु यद् R_1, संसाध॰ B ◇ त्र्यब्दतः] G; प्रवृतः AJ_7, अवृतः J_6R_2, अब्दतः $SJ_2J_4K_4PFK_5K_6$, पृष्ठतः α_1, पष्ठतः α_3, अष्टतः VJ_3, दृष्टतः K_2, भुतः γ_2W_2 *(unm.)*, भुत R_1 *(unm.)*, ॰येद् भुतः B 99c भट॰] $\mu VK_4K_5^{ac}$; हट॰ $GNJ_2PFK_5^{pc}\gamma$, नट॰ $R_2\alpha_3$, हठ॰ $SW_1MJ_4K_6$, हव॰ K_2J_3 ◇ ॰दोष॰] ॰भेद॰ α_1, ॰भेदैश् α_3 99d नट॰] भट॰ $J_2J_4K_4PJ_3\gamma$ ◇ ॰दोषस्य] ॰भेदस्य M, ॰भेदश्च α_3 ◇ चैव हि] जायते α_3 100b सुराधिपे] सुराधिप A, नराधिपे GB, सुरार्चिते $\alpha_1J_2J_4F$ 100c यो ऽस्मिन्] μF; यस्मिन् $GS\beta_1K_2PJ_3K_5K_6\gamma$, यस्मि R_2, यस्मिन्न् α_2, याश्म॰ α_3 ◇ शान्ते] अंते α_1, ॰न शां॰ α_3 ◇ परे तत्त्वे] $\mu R_2S\beta\gamma$; परतत्वे G, पतित्वा तु α_2, पतित्वा यो M, ॰ते पतित्वा α_3 100d योगे] μ; ज्योतिः J_2, योगी *cett.* ◇ योगी सुखात्मके] J_6J_7; योगी सुकात्मके A, योगसुखात्मनि G, योगे सुरात्मके $R_2\alpha_2$, योगे सुरार्चिते M, योगेश्वरात्मके *cett.* 101a प्रविष्टः] प्रविष्ट μJ_3R_1, प्रविष्टा $J_2J_4J_1$, प्रतिष्टा K_4, प्रविष्टाः J_5 101b पादौ] पादं $\mu GJ_2J_4K_4$ 101d द्वितीयं] द्वितीये SPJ_3B, द्वितीयो γ_1 ◇ भेदनं] *conj.*; मंथनं M, मथनं *cett.* 102a तृतीयं] तृतीये S, तृतीयो K_2 ◇ मथनं शस्तं] *conj.*; पानमुद्दिष्टं $\mu GR_2S\alpha_1VK_4PJ_3FK_5K_6\gamma$, पीनमुद्दिष्टं α_3, पामनमुद्दिष्टं J_2 *(unm.)*, यामनमुद्दिष्टं J_4 *(unm.)*, पातमुद्दिष्टं K_2 102b चतुर्थं] चतुर्थां A, चतुर्थे SK_2 ◇ च] μG; तत्॰ *cett.* ◇ प्रवेशनं] प्रवेशकं μ, प्रमेलनं G 102c ॰उद्घृष्य] $GSMJ_2J_4F^{ac}B$; ॰उद्हृष्य A, ॰उद्धृष्य $J_6J_7K_3F^{pc}K_6$, ॰उघृष्य R_2, ॰उद्घर्ष्य N, ॰उद्घर्ष्य W_1, ॰उद्घष्य K_1, ॰उत्कृष्य V, ॰उद्*ष्य K_4, ॰उदिष्टं K_2, ॰उष्टष्य P, ॰उर्द्घाष्य J_3, ॰उद्घश्य K_5, ॰उष्टस्य γ_1 102d उत्कर्षयेत्] उद्घर्षयेत् GNM, उद्धर्षयेत् W_1, उत्तच्चिपेत् J_1R_1 103a तद्] $\mu GS\alpha_3$; तु R_2, तं $\alpha_1\beta\gamma$ 103b ब्रह्मार्गलवि॰] μG; तृमार्गार्गल॰ R_2, त्रिमार्गार्गल॰ $S\alpha\beta_1K_2PJ_3FK_6$, त्रिभागार्गल॰ K_5, समार्गलम॰ J_1, समार्गल॰ $J_5W_2R_1$ *(unm.)*, परमार्ग॰ B *(unm.)* 103c भेदनं तद्] S; तं μ *(unm.)*, भेदनं त[*] G, भेदनं तं $R_2\alpha_1\beta_1PK_5K_6B$, भेदं न तं α_3, भेदनं ते K_2J_3, भेदनांते F, भेदनं त γ_1 ◇ वदन्ति स्म] वदति स्मां G 103d मथनं] ⊔⊔⊔⊔ μ ◇ तन्तुना] तंतुमत् G 104a लोहकील॰] लोहकेन G, लोहकोलं R_2 ◇ ॰प्रवेशेन] ॰प्रयोगेरा F 104b यदा] $R_2S\beta_1PJ_3\gamma$; यथा $\mu G\alpha K_2K_5K_6$, यधा F ◇ मथनम्] मंथनम् M ◇ आचरेत्] आरभेत् μK_2

मथनं तद्विजानीयाद्योगवृद्धिकरं प्रिये ॥१०४॥
उद्घाट्यार्गलमाकाशे जिह्वामूर्ध्वं प्रसारयेत् ।
प्रवेशं प्राहुरीशानि योगसिद्धिप्रवर्तकम् ॥१०५॥
ब्रह्मार्गलप्रभेदेन जिह्वासंक्रमणेन च ।
प्रत्ययः परमेशानि क्षणात्सत्यं प्रजायते ॥१०६॥
आदावानन्दभावत्वं निद्राहानिरतः परम् ।
संगमं भोजनं चैव स्वल्पमात्रं प्रजायते ॥१०७॥
पुष्टिः संजायते तेजोवृद्धिश्च भवति प्रिये ।
न जरा न च मृत्युश्च न व्याधिपलितानि च ॥१०८॥
ऊर्ध्वरेता महेशानि अणिमादिगुणान्वितः ।
यदि निश्चलभावेन योगमेवं प्रसाधयेत् ॥१०९॥
तदा प्रोक्तानिमान्सम्यक् फलान्लभति पार्वति ।
जिह्वाग्रे श्रीश्च वागीशा संस्थिता वीरवन्दिते ॥११०॥

104c मथनं] मंथनं MV ◇ तद्] μSB; तं *cett.* 104d योग॰] योगी $\mu\alpha_3$ ◇ ॰वृद्धि॰] ॰सिद्धि॰ α ◇ प्रिये] μMB; परेन् R_2, भवेत् $S^{pc}\alpha_2\alpha_3\beta_1PFK_5K_6\gamma_2W_2$, परं $S^{ac}K_2J_3R_1$ 105a उद्घाट्यार्गलं] उदर्घोर्गतम् A, उद्घार्गतम् J_6J_7 *(unm.)*, उभयोर्गलम् γ_2R_1 105b जिह्वामूर्ध्वं] जिह्वामूलं $\alpha_3J_1R_1$ ◇ प्रसारयेत्] प्रकारयेत् R_2 105c प्रवेशं] आवेशं F ◇ प्राहुरीशानि] प्राहुरीशानी AVJ_5W_2, परमेशानि G 105d ॰सिद्धि॰] ॰वृद्धि॰ G ◇ ॰प्रवर्तकम्] प्र**कं G, करं परं N, प्रवेशने W_1, प्रदायकं K_2 106a ब्रह्मार्गलप्रभेदेन] μ; प्रवेशे तालुमूलेन N, ब्रह्मार्गलप्रवेशेन *cett.* 106d क्षणात्सत्यं] क्षणार्धात्सं॰ μG 107a आनन्दभावत्वं] आनंदभावात्वं A, अनंदानुभवो G, आनंदभावश्च M, आनंदभावाति॰ J_5B, आनंदभावानि W_2 107b निद्रा॰] निंद्रा॰ A ◇ ॰हानिरतः] ॰हनिस्ततः G, ॰हानिस्ततः SF, ॰हारे ततः K_1, ॰हारं ततः K_3, ॰हारिताः J_4 *(unm.)*, ॰हानि इति J_3, ॰हानिः मतः J_5 ◇ परं] पदं μ 107c संगमं] μGW_1M; सगमे R_2, संगमे $S\beta_1PJ_3K_6J_5W_2B$, संगम α_3, संगमो K_2F ◇ भोजनं] भोजने K_5K_6 ◇ चैव] G; देवि *cett.* 107d स्वल्प॰] स्वल्पम् μ, जल्प॰ W_1M, स्वप्न॰ K_2B ◇ ॰मात्रं] अल्पं μ 108a पुष्टिः] $\mu\alpha_3$; सृष्टिस् G, तुष्टिः *cett.* 108b ॰वृद्धिश्च भवति] μ; देहसिद्धिर्भवेत् J_1R_1, देहवृद्धिर्भवेत् *cett.* 108c न जरा न च] नं जरा नं च A, न जरा तस्य M 108d व्याधि॰] $AM\beta\gamma$; व्याधिः J_6-$J_7GS\alpha_2\alpha_3$, *धिः R_2 ◇ ॰पलितानि च] α; ॰पलितं न च μR_2, पलितं तथा G, ॰पलितान्यपि $S\beta\gamma$ 109a ॰रेता] $GR_2S\alpha_1VK_2K_5K_6R_1B$; ॰येता A, ॰रेतो $J_6J_7\alpha_3J_2J_4K_4J_3F\gamma_2W_2$, ॰रतो P 109b ॰गुणान्वितः] μG; ॰फलोदयः R_2, ॰चतुष्टयां J_3, ॰समन्वितः *cett.* 109d योगमेवं] $GS\alpha_2FK_5$; योगी भावं μ, योगमेव M, योगमेतत् α_3, योग एव $\beta_1PJ_3K_6\gamma$, योग एवं K_2 ◇ प्रसाधयेत्] प्रसारयेत् μK_6, प्र**येत् R_2, प्रसादयेत् $J_2VK_4K_2P$ 110a तदा] यथा NM, तथा W_1, यदा α_3 ◇ प्रोक्तानिमान्] प्रोक्तमिमं G, फलानि प्रो॰ R_2 ◇ सम्यक्] सर्वं G, ॰क्तानि R_2, सम्यग् M, सस्य α_3, सत्यं J_1 110b फलान्लभति] μ; फलं भवति G, लभते पार्व॰ R_2, कामान्लभति $SVK_2PK_5K_6\gamma$, लभते वर॰ α_1, लभते काम॰ α_3, कामाल्लभंति J_2J_4, कामा लभ्रति K_4, कार्मान्लिभति J_3, कर्मान्लभति F^{ac}, कमाल्लभति F^{pc} ◇ पार्वति] ॰ति ध्रुवं R_2, ॰वर्णानि α_1 110c जिह्वाग्रे श्रीश्च] जिह्वाग्रे श्री AJ_7R_1 *(unm.)*, जिह्वाश्रीरस्य R_2, जिह्वाग्रस्थं च K_2 ◇ वागीशा] $\mu S\alpha_1\beta_1PJ_3FK_5$; वागीशे G, वागीशी $R_2\alpha_3K_6$, वागीशां K_2, वागेशि γ_1, वागेशी B 110d संस्थिता] संस्थिते G, संस्थितां K_2 ◇ वीरवन्दिते] मरवन्दिते G, वीप्सतः परं N

104cd *om.* G 107 *om.* NJ_1R_1

जिह्वामूलाधारभागे बन्धमृत्युः प्रतिष्ठितः ।
बन्धमृत्युपदं सर्वमुन्मूलय गणाम्बिके ॥१११॥
तदग्रेण विशेत्सोमधाम श्रीशम्भुसंज्ञितम् ।
अनेन देवि योगेन मनसाधिष्ठितेन च ॥११२॥
उन्मन्यावेशमायाति योगी तल्लयमाप्नुयात् ।
लयस्य प्रत्ययः सद्यः संभवत्यवि चारतः ॥११३॥
जिह्वाग्रे मन आधाय दृशा तद्धाम लक्षयेत् ।
मूलात्सुषुम्णामार्गेण पवनं चोर्ध्वमानयेत् ॥११४॥
ब्रह्मधामगतो योगी मनः शून्ये निवेशयेत् ।
ध्यायेदेवं परं तत्त्वं हेयोपादेयवर्जितम् ॥११५॥
आकाशगङ्गा स्रवति ब्रह्मस्थानात्सुशीतला ।
प्रपिबन्मासमात्रेण वज्रकायो भवेद्ध्रुवम् ॥११६॥
दिव्यदेहो भवेत्सत्यं दिव्यवाग्दिव्यदर्शनः ।

111a मूलाधार॰] $M\alpha_3J_5W_2$; मूलाधरे μ, मूले ध*र*ने G *(unm.)*, मूलाध** R_2, मूलधरा॰ $SW_1\beta_1K_2PJ_3K_5K_6$, मूलाधरा॰ FB, मूलाधारा॰ J_1, मूलाध्वार॰ R_1 **111b** ॰मृत्युः] μGSMF; ॰मृत्यु॰ $R_2W_1\alpha_3\beta_1K_2PK_5K_6\gamma$, ॰मृत्युं J_3 ◇ प्रतिष्ठितः] प्रतिष्टितं R_2, प्रतिष्ठिता α_3J_3 **111c** ॰पदं] $AJ_7K_5\gamma$; ॰प्रदं $J_6R_2S\alpha\beta_1K_2PJ_3FK_6$, ॰भयं G ◇ सर्वम्] सर्वेम् G, सर्वं $R_2W_1M\alpha_3$, सर्वे γ **111d** उन्मूलय] $\mu GSVK_2FK_5K_6\gamma$; उन्मूलति R_2, तन्मूलय W_1, मूलं मूल $M\alpha_3$, उन्पुलय J_2, उन्मूल J_4 *(unm.)*, उन्मुलय K_4, उन्मूय P *(unm.)*, ऊन्मूल्य J_3 *(unm.)* ◇ गर्णाम्बिके] μG; गुर्णांतिके MVK_2FK_5, गुर्णांकिते *cett.* **112a** ॰अग्रेर्ण] ॰अग्रे य R_2 ◇ विशेत्सोम॰] $S^{ac}\alpha_3$; विषा मोहं μ, विनाप्येकं G, वि*ना* माघं R_2, विशेत्सो हं S^{pc}, विनाशो हं W_1, विना मोघं M, विना मोहं β, विना मेवं J_1R_1, विना मेहं J_5W_2B **112b** ॰शम्भु॰] ॰शुभ॰ G ◇ ॰संज्ञितम्] ॰संज्ञकं $\mu\alpha_3F$ **112d** मनसाधिष्ठितेन च] *em.*; मनसा साधिते चले μ, *त्साधिष्ठिते जने G, ***साधितेन ते R_2, मनसाधिष्ठितेन ते $SW_1\beta_1K_2PFK_6\gamma$, मनसा साधितेन च α_3, षर्णमासैः साधितेन च M, दिनसप्तकमाचरेत् J_3, मनस्यधिष्ठितेन ते K_5 **113a** उन्मन्यावेशम्] आन्मन्यावेशम् G, उन्मन्यवश्यम् M, उन्मनीवशम् α_3 **113c** लयस्य] μG; लयनात् $R_2S\alpha\beta$, लंघनात् γ ◇ प्रत्ययः] प्रत्यया β_1 **113d** संभवत्य॰] μSK_6; संभवेत्व॰M, संपिवेच्च α_3, संभवंत्य॰ *cett.* **114a** मन आधाय] μ; मनसा ध्यायन् $G\alpha_3V$, *नसा ध्यायन् R_2, मनसा ध्यायेद् $SK_2J_3K_6\gamma$, मनसा ध्याये W_1J_4P, मनसा ध्यात्वा M, मनसा ध्याय J_2K_4, रसना ध्यायेद् F **114b** दृशा] $\mu SW_1J_2K_4PK_6$; तदा G, दृश्या R_2, दश MF, दशा $\alpha_3J_4VK_2$, दशां J_3, रसान् γ ◇ तद्धाम] $J_6J_7GSW_1\beta_1K_2PFK_6$; तद्वाम AJ_3, तद्वम R_2, धा[धा]म M, धातम α_3, वद्धाम γ **114c** मूलात्] मूला A ◇ सुषुम्र्णा॰] सुषुम्ना॰ K_3PFB **114d** पवनं] उन्मन्या G ◇ आनयेत्] उन्नयेत् M, चालयेत् K_3 **115a** ॰धाम॰] $\mu G\gamma$; ॰स्थान॰ J_3, ॰ध्यान॰ *cett.* **115c** ध्यायेदेवं परं] $SW_1\beta_1K_2PJ_3F$; ध्यायेत्परतरं μ, ध्यायन्परशिवं G, ध्यायेदेवं परे R_2, ध्यायेद्देवि परं $M\alpha_3$, ध्यायेद्देवं परं तत्वं K_6, व्यापदेवं परं J_1R_1, व्यापिदेवं परं J_5W_2, *व्यामि*देवं परं B **115d** ॰पादेय॰] ॰पादान॰ $\beta_1K_2PK_6\gamma$ ◇ ॰वर्जितम्] ॰वर्जितः $R_2J_3\gamma$ **116b** सुशीतला] सुशीतलं $\mu\alpha_3F$, सुलीलया M, सुशीतलः γ_2 **116c** प्रपिबन्] μ; प्रपिबेन् G, तापवेन् R_2, यः पिबेन् *cett.* ◇ ॰मात्रेर्ण] ॰त्रयेर्ण α_3 **117a** ॰देहो] ॰कायो μ **117b** दिव्यवाग्दिव्यदर्शनः] दिवादियत्वदर्शनं G, दिव्यकार्यादिदर्शनं M, दिव्यकायावदर्शनं α_3, दिव्यवाक् दिव्यदर्शनं γ_1

111a N *omits* 111–123, *replacing it with* गोरक्षसंहिता$_N$ 184–190, 192 and 197–198. W_1 *has the insertion but keeps* 111–123: *see description of sources for details.* **2.113d** विचारतः – 3 .8d ॰रूपिर्णी *om.* K_5 (f.11 *missing*) **115ab** *om.* R_2W_1

दिव्यबुद्धिर्भवेद्देवि दिव्यश्रवण एव च ॥११७॥
जिह्वाग्रे कोटिचन्द्राभां वागीशां परिभावयेत् ।
परामृतकलातृप्तां कवित्वं लभते क्षणात् ॥११८॥
जिह्वाग्रे संस्थितां लक्ष्मीं परामृतविमोदिताम् ।
ध्यायन्योगी महेशानि योगसाम्राज्यमाप्नुयात् ॥११९॥

[पञ्च सहजाः]

सहजाः पञ्च विख्याताः पिण्डे ऽस्मिन् †परमात्मके† ।
यदा संजायते देहो मातृदेहे पितृक्षयात् ॥१२०॥
तत्र सार्धं भवन्ति स्म देहे वृद्धिमुपेयुषि ।
आद्या कुण्डलिनीशक्तिः सहजा प्रथमा स्मृता ॥१२१॥
द्वितीया च सुषुम्णाख्या जिह्वा चैव तृतीयका ।
तालुस्थानं चतुर्थं च ब्रह्मस्थानं तु पञ्चमम् ॥१२२॥
उन्नीय सहजामाद्यां द्वितीयां सहजां न्यसेत् ।

117d दिव्यश्रवण] *em.* Sanderson; दिव्यः श्रवण SW_1, दिव्यश्रवणम् *cett.* **118b** वागीशां] वागीशीं $\mu GJ_2J_4FK_6$ ◇ परि°] μG; प्रवि° $R_2SW_1K_2PJ_3FK_6\gamma_1$, *om.* M, प्रति° α_3B, च वि° β_1 **118c** °तृप्तां] $\mu R_2S\alpha$; °तृप्त G, °तृप्ता $\beta_1K_2PK_6\gamma$, °तृप्ताः J_3, °तृप्तः F **118d** कवित्वं] कवितां μ ◇ क्षणात्] $\mu GR_2\alpha_3$; ध्रुवं *cett.* **119a** संस्थितां] संस्थिता $W_1K_3K_2J_3K_6\gamma$ ◇ लक्ष्मीं] लक्ष्मी $R_2K_2K_6\gamma_1$, लक्ष्मीः B **119b** °विमोदिताम्] $M\alpha_3$; °विमोदितः μ, °[.]मोदितां G, °विमोदिनीं R_2, °विमोहिनीं $SW_1\beta_1PF$, °विमोहिनी $K_2K_6\gamma$, °विमोहिता J_3 **119c** ध्यायन्] $\mu GM\alpha_3$; ध्याये R_2, ध्यायेद् $SW_1\beta\gamma$ ◇ महेशानि] महेशानीं G **120a** सहजाः] सहजा $K_3VK_2J_3FK_6\gamma$, सहजात् J_2K_4 ◇ विख्याताः] μGR_2SMK_1; विख्याता $W_1K_3J_2J_4VK_2PJ_3FK_6\gamma$, विख्यातां K_4 **120b** †परमात्मके†] μG; परमांकितो R_2, परिसांकिते S, परमांतिके α, परिमांतिते J_2K_4, परिमांतते J_4, परिमांतितो V, परमांकिते K_2FJ_1B, परिमांकिते $PK_6J_5W_2$, परिमाकिता J_3 **120c** देहो] $S\alpha_3\beta_1K_2PJ_3K_6\gamma$; देहे AR_2F, देहं J_6J_7, देह G, देवि W_1M **120d** °देहे] $\mu R_2S\alpha$; °देह° G, °देहो $\beta\gamma$ ◇ पितृक्षयात्] $R_2S\alpha\beta$; पितृक्षणात् μ, °परिक्षये G, पितक्षकात् γ **121a** तत्र सार्धं] $J_6J_7GR_2SPFK_6$; तत्रा सार्धां A, तत्तस्यार्धं α, तत्र सार्धा β_1, तं सार्धं K_2 *(unm.)*, तत्र सार्द्ध $J_3\gamma_1$, तत्र सार्धां B ◇ भवन्ति स्म] भवति स्म P, भवत्यस्माद् F **121b** देहे] μR_2; देह° *cett.* ◇ वृद्धिम्] बुद्धिम् γ ◇ उपेयुषि] $\mu\alpha_3$; उवेयुषे G, उपेयुषी R_2W_1MV, उपयुषी J_2, उपेयुषः SJ_3FK_6B, उपेयषी J_4, उपेयुषो K_4, उपेयषुः K_2, उपेयेषः P, उपेयसः γ_1 **121d** सहजा प्रथमा] *transp.* μ, [..]मा सहजा G ◇ स्मृता] स्थिताः A, स्थिता J_6J_7, मता J_3 **122a** च] μG; तु *cett.* ◇ सुषुम्णा°] सुषुम्ना° $S\alpha_3J_4P$ ◇ °ख्या] μGR_2W_1M, स्याज् SPJ_3FK_6B, स्यात् α_3, स्या $J_2VK_4K_2\gamma_1$, °स्थाज् J_4 **122b** जिह्वा] सिद्धा α_3 ◇ तृतीयका] तृतीयकं G, तृतीयागा J_2, तृतीयगा J_4K_4, तृतीयमा V, द्वितृतीयका J_3 *(unm.)*, तृतीयकाः γ_1 **122c** च] μG; स्याद् *cett.* **122d** तु] च $J_6J_7GJ_3$ **123a** उन्नीय] $GR_2SVK_4PJ_3FK_6$; उन्नध्या A, उन्नध्य J_6J_7, उन्निद्रा W_1M, तन्निद्रां α_3, उन्मन्नी° J_2, उन्मनी° $J_4\gamma$, उन्मतो K_2 ◇ सहजामाद्यां] $R_2S\alpha_3VPJ_3F\gamma$; सहजामाद्या A, सहजामाया J_6J_7, सहजामद्यां G, सहजावस्था W_1M, °य सहजायां J_2, °य सहजाद्यां J_4, सहजाद्यां K_4 *(unm.)*, सहजामायां K_2, सहमाद्यान्त K_6 **123b** द्वितीयां] GS, द्वितीया γ, द्वितीये *cett.* ◇ सहजां] SB; शहजे A, सहजे $J_6J_7R_2\alpha\beta_1K_2PJ_3F$, सहजा $G\gamma_1$, सहजो K_6 ◇ न्यसेत्] विशेत् μ

तृतीयां सहजामूर्ध्वं चतुर्थे सहजे विशेत् ॥१२३॥
चतुर्थं सहजं भित्त्वा सहजं पञ्चमं विशेत् ।
एतद्भेदं मया प्रोक्तं दुर्विज्ञेयं कुलेश्वरि ॥१२४॥

इति श्रीमदादिनाथप्रोक्ते महाकालयोगशास्त्रे
उमामहेश्वरसंवादे खेचरीविद्यायां द्वितीयः पटलः

123c तृतीयां] SαK$_6$; तृतीय° μJ$_4$J$_3$, तृतीया GR$_2$VK$_4$PFγ, तृतया J$_2$, तृतीम K$_2$ ◇ सहजाम्] साहजाम् A, सह*ज* G, सहजान्य् J$_4$ ◇ ऊर्ध्वं] *em.*; ऊर्ध्वा μ, र्द्धा च G, ऊर्ध R$_2$, उच्चैश् S$\beta\gamma$, ऊर्ध्वां W$_1$M, ऊर्ध्वे α_3 **123d** चतुर्थे] αJ$_4$F; चतुर्थ° μK$_2$J$_3$, चतुर्थं GJ$_2$VK$_4$PK$_6\gamma$, चतुर्ये R$_2$, चतुर्थां S ◇ सहजे] सहजा $\mu\gamma$, सहजं G, सहजां SK$_6$ **124a** चतुर्थं] चतुर्थ° μR$_2$VJ$_3$J$_5$W$_2$, चतुर्थीं G, चतुर्थां S, निगुह्यं N, चतुर्थे α_3 ◇ सहजं] सहजा A, सहजां J$_6$J$_7$GS ◇ भित्त्वा] नित्वा R$_1$ **124b** सहजं पञ्चमं] पंचमे सहजे SMK$_2$, सहजे पंचमे F ◇ विशेत्] भ्यसेत् A, व्रजेत् G, न्यसेत् K$_2$ **124c** एतद्] एवं R$_2$ ◇ भेदं मया] भेदरयं M, एव मया γ ◇ प्रोक्तं] प्रोक्ता R$_2$ **124d** °ज्ञेयं] °ज्ञेयाः R$_2$ ◇ कुलेश्वरि] कुलेश्वरी R$_2\alpha_3$K$_6$J$_5$W$_2$R$_1$, महेश्वरी K$_2$

124cd *om.* J$_3$ **124d** तत्सर्वं प्रयत्नेन गोपनीयं समाहितः *add.* V

तृतीयः पटलः

शिव उवाच

[कुण्डलिनीशक्तिः]

मूलात्कुण्डलिनीशक्तिं सुषुम्णामार्गमागताम् ।
लूतैकतन्तुप्रतिमां सूर्यकोटिसमप्रभाम् ॥१॥
प्रविश्य घण्टिकामार्गं शिवद्वारार्गलं शिवे ।
भित्त्वा रसनया योगी कुम्भकेन महेश्वरि ॥२॥
प्रविशेत्कोटिसूर्याभं धाम स्वायम्भुवं प्रिये ।
तत्रामृतमहाम्भोधौ शीतकल्लोलशालिनि ॥३॥
पीत्वा विश्राम्य च सुधां परमानन्दपूर्णया ।
बुद्ध्या तत्सुधया तृप्तमात्मदेहं विभावयेत् ॥४॥
अनेन दिव्ययोगेन जायते दिव्यदर्शनम् ।
खेचरत्वं भवेत्सत्यं सर्वरोगक्षयस्तथा ॥५॥
वञ्चनं कालमृत्योश्च त्रैलोक्यभ्रमणं तथा ।

Witnesses for the third paṭala:
$AJ_6J_7GR_2SNW_1MK_1K_3J_2J_4VK_4K_2PJ_3FK_5K_6J_1J_5W_2R_1B$;
D (32c–47d); H_1H_3 (19); H_2 (15, 18–19, 21ab, 26, 29cd, 30cd, 31c–32b)
μ=AJ_6J_7 ◇ α=$NW_1MK_1K_3$ α_1=NW_1M α_2=NW_1 α_3=K_1K_3 ◇
β=$J_2J_4VK_4K_2PJ_3FK_5K_6C$ β_1=$J_2J_4VK_4$ ◇ γ=$J_1J_5W_2R_1B$ γ_1=$J_1J_5W_2R_1$ γ_2=J_1J_5

1a मूलात्] μGR_2S; मूलां α_2, मूल॰ $\alpha_3\beta_1K_2PFK_6$, मूलं $J_3\gamma$ ◇ कुण्डलिनी॰] कुंडलिनीं α_2V ◇ ॰शक्तिं] ॰शक्तिः SK_2B; ॰शक्ति $W_1J_4J_3\gamma_1$ **1b** सुषुम्णा॰] सुषुम्ना॰ $J_6^{ac}GS\beta_1VPJ_3FB$ ◇ ॰मार्गम्] ॰मार्ग॰ G ◇ आगताम्] ॰संस्थितां G, आगता SK_2B, आश्रिता J_3, आगतः γ_1 **1c** लूतैक॰] तुलैक॰ γ_1, तूलैक॰ B ◇ ॰प्रतिमां] ॰प्रतिमा $J_2J_4K_4\gamma$ **1d** सूर्यकोटि॰] कोटिसूर्य॰ μG ◇ ॰प्रभाम्] ॰प्रभं A, ॰प्रभा K_4B **2a** प्रविश्य] प्रावेश्य K_2 ◇ घण्टिका॰] घटिका॰ $AJ_4K_2J_3\gamma_1$, घण्टका॰ G, पंथिका R_2 ◇ ॰मार्गं] ॰मार्गे $A\gamma$, ॰मार्गा R_2M, ॰मार्ग J_3 **2b** शिव॰] शिरो॰ R_2 ◇ शिवे] प्रिये M, शिवं α_3J_3, विशेत् K_6 **2d** महेश्वरि] कुलेश्वरि M **3a** प्रविशेत्] $J_6J_7SW_1\alpha_3PK_4FK_6$; प्रविंशेत् A, प्रविश्य G, ***त् R_2, प्राविशेत् NMJ_2J_4V, प्रवेश्य K_2, प्रावेशेत् J_3, प्राविशत् γ_2W_2B, प्राविश R_1 ◇ ॰भं] $\mu GR_2MJ_2J_4K_4$; ॰भां $S\alpha_2\alpha_3PJ_3K_6J_5W_2$, ॰भ्यां VJ_1R_1, ॰भा K_2B, ॰भः F **3b** ॰भुवं] $\mu G^{pc}R_2S\alpha_1J_4VK_4$; ॰भुवे $G^{ac}J_3K_6$, ॰भुवि α_3, ॰भवं J_2K_2, ॰भवे $P\gamma$, ॰भु*वे* F ◇ प्रिये] शुभे G, शिते F **3c** तत्रामृत॰] परामृत॰ G, तत्रामृतं MB, तत्रमृत॰ α_3, तयामृत॰ J_3 **3d** शीत॰] शिव॰ α_3 ◇ ॰शालिनि] MFB; ॰मालिनि AG, ॰मालिनी J_6J_7, ॰शालिनीं R_2SN, ॰शायिनी W_1, ॰शालिनी $\alpha_3\beta_1K_2PK_6\gamma_1$, ॰वारिणा J_3 **4a** विश्राम्य] $GS^{pc}\beta\gamma_1$; विश्रम्य $\mu R_2S^{ac}\alpha B$ ◇ च सुधां] सुधया G, वसुधां J_3 **4b** ॰पूर्णया] पू*र्व*या G **4c** बुद्ध्या] बुध्ये G ◇ तत्सुधया] त*च्छु*द्धया S, तच्छुद्धया J_3F ◇ तृप्तम्] μG; कृष्टम् SW_1, हृष्टम् R_2NMB, रच्चयम् α_3, *इष्ट*म् J_2, द्रष्टम् J_4K_6, दृष्टाम् $V\gamma_2W_2$, *om.* K_4, दष्टम् K_2, वृष्टम् P, दष्टःम् J_3, दृष्टम् F, षृाम् R_1 *[sic]* **4d** ॰देहं] $\mu GR_2S\alpha_2\alpha_3J_3F$; ॰देह MPK_4, ॰देहे $J_2J_4K_2K_6\gamma$, ॰चेहं V ◇ विभावयेत्] M; प्रभावयेत् μ, प्रबोधयेत् G, सुधापयेत् R_2, सुभावयेत् $S\alpha_2\alpha_3VJ_3F$, शुभावयेत् J_2K_2P, ॰षु भाववयेत् J_4 *(unm.)*, ॰षु भावयेत् K_4K_6, तु भावयेत् γ **5a** दिव्य॰] देवि μ **5b** ॰दर्शनम्] μGR_2VK_6; ॰दर्शनः *cett.* **5d** ॰क्षयस्तथा] ॰क्षयंकरं $\beta\gamma$ **6a** वञ्चनं] वचनं AJ_6, चंचनं J_7, मोचनं G ◇ ॰मृत्योश्च] *em.*; ॰मृत्युश्च μ, ॰मृत्युं च J_3, ॰मृत्यूनां *cett.* **6b** त्रैलोक्य॰] त्रैलोक्यं G, त्रैलोक्ये S ◇ ॰भ्रमणं तथा] क्रमते क्षणात् G

1ab *om.* M **1a – 8d** ॰रूपिणी *om.* K_5 (f.11 *missing*)

अणिमादिगुणोपेतः संसिद्धो जायते ध्रुवम् ॥६॥
योगीन्द्रत्वमवाप्नोति गतिरव्याहता भवेत् ।
नवनागसहस्राणां बलेन सहितः स्वयम् ॥७॥
जायते शिववद्देवि सत्यं सत्यं मयोदितम् ।
इडापिङ्गलयोर्मध्ये सुषुम्णा ज्योतिरूपिणी ॥८॥
वर्णरूपगुणैस्त्यक्तं तेजस्तत्र निरामयम् ।
प्रसुप्तभुजगाकारा या सा कुण्डलिनी परा ॥९॥
गङ्गा च यमुना चैव इडापिङ्गलसंज्ञके ।
गङ्गायमुनयोर्मध्ये तां शक्तिं संनिवेशयेत् ॥१०॥
ब्रह्मधामावधि शिवे परमामृतरूपिणीम् ।
तन्मयो जायते सत्यं सदामृततनुः स्वयम् ॥११॥
शिवधाम गता शक्तिः परमेशात्परं पदम् ।
तद्भोगतृप्तिसंतृप्ता परमानन्दपूरिता ॥१२॥
सिञ्चन्ती योगिनो देहमापादतलमस्तकम् ।

6c ◦गुणोपेतः] $GS\alpha V$; ◦गुणोपेतं $\mu J_2J_4K_4PFK_6$; गुणोपेतः R_2, गुणोपेतु K_2, ◦गुणोपेतां $J_3\gamma$ **6d** संसिद्धो] $J_6J_7R_2SMK_1VPJ_3FK_6$; संसिद्धि $AJ_2K_4\gamma_1$, प्रसिद्धो G, स सिद्धो α_2, संसिद्धा K_3, संसिद्धिं J_4B, संसिद्धिर् K_2 ◇ जायते] लभते AJ_7B, भवति M **7a** योगीन्द्रत्वमवाप्नोति] योगेंद्रतत्वमाप्नोति α_3, योगेंद्रत्वमवाप्नोति γ_2 **7b** अव्याहता] अव्यहता A, अव्याहाता J_2P, अवाहता J_4, अव्याहती J_3 **7d** बलेन] वदेत्तं $PF\gamma_2R_1$, वदे तं J_3W_2, वदेन K_6 ◇ सहितः] सहित GR_2-J_3FK_6, सहिता $J_2J_4K_4$ **8a** शिववद्देवि] शिवपदे पि α_3 **8d** ज्योतिरूपिणी] कांतिमत्यलं G, योनिरूपिणी K_2 **9a** ◦गुणैस्] $SW_1\beta$; ◦गणैः μ, ◦गुणैर् $G\gamma$, ◦गुणैः $NM\alpha_3$ ◇ त्यक्तं] $R_2S\beta_1PJ_3FK_5K_6$; साकं μ; युक्तं G, पूर्णो N, त्यक्त W_1, पूर्णं M, पूर्णैस् α_3, त्यक्तः K_2, युक्तैस् γ **9b** तेजस्तत्र] तेन तत्र W_1, वस्तुतस्तु M, तेज्ञस्तत्र K_5 ◇ निरामयम्] $\mu SMVJ_3$; निरायं R_2 *(unm.)*, निरालयं *cett.* **9c** प्रसुप्त◦] सुषुम्णा AJ_7, सुषुम्ण J_6^{pc}, सुषुम्न J_6^{ac}, सुषुप्त◦ G, प्र[..] R_2, प्रसुप्ता α_3V ◇ ◦गाकारा] ◦गाकाशे μ, ◦गाकारां J_4, ◦गाकारं K_2, ◦गाकार J_3, ◦गीकारा γ_1, ◦गीवेयं B **9d** या सा] यत्तत् μ, यसां R_2, माया M, या K_4 *(unm.)*, या सां W_2 **10b** ◦संज्ञके] μ; ◦संज्ञिके GSK_6, ◦संज्ञिता α_1J_3, ◦संज्ञिते $R_2\beta_1K_2PFK_5\gamma$, ◦संज्ञिका α_3 **10d** शक्तिं] शाक्ति AR_2, शाक्तिं MVB **11a** ◦धामा◦] ◦द्वारा◦ G **11b** परमामृत◦] परमानंद◦ GM ◇ ◦रूपिणीम्] μR_2K_5; ◦पूर्णया G, ◦रूपणीं J_3, ◦रूपिणी *cett.* **11c** तन्मयो] तन्मनो G ◇ सत्यं] शीघ्रं B **11d** सदा◦] परमा◦ μ *(unm.)*, परा◦ GM, तदा◦ K_2, सद्य◦ γ_1, सद्यो B ◇ ◦तनुः] ◦तनुं A, ◦तनु $J_6J_7R_2J_3J_5W_2$, ◦मयं G, ◦तमः K_2 **12a** शिवधाम] शिवागम◦ G, शिवधामा◦ $R_2\alpha_2$ ◇ गता] $AGR_2\alpha$; गतां $J_7J_6\beta_1K_2FK_5K_6$, गतीं P, गतं J_3, गतिं γ_1, गतिः B ◇ शक्तिः] $AGR_2S\alpha B$; शक्तिं $J_6J_7\beta_1PFK_5K_6J_1$, शक्तीं K_2, शक्ति $J_3J_5W_2R_1$ **12b** परमेशात्परं पदम्] परमेशास्पदं पदं μ, पर∗मस्पिदं परम् R_2, , परमेशत्पदं परं α_3 **12c** ◦भोग◦] ◦भाग◦ μ, ◦भाग्य◦ γ ◇ ◦संतृप्ता] ◦संदीप्तं G, ◦∗तत्वा R_2, ◦संतृप्ताम् α_2 **12d** ◦पूरिता] ◦रूपिता μ, ◦पूरितं GR_2, ◦पूरितः K_2 **13a** सिञ्चन्ती] J_6SMFK_5; सिचंति AK_6, सिंचंति $J_7GR_2J_2VK_4P$, संचिन्त्य α_3, सिंचिति J_4 *(unm.)*, शिंचिंत K_2, सिचिंती J_3, संचित्य γ

12d – 13a *om.* α_2

सुधया शिशिरस्निग्धशीतया परमेश्वरि ॥१३॥
पुनस्तेनैव मार्गेण प्रयाति स्वपदं शिवे ।
एतद्रहस्यमाख्यातं योगं योगीन्द्रवन्दिते ॥१४॥
[कालजयः]
उत्सृज्य सर्वशास्त्राणि जपहोमादि कर्म यत् ।
धर्माधर्मविनिर्मुक्तो योगी योगं समभ्यसेत् ॥१५॥
रसनामूर्ध्वगां कृत्वा त्रिकूटे संनिवेशयेत् ।
ब्रह्माण्डे ब्रह्मरेखाधो राजदन्तोर्ध्वमण्डले ॥१६॥
त्रिकूटं तं विजानीयात्तत्र लिङ्गं समुज्ज्वलम् ।
कालक्रमविनिर्मुक्तं दुर्विज्ञेयं सुरैरपि ॥१७॥
इडायां रात्रिरुद्दिष्टा पिङ्गलायामहः स्मृतम् ।
चन्द्रादित्यौ स्थितौ देवि नित्यं रात्रिदिवात्मकौ ॥१८॥
न दिवा पूजयेल्लिङ्गं न रात्रौ च महेश्वरि ।

15 *cit.* गोरक्षसिद्धान्तसंग्रह p.4 19 = हठप्रदीपिका 4.42

13c सुधया] μ; अथ सा $GR_2S\alpha\beta_1PJ_3K_5K_6$, ईष सा K_2, अधस्ताच् F, अथासाच् γ_2W_2, अथाच् R_1 *(unm.)*, अभ्यासाच् B ◇ शिशिरस्निग्ध॰] μ; शक्तिरश्मिस्थ G, शशिरश्मिस्था $R_2S\alpha$, चारीरस्था J_2 *(unm.)*, रींशक्तिस्थां J_4, शक्तिरश्मिस्था $VK_4K_5^{ac}$, च शरीरस्था K_2FK_6, च्च शरारस्था P, च शरीरस्थं J_3, [स्वशरीर]स्था K_5^{pc}, च शरीरस्थो γ **13d** ॰शीतया] μ; शीतला $GR_2S\alpha\beta$, शीतलां γ ◇ परमेश्वरि] $J_6J_7GSNMK_3P$; परमेश्वरी $AR_2W_1K_1\beta_1K_2J_3K_5K_6$, ता महेश्वरि J_1B, ता महेश्वरी $J_5W_2R_1$ **14a** पुनस्] प्राणस् γ **14b** प्रयाति] प्रयातः μ, पूजाति α_3 ◇ स्वपदं] स्वं पदं G, स्वयं α_3 *(unm.)*, स्वपुरं K_2 ◇ शिवे] μMJ_1R_1; प्रिये *cett.* **14c** रहस्यम्] रहसम् μ ◇ आख्यातं] देवेशि J_3 **14d** योगं] योगे $R_2\alpha$, योगी VK_6, मया K_5 ◇ योगीन्द्र॰] योगेंद्र॰ $R_2\alpha_3J_3\gamma_1$ ◇ ॰वन्दिते] ॰वन्दिताम् α_3, ॰वंदितं J_4K_6 **15b** कर्म] ॰कं च μG ◇ यत्] च $R_2M\alpha_3J_3H_2$, ॰जात् J_2J_4V **15c** ॰मुक्तो] ॰मुक्तं K_2 **16b** त्रिकूटे] $\mu R_2S\alpha$; भ्रूकुटीं G, त्रिकूटं $\beta\gamma$ **16c** ब्रह्माण्डे ब्रह्म॰] ब्रह्मरंध्रे ब्र॰ J_1R_1 ◇ ॰रेखाधो] $\mu R_2S\alpha_1VPJ_3FK_5K_6$; ॰रेखो*र्ध*ो G, ॰रेखायां α_3, ॰रेख्याधो J_2K_4, ॰रेखाधा J_4, ॰रोयोर्धा K_2, ॰ह्मरेखा J_1, ॰रेखाद्यो J_5, ॰रेखाद्यौ W_2, ॰ह्मरेख R_1, ॰रेखाद्ये B **16d** राजदन्तोर्ध्वमण्डले] $\mu GS\alpha$; ***तोर्धमंडलो R_2, दंतोर्ध्वमंडले प्रिये J_2J_4VP, दंतोर्ध्वं मंडले प्रिये K_4F, दतो यन्मंडलं शिवे K_2, दंतोर्ध्वमंडलं प्रिये J_3K_5, दन्तोर्ध्वे म्मण्डलं प्रिये K_6, तदूर्ध्वं मण्डलं प्रिये γ_2R_1B, तदूर्ध्वमंडलं प्रिये W_2 **17a** त्रिकूटं] भ्रूकुटीं G, त्रिकूटे R_2 ◇ तं विजानीयात्] αK_2; तं विजानीही A, तं विजानीहि J_6J_7, तत्र जानीयात् $GR_2S^{ac}\beta_1PJ_3FK_5K_6\gamma$, तद्विजानियात् S^{pc} **17b** तत्र लिङ्गं समुज्ज्वलम्] त्रिलिंगं सममुज्ज्वलं α_3 **17c** कालक्रम॰] *em.* SANDERSON; कलाकर्म॰ G, सर्वकर्म॰ M, कालकर्म॰ *cett.* ◇ ॰मुक्तं] ॰मुक्तो $S\alpha$, ॰मुक्तां J_5W_2 **17d** ॰ज्ञेयं] ॰ज्ञेयः α_1 **18a** इडायां] $\mu S\alpha VFK_5H_2$; इडया $GK_2\gamma$, इडाया $J_2J_4K_4PJ_3K_6$ ◇ रात्रिर्] $\mu GS\alpha K_2K_5H_2$; रात्रि $R_2J_4K_4$, रात्रिन् J_2V, रात्रिम् PJ_3FK_6B, रात्रम् γ_1 ◇ उद्दिष्टा] $J_6S\alpha_3J_2VPFK_5K_6B$; उद्दिष्टां $AJ_7\gamma_2R_1$, उत्त्विाप्ता G, *द्दिष्टं R_2, उदिता α_1, तदृष्टा J_4, तुद्दिष्टा K_4, उदिष्ट K_2, उदिष्टा J_3, उद्विष्ठां W_2 **18b** पिङ्गलायाम्] पिंगलायाः V, पिंगलया B ◇ अहः] अह $AR_2\alpha_3K_2J_3K_6$, अहा G, *रुः V ◇ स्मृतम्] स्मृतः $\mu J_4VK_2J_3$-J_1R_1, स्मृत J_5W_2 **18d** ॰दिवा॰] $\mu G\alpha_3BH_2$; दिना॰ *cett.* **19a** न दिवा] *transp.* $GW_1H_1H_3$, वासरे H_2 **19b** न रात्रौ] *transp.* μ, रात्रौ चै॰ $\alpha_3H_1H_2H_3$ ◇ च महेश्वरि] परमेश्वरि M, ॰व न पूजयेत् $\alpha_3H_1H_2H_3$

19b *and* **19d** *transp.* K_6

सर्वदा पूजयेल्लिङ्गं दिवारात्रिनिरोधतः ॥१९॥
अहोरात्रिमयं चेदं कालक्रमस्वभावजम् ।
कालक्रमनिरोधेन कालमृत्युजयो भवेत् ॥२०॥
कालक्रमविनिर्मुक्तां चिन्तयेदात्मनस्तनुम् ।
पूजयेद्भावपुष्पेण तर्पयेत्पङ्कजामृतैः ॥२१॥
एवं षण्मासयोगेन जायते ह्यजरामरः ।
सर्वज्ञत्वं लभेत्सत्यं शिवसाम्यो निरामयः ॥२२॥
तालुमूले समावेश्य रसनामूर्ध्ववक्त्रगाम् ।
तत्र जातां सुधां पीत्वा शीत्कारेण शनैः शनैः ॥२३॥
प्रपिबेत्पवनं योगी निरालम्बे पदे शिवे ।
मनः संयोज्य चोन्मन्या सहजं योगमाचरेत् ॥२४॥
अनेन योगी षण्मासाज्जायते ह्यजरामरः ।
चिबुकं योजयेद्देवि षोडशस्वरमण्डले ॥२५॥
भ्रूमध्ये चक्षुषी न्यस्य जिह्वामूर्ध्वं प्रसारयेत् ।
संप्राप्य कुम्भकावस्थामिडापिङ्गलरोधनात् ॥२६॥

19c सर्वदा] सततं $\alpha_3 H_2 H_3$ **19d** °रात्रि°] °रात्रौ $AK_2K_6\gamma_1 H_2 H_3^{vl}$, °रात्रं GH_3 ◇ °निरोधतः] निरोधवाः μ, न पूजयेत् H_2H_3 **20a** °रात्रिमयं] $\mu R_2\alpha_3$; °रात्रमयं $S\alpha_1\beta\gamma$, °रात्रमवि° G ◇ चेदं] $S\beta\gamma$; देवं $AJ_7\alpha_2\alpha_3$, वेदं J_6, °च्छेदं G, देव R_2, लिंगं M **20b** काल°] कालं J_4, कालः B ◇ °क्रम°] J_4; °कर्मश् PK_6, °कर्मं J_5W_2, °कर्म° *cett.* ◇ °स्वभावजम्] °स्वभावकं M, च भावजं $PK_6\gamma$ **20c** °क्रम°] J_4; °कर्म° *cett.* **20d** °मृत्युजयो भवेत्] °मृत्युजयं लभेत् μ, °मृत्युर्यथा भवेत् K_1, °मृत्यु यथा भवेत् K_3, °मृत्युर्जयो भवेत् $K_2PJ_3K_6\gamma_1$ **21a** °क्रम°] H_2; °धर्म° α_3, °कर्म° *cett.* ◇ °मुक्तां] GR_2MB; °मुक्तश् α_2, °मुक्तो $\alpha_3J_3H_2$, °मुक्ता V, °मुक्तं *cett.* **21b** चिन्तयेद्] चिंतयान्न् A, चिंतयन्न् J_6J_7 **21d** तर्पयेत्] $\mu GR_2SNM\alpha_3VK_5J_1B$; तर्पयं $W_1J_2J_4K_4K_2PJ_3FK_6J_5W_2R_1$ ◇ पङ्कजामृतैः] μG; तं कलामृतैः $R_2S\alpha_2VPJ_3K_5\gamma$, तां कलामृतैः M, तं कलामृतं α_3, तं कलामृतो J_2, तं कलामृतौ $J_4K_2K_4K_6$, तु कुलामृतैः F^{pc}, तु कलामृतैः F^{ac} **22c** लभेत्सत्यं] μ; भवेत्सत्यं G, भवेन्नित्यं *cett.* **22d** °साम्यो] °शाम्यं α_2, °साम्यं M, °स्यास्य α_3, °साम्ये γ_1 **23a** °मूले] °मूलं GW_1J_3 **23b** °वक्त्र°] °चक्र° $\alpha_3\gamma$ ◇ °गां] °कां μ, °गा α_3 **23c** तत्र जातां सुधां पीत्वा] $SM\beta_1PJ_3FK_5J_1R_1B$, तत्तत्र जातं तु पिवन् A, तत्तत्र जातं भु पिवन् J_6J_7, तत्र *मृ*तां सुधां पीत्वा G, तत्र जातासु पीत्वा सी N, तत्र जातां सु पीत्वा सीत् W_1, तत्र याता स्वुधां पीत्वा K_1, तत्र याता स्वधा पीत्वा K_3, तत्र जातं सुधां पीत्वा K_2, तत्र जातां शुधां पीत्वा K_6, तत्र जातं सुधां पित्वा J_5W_2 **23d** शीत्कारेण] सीत्कारेण $\mu S\alpha$ **24a** पवनं] μG; पंचमं $SJ_2VK_2PJ_3FK_5K_6\gamma$, पंचमे α_1, पंचसं α_3, श्राचर्मं J_4 **24b** पदे] पदे परे G *(unm.)* **24c** सम्योज्य] संयम्य K_2B ◇ चोन्मन्या] चोन्मन्यां M, यो नान्या α_3 **24d** सहजं] सिंहजं K_2, सहसं J_3 **25a** °मासाज्] °मासे α_3 **25c** चिबुकं] $S\alpha_2$; चिवुकं $AJ_7R_2\alpha_3\beta_1K_2PK_5K_6$, चिव्रुकं J_6, चुबुकं GB, चुवुकं M, चिबूकं J_3, चुंचुकं F, चंचुकं J_1R_1, चंवुकं J_5, चुंबुकं W_2 ◇ योजयेद्] च जपेद् α_3 **25d** °मण्डले] $\mu GR_2SMVK_2K_5K_6$; °मण्डलं *cett.* **26a** °मध्ये] °मध्य GW_1 ◇ न्यस्य] न्यस्त G **26d** °रोधनात्] μG; °रोधतः $R_2S\alpha_2\beta B$, °योगतः M, °रोधनं α_3H_2, °रोधितः γ_1

22c – 25b *om.* R_2 (*eye-skip to* °मरः) **24a – 25b** *om.* K_4 **25ab** *om.* G

मूलशक्तिं समुद्बोध्य भित्त्वा षट्सरसीरुहान् ।
तडित्सहस्रसंकाशां ब्रह्माण्डोदरमध्यमे ॥२७॥
धाम्नि शीतामृताम्भोधौ संनिवेश्य चिरं वसेत् ।
यदा ब्रह्ममये धाम्नि योगी वसति लीलया ॥२८॥
तदा निर्जीववद्देहे भा विस्फुरति तत्पदम् ।
अनेन देवि योगेन दिनसप्तकमाचरेत् ॥२९॥
यदा तदा स भवति जरामरणवर्जितः ।
माससमात्रप्रयोगेन जीवेदाचन्द्रतारकम् ॥३०॥
यदा ब्रह्मपुरं भित्त्वा योगी व्रजति लीलया ।
तदा शिवत्वमाप्नोति नित्यदेहमयं शिवे ॥३१॥
न पुनः पिबते मातुः स्तनं संसारचक्रके ।
[देहमोचनं कालवञ्चनं च]
यदा तु योगिनो बुद्धिस्त्यक्तुं देहमिमं भवेत् ॥३२॥
तदा स्थिरासनो भूत्वा मूलशक्तिं समुज्ज्वलाम् ।

32c – 47d *cit.* नारायणदीपिका *(D)* *ad* क्षुरिकोपनिषद् 12, ĀSS 29, pp.154–155

27b भित्त्वा] *em.*; भित्वा μ, भीटत्वा K_5^{ac} *(unm.)*, नीत्वा *cett.* ◇ °रुहान्] $\mu G \alpha_2 K_5 \gamma$; °रुहात् *cett.* 27c तडित्सहस्र°] सहस्रसूर्य° G ◇ °संकाशां] $\mu GNVK_2$, °संकाशा $R_2J_2J_4K_4PFK_5\gamma$, °संकाशो SW_1, °संकांशां M, °संकाशं α_3, °संकासं J_3, °शंकाशाद् K_6 27d °मध्यमे] °मध्यगे μSK_2, °मध्यगां GR_2, °मध्यगं α_3 28a धाम्नि] ध्यानी α_3, धानि K_4, धात्रि γ_1, धात्री B 28b वसेत्] $\mu GR_2SJ_2VJ_3K_5B$; विशेत् $\alpha J_2^{vl} FK_6\gamma_1$, वशेत् J_4K_2P 28c यदा] ब्रह्म° M ◇ ब्रह्ममये] ब्रह्ममयो GK_2, °मध्ये यदा M ◇ धाम्नि] धात्रि NW_2, धात्री B 28d योगी] योगः α_3 ◇ वसति] μG; सर्वत्र α_3, [..] R_2, गच्छति *cett.* 29a निर्जीववद्] नीजीववद् AG, निजीवये N, निज्जीवये W_1 ◇ देहे] $J_3F\gamma$; एहं A, देहं J_6J_7, देहो $GS\alpha_1J_2^{vl}VK_4PK_5K_6$, [..] R_2, वेहो α_3, देह J_2, एहो J_4K_2 29b भा वि°] μ; [..] R_2, भा P *(unm.)*, भाव γ_1, भावः B, भाति *cett.* ◇ °स्फुरति] स्पुरति S, स्फरजि J_2, स्मरति J_4K_2, स्फरति K_4J_3 29c देवि] देव° α_3, दैव° H_2 29d दिन°] सप्त° α_3H_2 ◇ °सप्तकम्] °सप्तक्र° R_2 ◇ आचरेत्] आश्रयेत् G, °मेण तु R_2 30a यदा] तदा μ ◇ तदा] पदं G ◇ स भवति] $J_6J_7S\alpha_2V$; संभवति $AR_2\alpha_3J_2K_4K_5K_6$, समाप्नोति G, संभवंति J_4 30c °मात्र°] °त्रय° $S\alpha H_2$ 31a °पुरं] °पदं G, °परं J_3 31b योगी] योगं α_3 31d नित्यदेहमयं] α_2; त्यक्त्वा देहमिमं μG, ****मिमं R_2, नित्यं देहमिमं K_6, नित्यदेहनिसं H_2, नित्यदेहमिमं *cett.* 32a न पुनः] पुनर्न R_2 ◇ पिबते] पिबति $R_2\alpha_2\alpha_3H_2$ ◇ मातुः] $M\alpha_3V$; *om.* R_2, स्तन्यं K_2, मातु *cett.* 32b स्तनं] स्तन्यं GF, स्तनौ $S\alpha H_2$, मातुः K_2 ◇ संसार°] स चार° K_6 ◇ °चक्रके] $S\alpha H_2$; °चक्रमा AJ_7, चंक्रमा J_6, °चक्रतः G, चच्क्रगः *(sic)* R_2, °चक्रमात् $\beta_1PJ_3K_5K_6\gamma_1$, °सागरे K_2, °चंक्रमात् FB 32c यदा] तदा μ ◇ तु योगिनो बुद्धिस्] $R_2SJ_4VPFK_5^{pc}K_6D$; तु योगिनो वृद्धिस् AJ_7, तु योगिनो व्रुद्धिस् J_6, तु योगिनो बुद्धिर् G, वाङ्मनोबुद्धिभिस् α_2, च वाङ्मनोवुद्धिस् M, तु वाङ्मनोवुद्धिस् α_3, तु योगीनो वुद्धिस् $J_2K_4K_5^{ac}$, तु योमिनो वुद्धि K_2, तु योगिनो बुद्धि J_3, तु योगिनो J_1R_1, तु योगीनो J_5W_2, तु योगिन्मे B 32d त्यक्तुं] $SMJ_2VK_4PFK_5K_6D$; त्यक्तं $\mu R_2\alpha_2\alpha_3J_4K_2$, मोक्तुं G, त्युक्तु J_3 ◇ इमं] इदं α_2 ◇ भवेत्] प्रिये μ 33a स्थिरासनो] स्थिरमना S^{ac} 33b मूल°] μGM; मूलां $R_2\alpha_2$, मूलाच् SFK_5K_6D, मूला $\alpha_3\beta_1K_2PJ_3\gamma_1$, मूर्छा B ◇ °शक्तिं] μGW_1MJ_4; श* R_2, छक्तिं $S\alpha_3J_2VK_4PJ_3FK_5K_6\gamma_2R_1D$, शक्ति NK_2B, छक्ति W_2

29a जायते नात्र संशयः तदानीं शववद्देहो *add.* G 29c – 30b *om.* M 30 *om.* $K_2PJ_3F\gamma$ 32c बुद्धिस् – 33a स्थिरासनो *om.* γ *(eye-skip to* भूत्वा*)*

कोटिसूर्यप्रतीकाशां भावयेच्चिरमात्मवित् ॥३३॥
आपादतलपर्यन्तं प्रसृतं जीवमात्मनः ।
संहृत्य क्रमयोगेन मूलाधारपदं नयेत् ॥३४॥
तत्र कुण्डलिनीशक्तिं संवर्तानलसंनिभाम् ।
जीवानिलं चेन्द्रियाणि ग्रसन्तीं चिन्तयेद्धिया ॥३५॥
संप्राप्य कुम्भकावस्थां तडिद्वलयभासुराम् ।
मूलादुन्नीय देवेशि स्वाधिष्ठानपदं नयेत् ॥३६॥
तत्रस्थं जीवमखिलं ग्रसन्तीं चिन्तयेद् व्रती ।
तडित्कोटिप्रतीकाशां तस्मादुन्नीय सत्वरम् ॥३७॥
मणिपूरपदं प्राप्य तत्र पूर्ववदाचरेत् ।
समुन्नीय पुनस्तस्मादनाहतपदं नयेत् ॥३८॥
तत्र स्थित्वा क्षणं देवि पूर्ववद्ग्रसतीं स्मरेत् ।
उन्नीय च पुनः पद्मे षोडशारे निवेशयेत् ॥३९॥
तत्रापि चिन्तयेद्देवि पूर्ववद्योगमार्गवित् ।

33c कोटिसूर्य°] सूर्यकोटि° K_5*D* **33d** चिरम्] छिवम् G ◇ आत्मवित्] आत्मनि SK_2PJ_3-$FK_6\gamma$, आत्मनः *D* **34b** प्रसृतं] प्रसतं R_2, प्रसृतां K_2, प्रमृतं P, प्रन्नुतं F, अमृतं γ ◇ आत्मनः] आत्मनि $S\alpha$, आत्मनां K_2, आत्मनं J_3 **34c** संहृत्य] संहत्य AJ_6J_3, हंसत्य J_7, संहृष्य J_4, संवृत्य γ_2, संदृत्य W_2 ◇ क्रम°] कर्म° $S^{ac}\beta\gamma$ **35a** कुराडलिनी°] कुंडलिनीं $GR_2\alpha_1D$ ◇ °शक्तिं] μGR_2MD; शक्तिम् α_2, शक्तिर् $SJ_2J_4K_4PJ_3FK_5K_6\gamma$, शक्ति α_3, शक्तिंर् V, शक्तिर्म K_2 **35b** संवर्तानल°] μGR_2D; आवर्तानल° $S^{pc}\beta\gamma$, आवृतानल° S^{ac}, आवर्तानिल° α_2, सवर्त्तान[ल]° M, सर्वत्रानिल° α_3 ◇ °निभाम्] °निभा SK_5B, °निभं α_3F **35c** जीवानिलं] $R_2S\alpha_1\beta_1FK_5K_6\gamma_1$; जीवानित्यं μ, जीवानलं GK_2J_3B, जित्वानिलं α_3, जीव*नि*लं P, जीवं निजं *D* **35d** ग्रसन्तीं] $GS\beta_1FK_5D$; ग्रसतीं AJ_7, ग्रसंती $J_6R_2\alpha_2K_2PB$, सिंचंतीं M, ग्रसंतं α_3, ग्रसंते J_3, ग्रसंति $K_6\gamma_1$ **36b** °वलय°] °ज्वलन° R_2D, °अनल° B ◇ °भासुरां] °भास्करां $AJ_6^{pc}J_7$, °भासुरं α_3 **36c** मूलाद्] μGSK_5K_6; मूलम् α, मूल° β_1, मूला $K_2PJ_3F\gamma D$ ◇ उन्नीय देवेशि] μG; उन्नीय देवेशी R_2, द्वितीयं देवेशि $S\beta B$, उन्निद्रयेद्देवि α_1, उत्तीर्य देवेशि α_3, द्वितीय देवेशि γ_1, °धाराद्यतिर्देवि *D* **37a** °स्थं] सं° μ, °स्थ° G, °स्थां α_2K_2, °स्था γ **37b** ग्रसंतीं] $\mu S\alpha_3VPFK_6$; ग्रसं*तीं* G, ग्रसंती $R_2W_1J_3B$, ग्रसंतं NM, ग्रसतां J_2J_4, ग्रसतीं K_4, ग्रसंति $K_2\gamma_1$ ◇ व्रती] R_2SW_1-$M\beta_1K_2J_3K_6BD$; च ताम् μ, प्रिये G, व्रतं NK_3, व्रताम् K_1, व्रतीं P, वति J_1R_1, व्रति J_5W_2 **37c** प्रतीकाशां] $J_6J_7GR_2K_2W_2BD$; °प्रतिकाशां AJ_2K_4, °प्रकाशं तत् S, °प्रतीकाशं $\alpha VPJ_3FK_5K_6$, °प्रतिकाशं J_4, °प्रकाशांत J_1R_1, °प्रकाशां J_5 *(unm.)* **37d** उन्नीय] J_6GSMD; उनीय A, उत्तीर्य *cett.* ◇ सत्वरम्] तत्परां G **38a** प्राप्य] प्रारा μ **38b** पूर्ववद्] सूर्यं यद् A, सूर्य यद् J_6J_7 **38c** समुन्नीय] समुत्तीर्य $\alpha_2\alpha_3$ ◇ पुनस्तस्माद्] पदस्थानाद् μ **38d** नयेत्] व्रजेत् M **39b** पूर्ववद्] पूर्व*व** G, पूर्ववर्° α_3, पूर्ववत् $P\gamma_1$, ग्रसंतीं K_5 ◇ ग्रसतीं] $SNVFK_6B$; धि सतीं A, धसतीं J_6J_7, अवतिं G, योगमा° R_2D, ग्रसती W_1, ग्रसतां M, °गसतां α_3, धमती J_2, धमति J_4, ध सती K_4, ग्रसन K_2, ग्रसंती P *(unm.)*, रसतं J_3, पूर्ववत् K_5, ग्रसति γ_1 ◇ स्मरेत्] °र्गवित् R_2D **39c** उन्नीय च] μG; उत्तीर्य तु α_2, तन्नादयत् α_3, समुन्नाय J_3, समुन्नीय K_5, अनाहते D_1, उन्नीय तु *cett.* ◇ पुनः] ततः M, नयेद् D_1 ◇ पद्मे] पादौ α_3, योगी D_1 **39d** षोडशारे] षोडशरि A, षोडशांते G, तत्र पूर्व° D_1 ◇ निवेशयेत्] निवाशयेत् A, व**येत् G, °वदाचरेत् D_1 **40a** तत्रापि चिन्तयेद्देवि] ततो विशुद्धादानीय D_1 **40b** पूर्ववद्] कुराडलीं D_1 ◇ योगमार्गवित्] योगमात्मवित् μ, पूर्ववच्चरेत् D_1

38cd *om.* *D* **39c – 40b** *om.* R_2D_2 (*eye-skip to* उन्नीय)

तस्मादुन्नीय भ्रूमध्यं नीत्वा जीवं ग्रसेत्पुनः ॥४०॥
ग्रस्तजीवां महाशक्तिं कोटिसूर्यसमप्रभाम् ।
मनसा सह वागीशी भित्त्वा ब्रह्मार्गलं क्षणात् ॥४१॥
परामृतमहाम्भोधौ विश्रामं सम्यगाचरेत् ।
तत्रस्थं परमं देवि शिवं परमकारणम् ॥४२॥
शक्त्या सह समायोज्य तयोरैक्यं विभावयेत् ।
यदि वञ्चितुमुद्युक्तः कालं कालविभागवित् ॥४३॥
यावद् व्रजति तं कालं तावत्तत्र सुखं वसेत् ।
ब्रह्मद्वारार्गलस्याधो देहकालप्रयोजनम् ॥४४॥
तस्मादूर्ध्वपदे देवि न हि कालप्रयोजनम् ।
यदा देव्यात्मनः कालमतिक्रान्तं प्रपश्यति ॥४५॥
तदा ब्रह्मार्गलं भित्त्वा शक्तिं मूलपदं नयेत् ।
शक्तिदेहप्रसूतं तु स्वजीवं चेन्द्रियैः सह ॥४६॥

41c – 42d *cit.* नारायणदीपिका *(D) ad* योगशिखोपनिषद् 2.3, ĀSS 29, p.485

40c तस्मादुन्नीय] तस्मात् भ्रूमध्यं G, तस्मादुत्तीर्य α_2, उन्नीय तस्माद् D ◇ भ्रूमध्यं] उन्नीय G, भ्रूमध्ये $J_4K_2K_6BD$ **40d** नीत्वा जीवं ग्रसेत्] नीरन्धीरं ग्रसे* R_2, नीरन्धीरं ग्रसन् D_1, नीरन्धरं ग्रसेत् D_2 **41a** ग्रस्त°] $\mu\beta_1K_2PFK_5K_6W_2B$; ग्रस° G, ग्रस्तं $R_2SW_1M\alpha_3D$, यस्तं N, यस्तु J_3 ◇ °जीवां] μG°; न्धीरं R_2D, °ज्जीवं V, °जीवा J_3B, जीवं *cett.* ◇ महाशक्तिं] $\mu GJ_4K_2K_5K_6$; महाशक्त्या R_2D, महाशक्तिः $SF\gamma$, महेशानि α, महाशक्ति $J_2VK_4PJ_3$ **41b** °प्रभाम्] $\mu GK_5K_6\gamma_1$; °प्रभं $R_2S\alpha\beta_1K_2PFD_1$, °प्रभुः J_3, °प्रभा BD_2 **41c** वागीशी] $\alpha_2VPK_5K_6$; वागीशि $\mu GS^{pc}MJ_2J_4K_4$, वागीशीं R_2F, वागीशे S^{ac}, वागीशं α_3, वागीशा $K_2J_3D_2$, वागीसी γ_1, वागेशी B, वागीश्या $D_1D_2^{vl}$ **41d** भित्त्वा] नीत्वा α_3 **42b** विश्रामं] विश्वासं μ, विश्रान्तिं D ◇ सम्यग्] न्धरणं M, तत्र D ◇ आचरेत्] कारयेत् D **42c** देवि] देवं R_2 **42d** शिवं] शिवे SK_2J_3F, शिवै $P\gamma_1$ **43a** सह समायोज्य] सहस्रमायोज्य $PJ_3\gamma$, सह मया योज्य K_5 **43c** यदि वञ्चितुम्] यदि मोचितुम् μ, यदिदं चिंतम G *(unm.)*, यदिदं विसम् α_3 ◇ उद्युक्तः] $J_6J_7R_2S\alpha\beta_1PK_5K_6B$; अयुक्तः A, यद्युक्तं G, उच्छक्तः K_2, उत्सुक्तः J_3, उद्यक्तः F, उद्योगं J_1, उद्योक्तं J_5W_2 **43d** कालं] कालः G ◇ °विभाग°] °विधान° M, °विभाव° F **44a** यावद्] कालः R_2, कालस् D ◇ व्रजति] भजति AJ_7, स यावद् R_2, जीवत K_2, यतीतं F, तु यावद् D ◇ तं कालं] व्रजति R_2D, तत्कालं $G\alpha_3K_2$ **44b** तत्र सुखं] तस्यां मुखं N, तस्यां सुखं W_1M, तत्संमुखं α_3 ◇ वसेत्] वशेत् $AJ_7\alpha_3K_2J_3F^{ac}$, भवेत् G, व*शे*त् K_6 **44c** °र्गलस्याधो] μW_1MK_5D; °र्गळस्याधः G, र्ग*याधो R_2, °र्गलायाधो $S\beta_1PF\gamma$, °र्गलःस्याधो N, °र्गलस्यादौ α_3, °र्गलाच्चादो K_2, °र्गलायाधौ J_3, °र्गलांयाधो K_6 **44d** देह°] देहे μK_5, देवि G ◇ °काल°] °लन्न° $NM\alpha_3$, °लन्त्य° W_1 **45a** ऊर्ध्वपदे] ऊर्ध्वपदं αD_2, ऊर्ध्वं पदं D_1 ◇ देवि] देयं D, देहं D_1^{vl} **45c** यदा] यदि α_3 ◇ देव्य्] दिव्य्° $G\alpha_1$, *दिव्य्*° J_4, देव्° J_3, D_2^{vl} **45d** प्रपश्यति] प्रविश्यति A, स पश्यति M, प्रसाश्यति J_2K_4, प्रशाम्यति J_4, प्रणाश्यति K_5 **46b** शक्तिं] μR_2SMVFK_5D; शक्ति° *cett.* ◇ °पदं] °पदे μM **46c** शक्ति°] शक्तिं AJ_6W_1 ◇ °देह°] देहा° μ, देहे W_1, दह PJ_3, मूल F ◇ °प्रसूतं] $R_2SJ_4VK_4PJ_3FK_6\gamma D$; °त्मसूनं μ, °प्रसू*नं* G, °प्रवाहस् N, प्रसृतं W_1, °प्रस्तुतं $M\alpha_3$, °प्रसुतं J_2, °प्रभूतं K_2, प्रसूतस् K_5 ◇ तु] *तं* G, तं M, च α_3, वै F **46d** स्वजीवं] $\mu GR_2M\alpha_3D$; स जीवश् $SJ_2J_4K_4PJ_3FK_5$, तं जीवं NK_6, सजीवं W_1B, सृजीवश् V, स जीवेश् K_2, सर्जाव γ_2, स जीव W_2, सुजीव R_1 ◇ सह] सहः $\mu J_2K_4PJ_3$

40cd *om.* S **40d** ग्रसेत् – **41a** जीवां *om.* γ_2R_1 **43c – 44b** *om.* R_1 **45ab** *om.* γ

तत्तत्कर्मणि संयोज्य स्वस्थदेहः सुखं वसेत् ।
अनेन देवि योगेन वञ्चयेत्कालमागतम् ॥४७॥

[देहत्यागः]
यदि मानुष्यकं देहं त्यक्तुमिच्छा प्रवर्तते ।
ततः परमसंतुष्टो ब्रह्मस्थानगतं शिवम् ॥४८॥
शक्त्या संयोज्य निर्भिद्य व्योम ब्रह्मशिलां विशेत् ।
व्योमतत्त्वं महाव्योम्नि वायुतत्त्वं महानिले ॥४९॥
तेजस्तत्त्वं महातेजस्यप्तत्त्वं जलमण्डले ।
धरातत्त्वं धराभागे निरालम्बे मनः पदे ॥५०॥
व्योमादिगुणतत्त्वेषु स्वेन्द्रियाणि निवेशयेत् ।
एवं सांसारिकं त्यक्त्वा परतत्त्वावलम्बकः ॥५१॥
अस्पृष्टः पञ्चभूताद्यैर्भित्त्वा सूर्यस्य मण्डलम् ।
परतत्त्वपदे शान्ते शिवे लीनः शिवायते ॥५२॥
न कल्पकोटिसाहस्रैः पुनरावर्तनं भवेत् ।
अनुग्रहाय लोकानां यदि देहं न संत्यजेत् ॥५३॥

47a तत्तत्कर्मणि] μVK_5K_6B*D*; तत्तत्कर्माणि $GSPJ_3F\gamma_1$, ततत्कर्मणि R_2K_2, तत्रोक्तेनापि α_1, ततोक्तिमूल° α_3, ततत्वर्मणि J_2K_4, ततंतुर्मणि J_4 ◇ संयोज्य] मार्गेण α_1, °पदं नयेत् α_3 *(unm.)*, संयोज्यं $J_4K_4PK_6\gamma_1$ **47b** स्वस्थदेहः] GF*D*; स्वस्य देहः μR_2, स्वस्थदेहं $S\beta_1K_2PJ_3$-K_5K_6, शक्तिमूलं N, शक्तिमूल° W_1M, छक्तिदेह° α_3, स्वसंदेहं J_1R_1, स्वसदेहं J_5W_2, स्वदेहं तु B ◇ सुखं वसेत्] $GS\beta_1K_5K_6\gamma$; सुखं चरेत् μ, ** वसेत् R_2, पदं नयेत् α_1, °स्य प्रश्रुतं α_3, मुखं वशेत् K_2, सुखं वशेत् PJ_3F, सुखं व्रजेत् *D* **47c** अनेन देवि योगेन] स्वजीवं चेंद्रियैः सह α_3 **47d** वञ्चयेत्कालमागतम्] वंचयेत्कालमार्गणं μ, तत्र कालसमागतः α_3 **48d** °स्थान°] °स्थानं $\mu\alpha_3K_2FK_6$ ◇ °गतं शिवम्] परं शिव α_3, °गतं शिवे J_3F **49a** निर्भिद्य] $GR_2SN\alpha_3VPJ_3$-K_5K_6; निर्भिन्न° μ, निभिद्य W_1, निर्भि*द्य*M, निर्जिद्य J_2K_4, निर्*भिद्य*J_4, निर्भिग K_2, निर्भेद्य F, नीभेदा γ **49b** व्योम] योग α_3 ◇ ब्रह्म°] °ब्रह्मा μJ_1 ◇ °शिलां] °सभां R_2, °शिवं α_3, °शिला K_2, °शिलं γ ◇ विशेत्] $\mu R_2\beta_1PK_5K_6$; वसेत् $GF\gamma$, व्रजेत् $S\alpha K_2$, वशेत् J_3 **49c** °तत्त्वं] °तत्व $\alpha_3\gamma_1$, °सत्त्वं K_2 **49d** महानिले] अथानिले μ **50a** महा°] तथा A, यथा J_6 ◇ °तेजस्य्] °तेजा° R_2, °तेजो α_3, °तेजः K_2F, °तेजस्व् γ **50b** अप्तत्त्वं] GVJ_3FK_5; आप्तत्वं μS, °पस्तत्व R_2, अंभसो α_1, यस्यत्वं α_3, अस्यत्वं J_2K_4, अपत्वं J_4K_6, जलं च K_2, असत्वं $P\gamma_1$, अतत्वं B **50c** धरातत्त्वं] महीतत्त्वं α, आपतत्त्वं γ_1, आपस्तत्त्वं B ◇ धराभागे] महीभागे α_1, महाभागे α_3 **50d** निरालम्बे] निरालंबं G ◇ पदे] GK_2B; परे $\mu SW_1M\beta_1PFK_5K_6\gamma_1$, परं $N\alpha_3J_3$ **51a** °गुण°] °पर° M **51b** स्वे°] चे° $W_1\alpha_3$ **51c** एवं] य* G ◇ सांसारिकं] μJ_4VK_5B; वंसावधिं G, सांसारकं R_2, संसारिकं $S\alpha_3J_2K_4K_2PFK_6\gamma_1$, शरीरकं α_2, शरीरं तु M ◇ त्यक्त्वा] पश्चात् N, त्यक्ता $M\alpha_3\beta_1K_2\gamma_2W_2$, त्यक्त्या R_1 **51d** पर°] परा μ, परं α_3J_4 ◇ °वलम्बकः] °वलंपकः A, °विलंवकः α_3, °वलंवकाः $J_2J_4K_4$, °वलंबकं γ_1, °वलंबनं B **52a** अस्पृष्टः] *conj.* Sanderson; अदृष्टः $\mu SK_2K_5K_6R_1$, अदृष्टं $GW_1J_2J_4$, अदृश्यः R_2, अदृष्ट° $NM\alpha_3K_4PF\gamma_2W_2B$, अदृष्टा V, अद्रष्टं J_3 ◇ पञ्च°] सर्व° S **52c** पर°] परं α_3 ◇ °तत्त्व°] $\alpha_3J_4\gamma$; °तत्वे μMV, °तत्त्वं G, **R_2, °तत्वो° $S\alpha_2J_2K_4K_2PFK_5K_6$, °त्वो J_3 *(unm.)* ◇ पदे] परे μG **52d** शिवे लीनः] शिवा लानः R_2 **53a** न कल्पकोटिसाहस्रैः] कल्पकोटिसाहस्रैश्च G, न कोटिकल्पसाहस्रैः α **53b** आवर्तनं] आवर्तिनो G, संवर्तनं α, आगमनं K_6

47cd *om.* α_1 **47c – 48d** *om.* G (*see addition at* 54b) **53a** स्रैः – **53d** यदि *om.* J_3

प्रलयान्ते तनुं त्यक्त्वा स्वात्मन्येवावतिष्ठते ।
इत्येषा खेचरीमुद्रा खेचराधिपतित्वदा ॥५४॥
जन्ममृत्युजरारोगवलीपलितनाशिनी ।
[खेचरीस्तुतिः शिवभक्तिश्च]
अनया सदृशी विद्या क्व चिच्छास्त्रान्तरे न हि ॥५५॥
खेचरीमेलनं देवि सुगुह्यं न प्रकाशयेत् ।
तस्याश्चाभ्यासयोगोऽयं तव स्नेहात्प्रकाशितः ॥५६॥
खेचरी नाम या देवि सर्वयोगीन्द्रवन्दिता ।
नैनां यो वेत्ति लोकेऽस्मिन्स पशुः प्रोच्यते शिवे ॥५७॥
नित्यमभ्यासशीलस्य अटतोऽपि जगत्त्रयम् ।
गुरुवक्त्रोपसंलब्धां विद्यामभ्यसतोऽपि च ॥५८॥
खेचरीमेलकाद्येषु नित्यं संसक्तचेतसः ।
न सिध्यति महायोगो मदीयाराधनं विना ॥५९॥

54b स्वात्मन्य्] आत्मन्य् α_3, स्वात्मन् γ_1 **54c** एषा] एवं $G\alpha$ **54d** ◦पतित्वदा] μ; ◦पतिस्त* G, ◦*पति*** R_2, ◦पतिस्तदा $S\alpha_1\beta\gamma$, ◦पतिस्तथा α_3 **55b** वली◦] वलि $AJ_6J_4VJ_3K_6$ ◇ ◦पलित◦] ◦दर्पवि◦ G **56a** ◦मेलनं] ◦मेलन A ◇ देवि] देवी $\alpha_2VJ_3K_6$ **56b** सुगुह्यं] सुगुप्तं μ, सगुह्य K_2, सगुह्यं γ ◇ न प्रकाशयेत्] $A\alpha_1$; न प्रकारयेत् J_6J_7, संप्रकाशितं G, ते प्रकाशितं $S\beta_1PFK_5K_6J_5W_2B$, तत्प्रकाशितं α_3, ते प्रकाशित K_2, ते प्रकाशितः J_3, ते प्रकाशिनी J_1R_1 **56c** तस्याश्] $G\alpha_1\beta_1PFK_5K_6$; तस्य μ, *स्य* R_2, तस्यां S, तस्या J_3 ◇ चाभ्यास◦] स्वाभ्यास◦ μ, अभ्यास◦ SJ_3 ◇ ◦योगोऽयं] ◦योगे यं A, ◦योगेन R_2J_4, ◦योगश्च α_1 **56d** स्नेहात्प्रकाशितः] दे* **** R_2, स्नेहेन कीर्तितः α_1, स्नेहात्प्रकाशितं J_2V, प्रीत्या प्रकाशितं J_3, स्नेहप्रकाशितः F **57a** खेचरी] मदिरा μ, खेचर्या α, खेचरो γ_2R_1 ◇ नाम या] न समा α, नाम यो J_1R_1 ◇ देवि] $\mu GS\alpha_1K_1J_2K_4K_2J_3FK_5^{ac}J_1R_1$; देवी $K_3J_4VPK_5^{pc}K_6J_5W_2B$ **57b** ◦योगीन्द्र◦] ◦योगेंद्र◦ $\alpha_3\gamma_1$ ◇ ◦वन्दिता] ◦वंदिते α **57c** नैनां] एनां $G\alpha_1$, तां न α_3, नयनां γ_1 *(unm.)* ◇ यो] *न*ो G **57d** पशुः] प्रभुः α_1 **58a** ◦शीलस्य] ◦शीलस्या G **58b** अटतो] आटतो AB ◇ ◦त्रयम्] ◦त्रये $W_1M\alpha_3$ **58c** गुरुवक्त्रोपसंलब्धां] μ; गुरु*व*क्त्रे पि लब्धस्य G, गुरुवक्त्रादसंलब्धा N, गुरुमन्त्रे च संलभ्य F, गुरुवक्त्राच्च संलभ्य *cett.* **58d** विद्यामभ्यसतो] विद्यामभशतो A, विद्यामभ्यस्यतो GK_5, विद्ययाभ्यासतो α_3 ◇ च] $\mu G\alpha_1$; वा *cett.* **59a** ◦मेलकाद्येषु] α_2; ◦मेलनादिश्च μ, ◦मेळनाद्येषु G, ◦मेलकाद्यैश्च $S\beta$, ◦मेलकामेषु M, ◦मीलकाद्येषु α_3, ◦मेलकाद्यौ श्री γ_1, ◦मेलकाद्यैः श्री B **59b** नित्यं] नित्य◦ R_2FK_6 ◇ संसक्तचेतसः] सप्रेमवेतसः μ, संसिक्तसेवतः J_3 **59c** सिध्यति] विद्यते G, सिध्यंति $J_4\gamma_1$ ◇ ◦योगो] ◦योगं μ, [..] R_2, ◦योगी $\alpha_2\alpha_3K_2J_3$ **59d** मदीया◦] मदिरा◦ μ, मदिदं G, गुरुरा◦ V, महीया◦ R_1

54b अनेन देवि योगेन वंचयेत्कालमार्गतः यदि मानुष्यकं देहं त्यक्तुमिच्छा प्रवर्तते ततः परमसंतुष्टो ब्रह्मस्थानगतं शिवं । मूलाधार त्रिकोणे वृषणगुदतले वह्निमायांतबीजं पाकस्तं **युक्तं रसनपरिगतं तन्मयं भाविता *ा । **त्यागं कवित्वं परपुरगमनं णं स्याज जीवेदाच*ंद्र*तारं मरणभयहरं सम्यगीशान धा । *add.* G **55–69** *This passage is significantly different in* G *and* μ: *see pp. 139–142 for editions of the passage as found in those witnesses and p. 7 for an analysis of the differences.* **56ab** *illegible* R_2 **56cd** *om.* $\alpha_3K_2\gamma$ **56d** एतद्योगो मयाख्यातः किं भूय श्रोतुमिच्छसि शंभोस् संभावनं लभ्य जयेच्चंद्रार्कतारकं *add.* G (≃ 68a, 68d, 69ab), शिवे सकलसिद्धिदा *add.* K_4 **57abc** *illegible* R_2 **58b – 59a** *illegible* R_2 **59d – 60b** *illegible* R_2

मत्प्रसादविहीनानां मन्निन्दापरचेतसाम् ।
पशूनां पाशबद्धानां योगः क्लेशाय जायते ॥६०॥
सर्वज्ञेन शिवेनोक्तां पूजां संत्यज्य मामकीम् ।
युञ्जतः सततं देवि योगो नाशाय जायते ॥६१॥
भक्त्या संतर्पयेद्देवि सर्वलोकमयं शिवम् ।
मय्येवासक्तचित्तस्य तुष्यन्ति सर्वदेवताः ॥६२॥
तन्मां संपूज्य युञ्जीत मत्प्रसादेन खेचरीम् ।
अन्यथा क्लेश एव स्यान्न सिद्धिर्जन्मकोटिषु ॥६३॥
सर्वे सिध्यन्ति मन्त्राश्च योगाश्च परमेश्वरि ।
मदाराधनशीलस्य मय्येवासक्तचेतसः ॥६४॥
तस्मान्मां पूजयेद्देवि सर्वयोगाभिवृद्धये ।
खेचर्यानन्दितो योगी योगं युञ्जीत तन्मयम् ॥६५॥

60a मत्॰] तत्॰ μ ◇ ॰प्रसाद॰] ॰प्रसाध॰ α_3, ॰प्रसादे PJ_3 ◇ ॰विहीनानां] ॰विहीनस्य G **60b** मन्निन्दा॰] तन्निंदा॰ μ, सदा सं॰ K_2 ◇ ॰परचेतसाम्] ॰परचेतसः G, ॰रतचेतसां S, ॰पारचेतसां J_2J_4V, ॰सारचेतसां K_2 **60c** पशूनां पाशबद्धानां] पशोः पाशप्रवंधस्य μ, पशोः पाशविबद्धस्य G **61a** सर्वज्ञेन] सर्वमेतच् G ◇ शिवेनोक्तां] J_6MK_2; छिवेनोक्तां G, शिवेनोक्त P, शिवेनोक्ते F, शिवेनोक्तं *cett.* **61b** पूजां] पूजा $K_3\gamma$ ◇ मामकीम्] $S\alpha J_4K_2J_3FK_6$; मादिरीं μ, मानवः G, मामिकीं J_2VK_4, मामिकां PK_5, मामिका γ **61c** युञ्जतः] $\mu\alpha_2$; यज्यतस् G, युज्यतः SJ_4VP-$J_3K_5^{pc}K_6$, पुंजतः M, पूजितः α_3, पुज्यतः J_2K_4, यज्यते K_2, पूज्यतस् F, युज्यत K_5^{ac}, पूज्यतः γ **61d** योगो] योगी γ **62a** भक्त्या संतर्पयेद्] $GR_2S\beta\gamma$; वारुण्या तर्पयेद् μ, भक्त्या संजायते α **62b** ॰मयं शिवम्] ॰मयं शिवे μF, ॰मये शिवे M **62c** मय्येवासक्तचित्तस्य] एकविंदुप्रदानेन μ, शिवध्यानपरे पुंसि G, मद्धानाशक्तचित्तस्य α_3 **62d** तुष्यन्ति] तृसंते A, तृप्यंते J_6J_7, तुष्यंते G, सर्वास्तु॰ K_5 ◇ सर्वदेवताः] कोटिदेवताः μ, सर्वदेवता $NK_3K_2J_3K_6\gamma_1$, ॰ष्यंति देवताः K_5 **63a** तन्मां] $\beta_1PJ_3K_5K_6B$; तस्मात् $\mu GS\alpha_1K_1F$, षण्मा॰ K_2, तन्मा γ_1 ◇ युञ्जीत] युंजीतः A, युज्यंतं G, संपूज्य α, पुंजीत J_2J_4, युजात J_3, प्रौजीत γ_2R_1, प्रोंजीत W_2 **63b** मत्प्रसादेन खेचरीम्] $SK_1J_2VPFK_6$; तत्प्रसादपवित्रितः μ, मत्प्रसादपवित्रितं G, ***देन खेचरीम् R_2, मत्प्रसादेन खेचरी $\alpha_1J_4K_2J_3\gamma$ **63c** क्लेश] क्लेशम् W_1K_1, क्रीय॰ K_2, क्तेश P ◇ एव स्यान्] संयाति N, आयाति W_1, संपत्तिर् M, आप्नोति K_1, पश्यंति K_3, ॰ते देवि K_2 **63d** सिद्धिर्] सिद्धि $W_1\gamma_1$, सिद्धिः J_3 ◇ जन्मकोटिषु] जन्मकोटिभिः $G\alpha$, खेचरीपदः J_3 **64b** योगाश्च] $\mu GM\alpha_3K_5$; यो[..] R_2, योगश्च $S\alpha_2\beta_1K_2PJ_3FK_6$, योगस्य γ ◇ परमेश्वरि] परमेश्वरी $\alpha_3VK_2J_3K_6\gamma_1$ **64c** मद्॰] मह्॰ $\mu P\gamma_1$, [.] R_2, सद्॰ K_3 **64d** मय्येवा॰] मयैवा॰ AJ_7, मय्यैवा॰ J_6, मध्याना॰ R_2, मद्धाना॰ α_3 **65a** तस्मान्मां पूजयेद्] GM; तस्मात्सां पूजयेद् R_2, तस्मात्पूजयते γ, तस्मात्संपूजयेद् *cett.* **65b** ॰योगा॰] ॰योग॰ $\alpha_1K_2J_3$, ॰रोगा॰ J_4, ॰योगान् B ◇ ॰भिवृद्धये] $\mu S\alpha_3\beta_1FK_5$; ॰भिवृच्छये G, ॰भिवृद्धयो R_2, ॰विवृद्धये α_1K_6, ॰स्य सिद्धये K_2, ॰निवृद्धये P, ॰निसिध्यये J_3, ॰निवर्द्धनी J_1R_1, ॰निवर्द्ध J_5 *(unm.)*, ॰निबर्द्धयत् W_2, ॰विवर्थयन् B **65c** खेचर्या॰] मदिरा॰ μ, खेचर्यां GN ◇ योगी] *om.* β_1, देवि $K_2\gamma$ **65d** योगं] योगो $AJ_2J_4K_4K_2PJ_3F\gamma$ ◇ तन्मयम्] नित्यदा μ, मन्मयं GR_2

---

61 *illegible* R_2 **62b** गौडी माध्वी च पैष्ठी च तथा कादंबरी वराः । कादम्बरी च द्रुमजा माध्वी मधुसमुद्भवा ।। पैष्ठी पिष्टसमुद्भूता गौडीक्षुरससंभवा । तासामेकतमां गृह्य तर्पयेत्सर्वदेवताः ।। असक्तः सुमहापूजां यदि कर्तुं च साधकः । कुर्याद् बिन्द्वेकदानं वा गुरुवाक्यावलम्बकः ।। *add.* μ *(for variants see page 139)* **62c–63a** *illegible* R_2 **63ab** *om.* K_3 **64b** सम्यक्पूजाप्रयोगेण मदिरानंदचेतसः । असंपूज्य पिवेद्देवि मदिरां यः स पापभाक् ।। *add.* μ, सम्यक्पूजाप्रयोगेन मध्याह्ने मत्तमानसः मामसंपूज्य योगेन पापं भवति नान्यथा *add.* G **64cd** *om.* G

विजने जन्तुरहिते सर्वोपद्रववर्जिते ।
सर्वसाधनसंयुक्तः सर्वचिन्ताविवर्जितः ॥६६॥
मृद्वासनं समास्थाय स्वगुरूक्तप्रकारतः ।
कुर्यादेकैकमभ्यासं गुरुवाक्यावलम्बकः ॥६७॥
अयं योगो मयाख्यातः सर्वयोगप्रसाधकः ।
तव प्रीत्या महेशानि किं भूयः श्रोतुमिच्छसि ॥६८॥
श्रीदेव्युवाच
शम्भो सद्भक्तिसंलभ्य जय चन्द्रार्धशेखर ।
त्वया श्रीखेचरीविद्या गुह्या साधु निरूपिता ॥६९॥

इति श्रीमदादिनाथप्रोक्ते महाकालयोगशास्त्रे
उमामहेश्वरसंवादे खेचरीविद्यायां तृतीयः पटलः

66b °वर्जिते] °वर्जितः α_3 **66c** °संयुक्तः] °संपन्नः S **67a** मृद्वासनं] $J_2VPJ_3FK_5K_6J_5W_2B$; मृद्वानसम् A, मृद्वास[नं] J_6, मृद्वासन $J_7J_4K_4$, मद्वर्गं च G, **सनं R_2, सिद्धासनं $S\alpha_1K_2$, रुद्रासनं α_3, सद्वासनं J_1R_1 ◇ समास्थाय] आस्थाय A *(unm.)*, समासाद्य α_1, समास्थाप्य γ_1 **67c** एकैकमभ्यासं] एकैकया देवि G, वैकैकमभ्यासं α_3 **67d** °वाक्या°] °मार्गो° α_3, °मार्गा° K_2 ◇ °वलम्बकः] °वलंबकं α_2V **68a** अयं योगो] एत योगं A, एतद्योगं J_6J_7 ◇ °आख्यातः] °आख्यातं μK_2, °आख्यातो γ **69a** शम्भो] शंभोः α_3, शन्तो J_3, शनो K_6 ◇ सद्भक्ति°] SK_3-$J_2VK_4PJ_3FK_5\gamma$; सद्भाव μW_1, संसि*क्त* R_2, स⊔क्ति N, यद्भक्ति M, सद्भक्तिं K_1K_2, मद्भक्ति J_4, स∗क्ति K_6 **69b** जय] जपं M, जयं $\alpha_3\gamma_1$ ◇ °चन्द्रार्ध°] चंद्रकं K_1, चंद्रक K_3, °चंद्रार्क° γ ◇ °शेखर] खेचरी α_3, °शेखरे $J_2J_4K_4K_2W_2$, °खेचरः V, °शेखरा K_6, °शेखरं γ_2R_1 **69c** श्री°] च G **69d** गुह्या साधु निरूपिता] $S\alpha_1\beta$; °साधनं गुह्यमीरितं μ, सारवत् गुह्यतामियात् G, गुह्या सा च निरूपिता α_3, गुह्यगुह्यनिरूपिता J_1, गुह्यद्गुह्यनिरूपिता J_5W_2, गुह्यागुह्यनिरूपिता R_1, गुह्याद्गुह्या निरूपिता B

66cd *om.* μG **67b** संतर्प शिवमीशानं सर्वदेवोत्सवप्रदं मत्प्रसादेन महता सर्वविज्ञानवान् भवेतसक्त-*स्सु*महापूजां यदि क*र्तुं* च साधकः *add.* G **67cd** *om.* μ ◇ संतर्प्य शिवमीशानं देवीं देवांश्च सर्वशः । तत्प्रसादेन लभते सम्यग् ज्ञानमखण्डितं ।। *add.* μ **68a–69b** *om.* G (*see addition at* 56d) **68ab** *om.* $R_2\alpha_3$ **68bc** *om.* μ **68d** इति श्रीमत्स्येंद्रसंहितायां षोडशः पटलः ।। *add.* μ **69d** *illegible* R_2

चतुर्थः पटलः

[सिद्धौषधानि]

अथ ते संप्रवक्ष्यामि सुदिव्यान्यौषधानि च ।
औषधेन विना योगी न क्व चित्सिद्धिमेष्यति ॥१॥
भिक्षूत्तमाङ्गपरिकल्पितनामधेयं
तत्पत्रपुष्पफलदण्डसमूलचूर्णम् ।
तक्रारनालपयसा मधुशर्कराद्यै
र्दद्यात्पृथक्कवलितं रसमण्डलानि
†पालित्यहानिमतिसत्त्वमुदारवीर्यम्
उत्साहरोगहरणानि च सम्यगेव† ॥२॥
कर्णे वराहो नयने गरुत्मान्

Witnesses for the fourth paṭala:
$AJ_6J_7SNW_1MK_1K_3J_2J_4VK_4K_2PJ_3FK_5J_1J_5W_2R_1B$; K_6 *(up to* 2a); O *(verse* 4)
$\mu=AJ_6J_7$ ◇ $\alpha=NW_1MK_1K_3$ $\alpha_1=NW_1M$ $\alpha_2=NW_1$ $\alpha_3=K_1K_3$ ◇
$\beta=J_2J_4VK_4K_2PJ_3FK_5K_6C$ $\beta_1=J_2J_4VK_4$ ◇ $\gamma=J_1J_5W_2R_1B$ $\gamma_1=J_1J_5W_2R_1$ $\gamma_2=J_1J_5$

1a अथ ते] μ; अथातः *cett.* **1b** सुदिव्यान्य्] $S\alpha_1K_1J_2B$; सुदिव्यान् μJ_4, सुदिव्यौन्य् K_3, ते दिव्यान्य् $VK_2K_5K_6$, दिव्यान्य् K_4 *(unm.)*, त दिव्यान्य् P, मे दिव्यान्य् J_3, देवि दिव्य् F, दिव्यानि γ_2, दिनि W_2 *(unm.)*, दिव्या R_1 *(unm.)* ◇ च] $\mu\alpha J_1R_1$; तु *cett.* **1c** योगी] योगं α_3 **1d** क्व] कश् α_3, किं J_4 ◇ एष्यति] $J_6S\alpha\beta_1PJ_3FK_5K_6$; इर्ष्याति A, इष्यसि J_7, इच्छति K_2, इष्यति γ_1, आप्नुयात् B **2a** भिक्षू॰] भिक्षण॰ μ, साक्षा॰ α_3, भिक्षु॰ J_2K_4, मिक्षु॰ J_4, भिक्ष॰ PR_1 ◇ ॰त्तमाङ्ग॰] ॰तमांग॰ A, ॰त्तमंग॰ α_3, ॰तंमाग॰ J_4, ॰त्तमां γ *(unm.)* ◇ ॰धेयं] $S\alpha_1\gamma$; ॰धेय μK_5, ॰धेया $\alpha_3J_2K_4$, ॰ध्येया J_4, ॰धेय VF, ॰ध्येयं K_2, ॰ध्येय P, ॰मध्ये J_3 **2b** तत्॰] यत्॰ J_3 ◇ ॰पत्रपुष्प॰] ॰पुष्पफुलं K_2, ॰पत्रापूष्प॰ J_3, ॰पुष्पपत्र॰ B ◇ ॰फल॰] ॰फलं VP, ॰वस॰ K_2 ◇ ॰दण्ड॰] ॰मूल॰ α_3 ◇ ॰चूर्णम्] ॰पूर्णं α_3 **2c** तक्रा॰] तत्का॰ S, तिक्ता॰ α_3, तक्ता॰ J_2VB, त्वक्रा॰ K_2 ◇ मधु॰] घृत॰ M ◇ ॰आद्यैर्] μF; ॰आज्यैर् *cett.* **2d** दद्यात्] $\mu S\alpha_1J_2VPFK_5$; यादः α_3, दृद्यात् J_4, तद्यात् K_4, देया K_2, दद्या J_3, दद्यत् γ_2W_2, चह्म R_1, दध्यत् B ◇ पृथक्॰] क्व चित् α_3 ◇ ॰कवलितं] $\mu SNMJ_2VPFK_5\gamma$; ॰ववलितं $W_1J_4K_4$, ॰क्रमगवं K_1, ॰कमगवं K_3, ॰वलित्त्वं K_2 *(unm.)*, ॰ववलिने J_3 **2e** पालित्य॰] $J_6J_7W_1M\alpha_3J_2VK_4$; पलित्य॰ A, पलित॰ SJ_3, पालिस॰ N, पालित॰ J_4P, पलि॰ K_2 *(unm.)*, वलीपलित॰ F *(unm.)*, मालिन्य॰ K_5, पलितं γ ◇ अतिसत्त्वम्] $\mu S\alpha J_2J_4VPJ_3FK_5$; अलिसत्वम् K_4, असत्त्वम् K_2 *(unm.)*, अतियतित्वम् γ_1 *(unm.)*, अयतित्वम् B **2f** उत्साहरो॰] $\mu\alpha$; उत्साहसे॰ S, उत्सापयेद् J_2, उत्प्रापयेद् J_4, उत्थापयेद् VPJ_3FK_5, उछापयेद् K_4, उत्थायएद् *(sic)* K_2, उत्थाय यो J_1, उत्थाप यो J_5W_2, उ*त्थ*ाय यो , उत्थाप्य यो B ◇ ॰गहरणानि च] J_6; ॰गहरिणानि च AJ_7, ॰कगमानानि च S, ॰गगहनानि च NW_1K_1, ॰गहनननानि च M *(unm.)*, ॰गगहना*नि* K_3, गहनतानव $J_2J_4VK_2PK_5\gamma$, गहनतानाव K_4 *(unm.)*, गगनताथने J_3, दहनतानव F ◇ सम्यगेव] $\mu J_2J_4K_4PJ_3F$; सर्वमेव $S\alpha$, संगमेव V, सम्यगेवा K_2, संम्यगेव K_5, सभ्यगेव γ_2R_1, सभ्यगे च W_2B **3a** कर्णे] $\mu S\alpha_1J_2VK_4K_2K_5$; कर्णो α_3J_4, कर्णौ PFJ_1, कर्णौं J_3, कणौ J_5W_2, वर्णो R_1, कर्णा B ◇ वराहो] वराहेः N, वराही J_2J_4, वराहुर् K_2, चराहो PJ_3F, वरोधो B ◇ नयने] नद्यने α_3 ◇ गरुत्मान्] AJ_6MK_5; गरुच्यान् J_7, गजस्यान् S, गरूत्मान् α_2J_4V, नवात्मा α_3, गरुत्मा K_4, रुगमान् K_2, गरुपान् ·PF, गरूपान् J_3, गरुडयान् γ_2R_1 *(unm.)*, गरुड्यान् W_2, गरुड्पान् B

2a परिकल्पित] प *end of K_6: f.22 damaged*

नखाश्च दन्ताः किल वज्रतुल्याः ।
युवा महामारुतसाम्यवेगो
जीवेच्च यावद्धरणीन्दुताराः ॥३॥
वाराहीकन्दचूर्णं घृतगुडसहितं भक्षयेत्पुष्टिवृद्धी
तक्रे दुर्नामनाशस्त्वथ पुनरपि गोक्षीरके कुष्ठनाशः ।
तच्चूर्णं शर्कराद्यैर्मधुमपि च पयः पाययेच्च द्विकालम्
द्वौ वर्षौ कृष्णकेशी हतवलिपलितः †कृष्णभेदी शरीरे† ॥४॥
एरण्डतैलसंयुक्तं गुग्गुलुं त्रिफलायुतम् ।
गन्धकं भक्षयेत्प्राज्ञो जरादारिद्र्यनाशनम् ॥५॥
अश्वगन्धा तिला माषाः शर्करा विश्वसर्पिका ।

---

4 *cit.* "खेचरीविद्या" (O) f.8v

3b नखाश्च] ग्रखंड° μ ◇ दन्ताः] दंतश् μ, दंताश् α_3, दंता $\beta_1PJ_3\gamma_2$, देता W_2 ◇ किल वज्रतुल्याः] $S\alpha_1J_2VK_2FK_5$; च भवेच्च वज्रं μ, च पुनर्भवेयुः α_3, किल वज्रतुल्यः J_4K_4, किल वज्रतुल्या P, खिल वज्रतुल्या J_3, किल वज्रतुल्यं γ_1, किल च न तुल्याः B **3c** युवा] वायु R_1 ◇ °साम्य°] °तुल्य° MK_5, सम्यग् $\beta_1PJ_3F\gamma$ ◇ °वेगो] $J_6J_7S\alpha K_2K_5$; °वेगा A, एव β_1J_3-$F\gamma$, ग्रव P **3d** जीवेच्च] μM; जीवेत्तु $SJ_2VK_4PFK_5$, जीवेत्स N, जीवेंदु W_1, जीवेत α_3B, जीवेत् J_4 *(unm.)*, जीवे तु K_2J_3, जवे च γ_2, जीवे च W_2, जवे*च्च*R_1 ◇ यावद्] पार्वं K_2 ◇ धरणीन्°] $\mu SW_1M\alpha_3$; वरणीं° N, धरणी° $J_2K_4K_2PFK_5$, हरणी° J_4, धरस्मी° V, वरणां° J_3, धरिणा° γ_1, वरिणा° B ◇ °दुताराः] $\mu S\alpha$; °हुताशः $J_2K_4PFK_5B$, °हुतासः J_4K_2, °हुतांशः V, °गतासः J_3, °हताश γ_2R_1, °हुताश W_2 **4a** वाराही°] चाराही° α_2 ◇ °कन्द°] °स्कन्द° K_1, °स्कद° K_3 ◇ °घृत°] °शघृत° J_2K_4 *(unm.)*, °शंघृत° J_4 *(unm.)* ◇ भक्षयेत्] भक्षयेद् α_3 ◇ °वृद्धी] SN; °वृध्यौ μ, °वृद्धिस् $M\beta_1O$, °वृद्धि W_1, °वृध्या K_5 **4b** तक्रे दुर्नाम°] μ; तक्रैर्दुर्नाम° SN, तक्रैर्दुनाम° W_1, तक्तें दूनाम° M, तर्क्रे दुर्नाम° J_2J_4V, तक्रें दुर्नाम° K_4, तक्रैन्दुर्नाम° K_5, तक्रे दुर्माम° O ◇ °नाशस्त्वथ] $\mu S\alpha_2K_5O$; नाशस्तथ M, नासस्त्यथ J_2VK_4, न समय J_4 ◇ कुष्ठ°] SMK_5^{pc}; कुष्ट° $\mu\alpha_2J_2J_4K_4K_5^{ac}O$, कृष्ट° V **4c** तच्चूर्णं] $\mu S\alpha_1VK_5$; तच्चूर्ण J_2, तचूंर्णं J_4, तद्वर्ण K_2, तद्वर्णं K_4PJ_3F, तद्वन्मधुशार्करादुग्धवर्णं γ *(unm.)*, तद्वर्सां O ◇ °शर्क°] °संक° K_2 ◇ °राद्यैर्] °राज्यैर् $S^{pc}W_1^{ac}MJ_3$ ◇ मधुमपि च पयः पाययेच्] μ; मधुयुतमपि यः सेवते S, मधुरपि च यः सेवयेत् N *(unm.)*, मधुरपि च यत्सेवयेत् W_1 *(unm.)*, मधुरपि च पयः सेवते M, मधुरपि च पी*य*ते J_2 *(unm.)*, मधुरपि च पुन पीयते J_4, मधुरपि वयज सत्ते V *(unm.)*, मधुरपि च पयते K_4, मधुर पिवेतयोमिनः K_2 *(unm.)*, मधुरपि वययते P *(unm.)*, मधुर पिविते J_3 *(unm.)*, मधुरपि पिबते F *(unm.)*, मधुरपि वसते K_5 *(unm.)*, मधुरपी पिवेते γ_2R_1 *(unm.)*, मधुरपी पिबसे W_2 *(unm.)*, मधुरपी पिवसेत् B *(unm.)*, मुधुरमपि पयः पीयते O ◇ च द्विकालम्] μ; सर्वकाल γ_1, सर्वकालं *cett.* **4d** द्वौ] द्वि° $F\gamma$, व° O ◇ वर्षौ] वर्षो μK_4, कर्षौ $S\alpha_2$, °र्षाभ्यो O ◇ °केशी] °केशो SMO, °केशा γ ◇ हत°] वलि° μ, दुत N, *द्रु*त W_1 ◇ °वलि°] °पलि° μ, °वलीत° J_4 *(unm.)*, °वहलि° V *(unm.)*, °वल° K_2, °वली° $K_5^{ac}W_2B$ ◇ °पलितः] α_1K_5O; °तहरो μ, °पतितः S, °पलीता $J_2J_4K_4$, °पलिता VK_2J_3, °मलीताहतवलिमलिता P *(unm.)*, °पलितं F, °पलित γ ◇ †कृष्ण°†] वर्ष° μ, कार्श्य° $S\alpha_2$, *चां*° J_4 *(unm.)*, चष्ण° K_4, कृष्ट° K_2 ◇ †शरीरे†] μMJ_3K_5O; °शरीरं *cett.* **5a** °तैलसंयुक्तं] °फलतैलेन μ **5b** गुग्गुलुं] FB; त्रिफला μ, गुग्गुलं *cett.* ◇ °त्रिफलायुतम्] गुग्गुलेन च μ **5c** प्राज्ञो] प्राज्ञे VK_5 **5d** जरा°] वली° M, मासे J_1 ◇ °दारिद्र्य°] $S\alpha_2FK_5B$; °दारिद्र° $AJ_7J_2VK_4K_2J_3W_2$, °दारिड्य° J_6, °पलित° M, °दरिद्र° J_4, °दारिद्रा° P, नदज° J_1R_1 *(unm.)*, द J_5 *(unm.)* ◇ °नाशनम्] °रामर J_1R_1, *om.* J_5 **6a** °गन्धा] °गंध α_2, °गंधास् M ◇ °तिला°] °तिल° $\alpha_2\alpha_3$ *(unm.)* ◇ °माषाः] μSM; °माष° $\alpha_2\alpha_3\gamma$, °माषा° β **6b** °विश्वसर्पिका] S; °विश्वसर्पिषाः μ, °स्वसर्पिध्यानं α_3 *(unm.)*, °किश्वसर्पिषा K_4, °विश्वसर्पिषा *cett.*

4ab *om.* $K_2PJ_3F\gamma$ **4a** पुष्टिवृद्धिस् – **5d** *om.* α_3

मासमात्रप्रयोगेन न रोगो मरणं भवेत् ॥६॥
पञ्चभिः पञ्चमासेन प्राप्यते ऽमरता प्रिये ।
गन्धकत्रिफलाकुष्ठं मधुरत्रयमेलितम् ॥७॥
भक्षयेत्प्रातरुत्थाय षण्मासाद्वलिपालिहा ।
पारदं गन्धकं देवि तालकं च मनःशिलाम् ॥८॥
कुनष्टिकायष्टिरजो रुद्राख्यं मुण्डिकारजः ।
त्रिमधुप्लुतमास्वाद्य वत्सरात् खेचरो भवेत् ॥९॥
भृङ्गं समूलं परिशोष्य चूर्णं
कृष्णांस्तिलांश्चामलकं तदर्धम् ।
मधुत्रयैः स्वाद्य सदैव वर्षान्
न व्याधयो नापि जरा न मृत्युः ॥१०॥

6c मास॰] षण्मास॰ α_3 *(unm.)* ◇ ॰मात्र॰] ॰त्रय॰ MVJ_3 **6d** न रोगो मरणं भवेत्] नरो मरवरं लभेत् μ, नरः परमपदं लभेत् α_3 *(unm.)* **7b** प्राप्यते] $\mu\alpha_3$; प्राप्नोति *cett.* ◇ ऽमरता] μ; परमां $SNMJ_4VK_4K_5$, परमं W_1F, मरतां α_3, परमा $J_2K_2P\gamma$, परम J_3 **7c** गन्धक॰] $V\gamma$; गंधकं *cett.* ◇ ॰कुष्ठं] J_6SMFW_2; ॰क्रुष्टं A, ॰कुष्टं $J_7\alpha_2K_1\beta_1K_2P\gamma_2R_1B$, ॰कुष्ठ K_3, ॰युष्टं J_3, ॰कुष्ट K_5 **7d** मधुरत्रय॰] मधुश्रय॰ γ *(unm.)* **8b** वलिपालिहा] $\mu\alpha_1J_2K_4K_5^{pc}$; वलितादिहा S, वलिपालिताद् α_3, वलिपालितहा J_4 *(unm.)*, वलितापही V, वलिपल्लिहा K_2, वलित्पलिथा P, वलिपलितिहा J_3 *(unm.)*, वलिपलितहा FW_2 *(unm.)*, वलीपालिहा K_5^{ac} *(unm.)*, वलिपलिहं तदा γ_2 *(unm.)*, वलिदंतदा R_1, पलितापहं B **8d** तालकं] तारकं AN ◇ ॰शिलाम्] $S\alpha_2K_1\gamma$; ॰शिला $AJ_6MK_3\beta_1K_2PFK_5$, ॰शिलाः J_7J_3 **9a** कुनष्टिका॰] β_1K_2PF; कुपष्टिका A, कुयष्टिका J_6J_7, कुष्ठं च ना॰ S, कुवंगना॰ α_2 *(unm.)*, कुवंगन॰ M, कनिष्टिका α_3, कनिष्टीका J_3, कुष्टिका॰ K_5 *(unm.)*, जवासा च γ ◇ यष्टिरजो] $J_6J_7\beta_1PFK_5$; यष्टिरजौ A, ॰डिकायष्टि॰ S, ॰टिकायष्टि॰ α_2, ॰मटिकायष्ति॰ M *(unm.)*, यष्टिरयो K_1, यष्तिरयो K_3, नष्टरुजो K_2, नष्तिरजो J_3, जेष्टिरजो γ_1, ज्येष्टिरजो B **9b** रुद्राख्यं] $\beta_1PJ_3K_5\gamma$; रुद्राक्षं μF, ॰रजोरु॰ $S\alpha_1$, मद्राक्षंम् K_1, मडाक्षं K_3, रुद्राख्या K_2 ◇ मुण्डिका॰] $\mu J_2VK_4PFK_5^{pc}J_1B$; ॰[द्रा]क्षमुं॰ S, ॰द्राक्षमुं॰ α_2, ॰द्राक्षमु॰ M, मदुका॰ α_3, मुडिका॰ $J_4J_5W_2R_1$, मुंडका॰ K_2, मुद्रिका॰ J_3, मुंडीका॰ K_5^{ac} ◇ ॰रजः] μ; ॰डिका $S\alpha_2$, आ[डि]का M *(unm.)*, ॰रजाः α_3, रसः $J_2VK_4K_2FK_5^{pc}\gamma$, रस $J_4K_5^{ac}$, रतः P, सरः J_3 **9c** त्रिमधु॰] $\mu\alpha_3$; मधुर॰ S, मधुरा॰ α_1, त्रिमधुरा॰ $\beta_1K_2PJ_3K_5\gamma_1$ *(unm.)*, त्रिमध्या F, त्रिमध्वा B ◇ ॰प्लुतम्] ॰त्रयम् S ◇ आस्वाद्य] μ; आसाद्य *cett.* **9d** वत्सरात्] $AS\alpha J_2J_4VPFK_5$; वत्सरा $J_6J_7J_3$, वसरा K_4, वत्सराद् K_2, वद्वत् γ_2R_1 *(unm.)*, वद्धत् W_2 *(unm.)*, ब*द्ध*वत् B ◇ खेचरो] μK_3; सबलो $SNVK_4FW_2$, प्रबलो W_1, सवलो $MJ_2PK_5\gamma_2R_1$, एव चरो K_1 *(unm.)*, सवलोक J_4 *(unm.)*, वत्सली K_2, वत्सलो J_3, सबली B **10a** भृङ्गं समूलं] मृगं समूलं γ_2R_1, मृगसंमूलं W_2, मृगस्य मूलं B ◇ परिशोष्य] परिपेष्य SW_1M, परिपेष्ट्य N, परिशोध्य K_1, शोष्यं K_5 *(unm.)* ◇ चूर्णं] $J_6J_7SNM\alpha_3J_4K_2J_3F$; चूर्ण AW_1, क्षिप्ता J_2, वंशैवचूर्णं V *(unm.)*, च शैवचूर्णं K_4 *(unm.)*, च शैलचूर्णं PK_5 *(unm.)*, शैलं γ **10b** कृष्णांस्] $S\alpha_2$; कृष्णास् μMPJ_3F, कृष्णं α_3, चूर्णंस् J_2, क्षिप्त्वा J_4, कृष्णा VK_2K_5, क्षप्राष्णास् K_4 *(unm.)*, कृष्णाति γ *(unm.)* ◇ तिलांश्] *em.*; तिला μVK_4, तिलान् $S\alpha_2$, MK_2F, तिलं α_3, तिलां $J_2J_4PJ_3K_5$, शिलाजित γ_2R_1B *(unm.)*, ति*शिलाजित W_2 *(unm.)* ◇ चामलकं] ह्यामलकं μ, आमलकं $S\alpha_2$, वामलकं γ_1 ◇ तदर्धं] तदर्धे A, तदर्ध $NJ_2J_3R_1$, दधि च α_3, तदर्थं B **10c** मधु॰] मधुर॰ $\beta_1K_2P\gamma$ *(unm.)* ◇ ॰त्रयैः] $J_6S\alpha\beta$; ॰त्रये A, ॰त्रयै J_7, ॰त्रय॰ γ ◇ स्वाद्य] $S\alpha\beta_1K_2PJ_3F$; खाद॰ μ, खाद्य $K_5\gamma_1$, खाद्यं B ◇ सदैव वर्षान्] ॰ति यस्त्रिवर्षं μ, नरोत्तमा α_3 **10d** न व्याधयो नापि] निव्याधोपरोगा न K_1, निव्याधोयरोगा न K_3

6c हस्तिना सह युध्यते । त्रिफला पुष्करो ब्राह्मी निःसाकोतिललंसनी पुनर्नवा वृद्धतारा †न ययुः† स्नेहमिश्रिता । षण्मासाहारयोगेन *add.* μ **6d – 7a** *om.* J_4 **7d** घृतमधुशर्करा *add.* W_1^{mg}

निर्गुण्डीपत्रमेकैकं त्रिकालं परिभक्षयेत् ।
द्वादशाब्दे भवेद्देवि जरामरणवर्जितः ॥११॥
निर्गुण्ड्यमलमुण्डीनां समं संसाधयेद्रजः ।
शर्कराघृतमध्वक्तं वत्सराद्वलिपालिहा ॥१२॥
माषकं गन्धकं स्वर्णं तालकं रुद्रलोचनम् ।
मधुत्रययुतं वर्षादजरामरणप्रदम् ॥१३॥
रसं शाल्मलिनिर्यासं गन्धकं मधुरत्रयैः ।
भक्षयेत्प्रातरुत्थाय षण्मासादजरामरः ॥१४॥

इति श्रीमदादिनाथप्रोक्ते महाकालयोगशास्त्रे
उमामहेश्वरसंवादे खेचरीविद्यायां चतुर्थः पटलः

11a निर्गुंडी°] निर्गुंठा° α_3 ◇ एकैकं] $\mu W_1\alpha_3$; एकं तु $SMVK_2PJ_3K_5\gamma$, एकं यस् N, एकं $J_2J_4K_4F$ *(unm.)* **11b** परिभक्षयेत्] परिभावयेत् μ **11c** °अाब्दे] °आशाद् μ, °आब्दाद् α_3, °आब्देन J_2J_4 *(unm.)* **12a** निर्गुण्ड्य्°] $\mu S\alpha_2$; निगुंड्य्° M, निर्गुंठ्य° K_1, निगुड्य्° K_3, निर्गुंड्° βB, निगुंड्° J_1, निगुड्° J_5W_2 ◇ °अमल°] α_2; °अनल° μ, °आमल° SMK_4, °आनल° α_3, °ईमल° $J_2VK_2PJ_3FK_5$, °ईमूल° J_4J_1, °इमूल° J_5W_2, °ईमूलं B ◇ °मुण्डीनां] $J_2J_4K_4K_2$-J_3FJ_1; °मुडाना A, °मुंडानां J_6J_7, °कीमुंडी SW_1, °मुंडी N *(unm.)*, °मुंडानां M, °निर्मुंडी α_3, °मुंठानां V, °मुडीनां P, °तुंडानां K_5, °मुडिनां J_5W_2, °मुडिना B **12b** समं] साम्यं $\mu\alpha_3$, समा K_2W_2B, समां γ_2 ◇ रजः] $\mu\alpha$; रसं SJ_2, रसः $J_4VK_2PJ_3K_5\gamma$, रस K_4 **12c** °मध्वक्तं] μ; °मध्वेकं $SJ_2J_4K_4J_3$, °मध्येक N, °मध्वेक W_1, °मध्येकं $MVK_2PK_5\gamma$, °मध्वर्कं α_3, °मध्वैकं F **12d** वलिपालिहा] $\mu S\alpha_1\beta_1P$; पलितापह K_1, पलितापहं K_3, वलिपल्लितहा K_2 *(unm.)*, वलिपलीतहा $J_3\gamma_1$ *(unm.)*, वलीपलितहा F *(unm.)*, वलिपालीहा K_5 *(unm.)*, वलितपलितहा B *(unm.)* **13a** माषकं] S; माषान्य° A, माषान्न° J_6J_7, षण्माषं N, षण्माष W_1, षण्मासं MJ_4, षण्मास α_3, णमाषसं J_2^{ac}, मासंद् J_2^{pc} *(unm.)*, माषमुद् V, मासामद् K_2, माषमद् PJ_3FK_5, माषाद् γ *(unm.)* ◇ गन्धकं] °मुद्गकं AJ_7, मुहकं J_6 ◇ स्वर्णं] स्वर्णो J_6V **13b** तालकं] तारकं N, तिलकं α_3 ◇ रुद्र°] भद्र° AJ_7 **13c** मधु°] मधुर° $\alpha_3K_2\gamma$ *(unm.)* ◇ वर्षाद्] वर्षाज् μ, चूर्ण α_3, वर्षाद्य् N **13d** अजरामरणप्रदम्] जरामरफलप्रदं μ, अजरामरणप्रदा J_6, अजरामरपदप्रदं α_3 *(unm.)*, अजरामरणं पदं γ_1 **14a** रसं] रस° $MK_3J_2J_4K_4K_2P$ ◇ °निर्यासं] निर्यास° α_3, निर्यातं K_2J_3 **14b** °त्रयैः] $\mu\alpha_3$; °त्रयं *cett.*

11d कुमारीपत्रमेकैकं त्रिकालं परिभक्षयेत् द्वादशाब्दा भवेद्देवि जरामरणवर्जितः *add.* μ **12** *om.* R_1 **13b** मधुत्रययुतं वर्षादजरामरणप्रदा उपामृद्गंधकं स्वर्णं तालकं भद्रलोचनं *add.* J_6J_7 **14b** आज्यं गुडो माक्षिकं च विज्ञेयं मधुरत्रयं *add.* γ

The *Khecarīvidyā*
An annotated translation

Chapter I

"Now,[190] o goddess, I shall teach the magical science[191] called Khecarī[192] by means of which, when it is understood,[193] one becomes ageless and undying in this world. Seeing this universe stricken by death, disease and decrepitude, my dear, one should steel one's resolve and take refuge in Khecarī. To him should one pay homage and turn to as guru with [one's] whole heart,[194] o goddess, who here on earth knows Khecarī, the destroyer of decrepitude, death and disease, in letter and spirit,[195] and practice.[196]

[Melaka]

The mantra of Khecarī is hard to obtain and so is its practice. The practice[197] and *melaka*[198] are not perfected at the same time. [The yogin] intent on just the practice might not attain *melaka* in this life. Through [carrying out] the practice, o goddess, he obtains [*melaka*] sometime in a subsequent life. *Melaka,* however, is not achieved even after one hundred lives [without carrying out the practice].[199] Carrying out the practice, which has been obtained by means of the correct emotional attiude, after many lives the yogin attains *melaka*, o goddess, sometime in a later life. Now when, o supreme goddess, the desirous [yogin] attains *melaka*, then he attains the *siddhi*:[200] which is described in the textual tradition. When [the yogin] attains *melaka*, both in letter and spirit, then, freed from the terror of transmigration, he becomes Śiva.

[This text]

Without [this] text, even gurus cannot understand [the mantra of Khecarī]. So, my dear, this very, very precious text must be obtained. As long as one does not have this text one shall wander about the earth. When it is obtained, o goddess, then *siddhi* is in [one's] hand. Without [this] text there is no *siddhi* even for one who wanders about the three worlds. So [the yogin], o goddess, should always worship Śiva, recognising [him] as the giver of *melaka*, the giver of the text, and the bestower of its practice.

I have taught many tantras, o goddess, [but], o you who are worshipped by the gods, in them the Khecarī *siddhi*, which destroys death, is not taught. *Mahākāla*[201] and *Vivekamārtaṇḍa*[202] and *Śābara*[203] and *Viśuddheśvara*[204] and *Jālaśamvara*:[205]

in these excellent tantras[206] the practice of [Khecarī] is proclaimed. *Melaka* and the other [results obtained] by means of Khecarī [are proclaimed in these tantras] sometimes clearly, sometimes unclearly. In this divine best of tantras *melaka* and the other [results] are proclaimed. Out of fondness for you I have taught here everything that there is to be known in the Khecarī doctrine[207] that might be hard to know. Therefore [the yogin] should procure this amazing text told by me; it has not been made public and is to be kept secret, o great goddess.

He alone is a guru who speaks the nectar of the teaching born from the lotus of my mouth; moreover, he who knows its implicit meaning is said to be the best [guru]. There is no guru better than him.

Having obtained this secret text one should not proclaim it to others.[208] After due consideration, it is to be taught to those who live on this path. He who makes this supreme text public to all and sundry will be quickly eaten by Yoginīs, o goddess, at the order of Śiva.[209] One should not untie its knot,[210] o goddess, without [performing] a *kaula* libation.[211] [After it has been] worshipped, placed upon an auspicious cloth and well scented with divine incense,[212] one should recite it in a place free of people to a yogin skilled in yoga. Distress [arising] from fire, illness, malign astrological influences and enemies undoubtedly arises in a house where this text is found unworshipped.[213] The family deities that bestow all wealth are present in the house where this book is worshipped, o Pārvatī. Therefore the wise man should protect [this book] with every effort. The yogin who wants these *siddhi*s described by me should guard this book with all [his] being.[214] I myself am the guru of him in whose possession the book is found, o goddess. The advantages and disadvantages [resulting] from the protection of [this] book have been clearly described by me, o great goddess.

[The Khecarī mantra]

Now hear [the mantra and practice of] Khecarī. And one should go, o goddess, to where there is a guru who has perfected the divine yoga and, after receiving the *vidyā* called Khecarī spoken by him, one should begin by scrupulously and tirelessly carrying out the practice described by him.

I shall proclaim the Khecarī mantra, which grants success in yoga, o goddess. Without it a yogin cannot enjoy Khecarī *siddhi*. Practising the yoga of Khecarī by means of the Khecarī mantra preceded by the Khecarī seed syllable, [the yogin] becomes lord of the Khecaras and dwells amongst them forever.[215]

The abode of the Khecaras[216] [and] fire,[217] adorned with the mother[218] and the circle,[219] is called the Khecarī seed-syllable.[220] By means of it yoga is successful.

The great Caṇḍā, which is known as the peak, bearing the flaming, fiery thunderbolt [and] joined with the previously described seed-syllable, is called the Vidyā [and] is extremely hard to obtain.[221]

[Now] I shall teach the six-limbed mantra.[222] [The yogin] should correctly[223] perform [the mantra-repetition] with it interspersed with the six [long] vowels, o goddess, in order to obtain complete success.[224] One should take the ninth letter

back from Someśa. The thirtieth letter from there, which is in the shape of the moon, is declared [to be next]. The eighth syllable back from there is next, my dear. Then the fifth from there, o goddess. Then the first syllable after that is the fifth [syllable of the mantra]. Then Indra joined with an *anusvāra*. This [mantra] is called Kūṭa.[225] It is to be obtained from the teaching of a guru and bestows fame in all worlds. Illusion, born of the body, with many forms [and] residing in the faculties,[226] does not arise even in sleep for the controlled [yogin], as a result of the continuous twelve-fold repetition [of this mantra]. The glorious Khecarī *siddhi* arises automatically for him who, totally self-controlled, recites this [mantra] five 40
hundred thousand times.[227] All obstacles are destroyed, the gods are pleased and, without doubt, wrinkles and grey hair will disappear.

After thus obtaining the great mantra [the yogin] should then carry out the practice; otherwise, o goddess, he suffers and [there is for him] no *siddhi* in the sphere of Khecarī. If [the yogin] does not obtain [this] nectarean mantra during the observance of the practice, then he should recite [it] having obtained it at the beginning of *melaka*.[228] Without this [mantra], o goddess, [the yogin] can never enjoy success. When this text is obtained then [the yogin] should resort to the mantra. Then, my dear, he quickly obtains the *siddhi* described therein.

[The physical practice]

In the manner described by his guru, [every day] for seven days the knower of *ātman* 45
should rub the base of the palate and clean away all impurity.[229] He should take a very sharp, well-oiled and clean blade resembling a leaf of the Snuhī plant and then cut away a hair's breadth [of the frenum] with it.[230] After cutting, he should rub [the cut] with a powder of rock-salt and *pathyā*.[231] After seven days he should again cut away a hair's breadth.[232]

[The yogin], constantly applying himself, should thus practise gradually for six months. After six months the binding tendon at the base of the tongue[233] is destroyed. Then, knowing the rules of time and limit,[234] the yogin should gradually pull upwards the tip of the tongue [235] having wrapped it in cloth.[236]

Then, in six months, after regular drawing out[237] [of the tongue], my dear, it 50
reaches [upwards] between the eyebrows, obliquely to the ears, and downwards it is gradually made to reach the base of the chin.[238] Then, only after three years, upwards it easily reaches the hairline, sideways the temples, my dear, [and] downwards the Adam's apple.[239] After three years more it covers the end of Suṣumṇā,[240] o goddess; obliquely it reaches the region above the nape of the neck [241] [and] downwards the hollow [at the base] of the throat.[242]

The practice must only be carried out gradually, not all at once.[243] The body of him who tries to do it all at once is destroyed. For this reason the practice is to be 55
carried out very gradually, o beautiful lady.

When the tongue reaches the aperture of Brahmā[244] by the external path, then [the yogin], o goddess, should rub with the tip of his finger the bolt [of the doorway] of

Brahmā ,[245] [which is] hard for even the gods to pierce,[246] [and] insert [his] tongue there. Practising thus for three years the tongue enters the door of Brahmā.[247]

[Churning]

When the door of Brahmā is entered [the yogin] should duly begin churning.[248] Some wise [yogins] achieve *siddhi* without churning. For [the yogin] who has perfected the Khecarī mantra success is achieved without churning. By doing both mantra-recitation and churning [however, the yogin] quickly obtains the result.

60 By means of a strong and smooth thread,[249] [the yogin] should insert a small probe of either gold, silver or iron into the nasal cavity. Fixing the breath in the heart [and] sitting in a steady pose, he should gently perform churning with his eyes focussed between his eyebrows.[250] By doing just this much the state of churning arises after six months. For the yogin who has completely restrained his *jīva*[251] [and] who has become identical with the object of contemplation, the state [of churning] arises as [easily as does] the deep sleep of children. Churning is not meant [to be done] constantly;[252] [the yogin] should practise it every month. But [the yogin] should always move his tongue around the pathway, o goddess.[253] [By practising] in this way complete success [arises] at the end of twelve years,[254] o great goddess. In [his] body he sees the entire universe as undifferentiated from himself.[255]

[The drinking of *amṛta* and its rewards]

65 [The yogin] should know the great pathway[256] in the skull[257] in the region above the uvula[258] between the eyebrows [to be] the Three-peaked Mountain,[259] [which is] honoured by the perfected ones [and] resembles a chickpea sprout.[260] He should fix his mind there. Licking with his tongue the supreme *amṛta* flowing there [and progressing] gradually on the path of the practice, [the yogin] should drink *[amṛta]* for four years, my dear. Grey hair and wrinkles are destroyed, supreme success arises and, as the knower of the meaning of all scriptures, [the yogin] lives for a thousand years. Success in sciences such as finding buried treasure, entering subterranean realms,[261] controlling the earth[262] and alchemy arise for the yogin after five years, o Pārvatī.

70 Duly drinking the flowing *amṛta* liquid with [his] tongue, the resolute yogin should curb his diet for twelve years, [living] as an ascetic.[263] By this application of the practice, the great yogin, free of grey hair and wrinkles [and] with a body as incorruptible as diamond lives for one hundred thousand years. With the strength of ten thousand elephants, my dear, he has long-distance sight and hearing. Capable of punishing and rewarding [people], he becomes powerful with respect to everything. These *siddhi*s, o goddess, only arise between the eyebrows.[264]

Placing the tongue in the ether,[265] [the yogin] should clench [his] teeth;[266] making the mouth [like] the hollow of a crow's beak,[267] he should drink the *amṛta* therein.

By drinking [the *amṛta*] he truly becomes free of old age and death after a year. He becomes a Khecara[268] and lives as long as the moon and the stars. The 75
best adept quickly attains absolutely all the magical powers[269] that are found in the three worlds, such as those of magical sandals,[270] the magical sword,[271] power over zombies,[272] magical elixirs, realgar,[273] invisibility,[274] access to the treasures of the subterranean realms [275] and power over male and female genies.[276]

Chapter II

[The *kalās* at the gateway of Brahmā]

O great goddess, at the barely perceptible bolted gate of Brahmā there is a great tetrad of *kalās*[277] consisting of the four aims of man.[278] On the eastern side is [the *kalā*] called Kṛtā, in the south Guptā, on the western side Śivā [and] in the north Parāparaśivā.[279]

When the yogin pierces that gateway with the tip of his tongue and drinks the *amṛta* from the eastern *kalā,* after a month he becomes a master of *dharma.* When the yogin licks with his tongue the *amṛta* at [the *kalā* called] Guptā in the south, there is no doubt that after just one month he becomes the lord of wealth in bodily form. When he drinks with [his] tongue the *amṛta* created in the western *kalā* of [the tetrad], then after a month the great yogin becomes the lord of pleasure. When he drinks the *amṛta* created in the northern *kalā*, then he obtains dominion over the highest gods.[280] When the lord amongst yogins drinks the great *amṛta* which is lying in the region above [the four *kalās*] at the opening of Brahmā, he becomes Śiva, liberated while living. When he practises every month for twelve years,[281] the yogin, free from all disease, omniscient, and worshipped by sages, becomes like Śiva, ageless and undying in this world.

After the yogin has repeatedly drunk the *amṛta* from the four *kalās*, o great goddess, he should then insert [his] tongue into the place of Brahmā and drink the *amṛta* [which is] very sweet, cool, pleasant, milk-coloured and free from froth. After just one month's practice, [the yogin] automatically becomes like a god. In two months he knows completely the meaning of all sacred texts, o Pārvatī. After three months, o goddess, he truly becomes free [and] like Śiva. After four months, great goddess, omniscience arises. In five months [he becomes] a great adept and is able to see the three worlds. In six months, filled with the goodness of the quality of ultimate bliss, [the yogin] becomes liberated while living; in this there is no doubt, o Parāparā. In the seventh month, with happy mind, he constantly associates[282] at will with great ghouls, ghosts, snakes and demons. In the course of the eighth month communion with the gods arises.[283] In the ninth month, the powers of becoming invisible and infinitesimal arise. In the tenth [month], the ability to assume any form at will, [which is] manifest to all the worlds, [arises]. In the eleventh [month], o goddess, knowing the past, present and future [and] as an almighty lord of the universe, [the yogin] becomes like Śiva. This that I have spoken is the truth.[284]

[The *kalā*s at Kedāra]

It is taught that Kedāra is where the *cūlitala* has been declared to be, o goddess.[285] Eight *kalā*s of Soma are described there, o you who are worshipped by the extreme adepts.[286] The first is Amṛtā,[287] o goddess, the second is called Mānadā; [then there are] Pūṣā and Tuṣṭi and Puṣṭi and Rati and Dhṛti, and the eighth is Śaśinī; all are oceans of the great *amṛta*. And when the yogin points [his] tongue towards that place then an eightfold stream of icy liquid flows there. Through contact with the flow of that [liquid], diseases of the body are destroyed. After eight months [of this practice] the yogin becomes a Khecara.[288]

[The *kalā*s at the Orb of Soma]

Verily, the place between the eyebrows is called the Orb of Soma.[289] A group of four *kalā*s is taught [to be] there, a seat of the great *amṛta*. [They are], by name, [the *kalā*] called Candrikā, and Kānti and Jyotsnā and Śrī. [The yogin] should insert his tongue there and drink [the *amṛta*] over and over again.[290] In four months the yogin becomes free from danger;[291] truly his body becomes as hard as diamond from drinking the flow of *[amṛta]*.

[The *kalā*s at the Diamond Bulb]

Above that is a rock, the Orb of the Khecaras,[292] known as the Diamond Bulb.[293] [The yogin] should recognise [it to be] at the top of the forehead; there, o goddess, is a triad of *kalā*s: Prīti, Aṅgadā and Pūrṇā. He should insert his tongue there. He should drink with his tongue the cool flowing *amṛta* of that milky stream. In three months, o goddess, [the yogin] becomes free from all disease, impervious to attack by all cutting weapons, unyielding to all methods [of hostile magic][294] [and] inconceivable by means of all the mundane sciences with their ugly objects. By the power of the Diamond Bulb he truly becomes like Bhairava.

[The *kalā*s at the Royal Tooth]

Below the nostrils and above the lips [295] is the great place [called] the Royal Tooth.[296] There, o goddess, is a pair of *kalā*s, Pūrṇāmṛtā and Śītalā. Holding the breath, [the yogin] should touch [them] with the tip of [his] tongue. A sweet, cool fluid is produced there, o goddess. Focussing his mind there, the ascetic should drink [the fluid] for three months. He becomes ageless and undying, free from all disease.

[The *kalā*s at the Base and Kuṇḍalinī]

The place between the anus and the testicles is called the Base.[297] Five *kalā*s are spoken of there, from which drips the supreme *amṛta*. Sudhā, Sudhāmayī, Prajñā, Kālaghnī, Jñānadāyinī:[298] [these] five *kalā*s are praised as streams of nectar, bestowing all *siddhi*s. The supreme feminine divinity is situated there, o goddess, the primordial Kuṇḍalinī. By contracting that region[299] [and] holding the breath, o you who are worshipped by the gods, [the yogin] should unite the cool *amṛta* situated there with the goddess of the Base. Leading [them] by way of the central channel [up] from the Svādhiṣṭhāna and other lotuses, he should think of [himself] as being sprinkled by the rain of that nectar up to his skull.[300] Taking the *amṛta* situated there, the great goddess Śrīkuṇḍalī goes by way of the central channel to the top of the abode of Brahmā, bathed in a surfeit of the nectar produced from the five *kalā*s of the Base. [The yogin] should imagine [her] pervading [his] body from his feet to his head. In five months of using [this technique], absorption into the five elements arises.[301] Through practising [it] in the morning, in the evening and at midnight[302] he truly becomes equal to Śiva.

[The *kalā*s at the Svādhiṣṭhāna]

That which is the place of the penis,[303] o goddess, is called the Svādhiṣṭhāna. There is said [to be] a triad of *kalā*s there, replete with the divine *amṛta*. They are called Susūkṣmā, Paramāhlādā and Vidyā. Holding his breath and awakening the goddess as before, he should lead [her up] as far as [his] skull and inundate his body [with *amṛta*]. In the course of three months the yogin attains the reward that has already been described.[304]

[The *kalā*s at the Bamboo Staff]

That which is between the anus and the penis is called the Bamboo Staff.[305] A tetrad of *kalā*s is taught [to be] there, consisting of the essence of the great *amṛta*. [They are] Suśītā, Mahātṛpti, Palitaghnī and Valikṣayā. [The yogin] should awaken the goddess there and inundate [his] body [with *amṛta*] as before; after four months of [this] practice he shall obtain the reward described earlier.

[The Iḍā and Piṅgalā Channels][306]

Piṅgalā is the channel of the sun; Iḍā is the channel of the moon.[307] The sun is called the bearer of poison, the moon is the bearer of nectar.[308] Practice is enjoined in that which is called the channel of the sun and in the channel of the moon; and concentration [is enjoined] in the channel of the moon.[309] The yogin should practise breath-retention. He should fill his body with air by way of the channel of the moon; expulsion [of air] by way of the channel of the sun is enjoined for improvement of the body.[310]

[The place of the ultimate *amṛta*]

I have taught you this four-fold place of *kalā*s, o goddess.[311] Now I shall teach the great place of the ultimate *amṛta*.[312] The Diamond Bulb in the forehead sparkles like the shining moon;[313] in its centre is the syllable *laṃ* and it is square. The deity there is the great Śiva. Gods [and] yogins worship [him] together with his consort.[314] At the *cūlitala*,[315] o great goddess, is a triangular *maṇḍala*, as bright as one hundred thousand suns. In the middle [the yogin] should visualise the great god Śiva, consisting of a *liṅga*, o goddess, with the syllable *raṃ* at the centre, embraced by his consort [and] surrounded by a troop of deities, o supreme goddess. In the right temple, o most fortunate goddess, is that which is encircled by six dots, containing the syllable *yaṃ* and smoke-coloured. There [the yogin] should visualise, o goddess, the god Maheśvara in the form of a *liṅga* together with [his] consort and surrounded by his troop of attendants. In the left temple, o goddess, is a [semi-]circle, looking like a half–moon, together with a lotus. It contains the syllable *vaṃ*, and in the middle there is a solid *liṅga* full of nectar, as white as cow's milk, [and] as bright as the autumn moon. It is together with its consort and is served by the entire host of gods and goddesses.

Thus have I described stations in the four directions, o goddess. In the middle of them is a great circle which contains the syllable *haṃ*. There, o Pārvatī, is situated the Supreme Lord, great Śambhu, together with his consort. He is in the form of a *liṅga*, together with [his] host, and is as bright as ten million suns. At the forehead is the lord of earth, at the back of the head is the lord of fire, in the right temple is the lord of air, in the left is the lord of water, o goddess, [and] in the middle is the lord of ether. I have described the five stations of Śambhu.[316]

Above the head of the god [who is] the lord of ether is a vessel full of the divine *amṛta*,[317] four fingers broad, with a door closing it at its base, a great rock with the moon above it[318] in the middle of an orb of light, as bright as ten million moons, impenetrable, the seat of *amṛta*. Immersed in the cool *amṛta* is a *liṅga*, o goddess, like a speck of dust, as bright as ten million moons, perfect,[319] [and] destroying the darkness of ignorance. Going beyond the five [*amṛta*-]stations, in order to obtain the ultimate substance,[320] [the yogin], holding the breath, should extend the goddess of speech,[321] with her mouth upwards,[322] together with [his] attention, to the doorway at the base of the pot of the ultimate *amṛta*.[323] Having reached [there] together with [his] mind, truly the yogin, restraining the flow of his breath, should playfully open the bolt with [his] tongue. There the yogin should drink the drink of yoga, [which is] hard for even the gods to obtain: the icy, milky *amṛta*, sweet [like] cool sugar-cane juice. Satiated by a surfeit of that nectar and having entered the supreme state, the yogin should obtain there in the skull union with the supramental state,[324] and eat, by means of yoga, the meat that consists of *nāda* and *bindu*.[325]

This rare secret has been proclaimed, o goddess. Truly, after six months [the yogin] obtains the reward which the omniscient Śiva has taught in the scriptural transmission; in this there is no doubt. He who desires [Khecarī] *siddhi* must not say anything to anyone who, [although] he has attained all [other] *siddhi*s, does not know this yoga, o goddess.[326] One should not cause this text to be given to those who delight in deceit and dishonesty, who do not recognise the guru as a god, and who do not know the observances taught in scripture.[327]

[Massaging the body with *amṛta*][328]

At the root of the tongue is situated, o goddess, the all-glorious fire. At its tip is the sun; the moon is situated in the middle of the forehead. *Siddhi* arises for him who correctly understands this.[329]

Having churned[330] and zealously awakened[331] the orb of fire, [the yogin] should
turn [his] tongue, on the tip of which is situated the sun, to the orb of the moon
at the forehead, which has liquefied due to the heat of that [fire].[332] [The yogin] 75
should gather in a vessel[333] that cool supreme *amṛta* [when it has] dripped from
the moon and emerged from the nostrils,[334] o goddess. By rubbing the body with
that *[amṛta]*, truly the channels of the body become purified.[335]

[The yogin] should stir up the essence of immortality which is produced at the anus and penis[336] and has emerged into a vessel, with the *amṛta* from the armpits,[337] embellished with fluid from the lower lip.[338] Rubbing the body with that, the yogin truly becomes free from disease in this life, mighty [and] free of wrinkles and grey hair.

Rubbing the root of the tongue, [the yogin] should massage his body with the great fluid that is produced there. Within half a year the tongue becomes four finger-breadths longer; in this there is no doubt.[339]

[Khecarīmudrā]

Pushing the tongue upwards with the fingers of the right hand, o goddess, [the 80
yogin] should push aside[340] the uvula with the fingers of the left hand.[341] Churning the place of fire, [the yogin] should gently turn the tongue above the uvula[342]
to the place of Śiva at the *kalās*[343] above the Three-peaked Mountain.[344] This
khecarīmudrā that I have taught you destroys death.

[The problems of *bhaṭa* and *naṭa*][345]

Four types of *bhaṭa* and likewise [four] types of *naṭa*[346] arise to obstruct him who practises thus. Drying up of the body,[347] sloth induced by hunger,[348] itchiness and pallor: these are the signs of *bhaṭa*. Listen to their remedies.

Having made the mind empty [the yogin] should rub [his] body with the essence 85
of immortality[349] for three months; by means of this this the body is nourished.[350]
He should rub [the body] three times in the day and three times at night.[351] By
pointing the tongue upwards towards the place of the Diamond Bulb[352] and licking
the nectar [produced] there, sloth induced by hunger truly disappears. By taking the
nectar [produced] there [and] the *amṛta* [from the anus and penis][353] and rubbing
the body [with them], both pallor and itching truly disappear.

The four varieties of *naṭa* have many manifestations, my dear. Eye-disease, trembling of the body,[354] fever and dizziness:[355] [thus] have I told [you] one type [of
naṭa]. Now hear the second: tooth disease, lack of strength and loss of suppleness
of the body. Now hear the third type [of *naṭa*], o goddess: high fever,[356] headache 90
and imbalance of the phlegmatic humour. [Now] may the fourth [type of *naṭa*]

be determined: vomiting, breathing trouble, blindness[357] and sleep that cannot be overcome.

Listen to the remedies of those [four types of *naṭa*]. [The yogin] should lead
Kuṇḍalinī from the Base into Suṣumṇā.[358] Making the tongue motionless and
pointing it upward, he should hold his breath. From the disturbance of Kuṇḍalinī,
o great goddess, a great sound arises.[359] When [the yogin] hears that sound then
he is said to be liberated [from the problems of *naṭa*]. He should visualise his body
as sprinkled with *amṛta*, o supreme goddess. By this [practice], o goddess, he be-
95 comes freed from the first problems [of *naṭa*] in a month. When he practises with
this method for two months, then he hears in his ears[360] the sound of the roar of
a great elephant.[361] He should visualise [his] body as before; he is freed from the
second [type of] problems [of *naṭa*]. After three months, having heard the sound
of Brahmā,[362] he should visualise [his body sprinkled with *amṛta*] as before; he is
freed from the faults of the third category. In this there is no doubt. In the fourth
month, hearing the sound of thunder called Aghora[363] and practising as before,
[the yogin] is freed from the problems of dizziness. Firm in his conviction, [the
yogin] should thus carry out the meditation and practice three times daily; truly,
after three years he becomes ageless and undying.

[The stages of the practice]

I have told [you] the remedies for the four faults of *bhaṭa* and for the problem[s]
100 of *naṭa*. [Now] hear more, o queen of the gods. I bow at the feet of that yogin
who, knowing all the categories of reality,[364] has entered into this peaceful supreme
reality,[365] the blissful yoga, o goddess.

The first [stage] is loosening,[366] o goddess; the second is piercing; churning is said
to be the third; the fourth is insertion.[367] After rubbing the base of the palate,
[the yogin] should pull out the tongue; he should know that to be loosening.[368]
The cleaving asunder of the bolt of Brahmā is called piercing.[369] When [the yogin]
practises churning by means of a thread and churning by inserting an iron pin he
should understand that to be churning,[370] which brings progress in yoga, my dear.
105 Having opened the gateway, [the yogin] should extend his tongue upwards into the
ether.[371] [This] is called insertion, o goddess. It brings about success in yoga.[372]

By breaking the bolt of Brahmā[373] and inserting the tongue, truly evidence of
success arises instantly, o supreme goddess. At first [there arise] a condition of
bliss[374] and a decrease in sleep;[375] social intercourse[376] and food-consumption[377]
diminish. Well-being arises and the lustre [of the body] increases, my dear; [there
are] no ageing and no death and no diseases and no grey hair. With his seed turned
upwards,[378] o great goddess, [the yogin] is endowed with the [eight] powers whose
110 first is minuteness.[379] If, with fixed mind, [the yogin] masters yoga thus, then, o
Pārvatī, he duly obtains these rewards that have been described.

On the tip of the tongue are situated Śrī[380] and Vāgīśā,[381] o you who are honoured by the heroic adepts; in the area at the base of the root of the tongue is situated the fetter of death.[382] Completely eradicate the place of the fetter of death, o mistress of the host![383] With the tip of the tongue [the yogin] should enter the place of Soma called Blessed Śambhu.[384] By this yoga, o goddess, and with a controlled mind, the yogin enters the supramental state [and] achieves absorption in it.[385] Evidence of absorption is sure to arise immediately.

Applying his mind to the tip of the tongue, he should focus on that place with [inner] vision.[386] The yogin should lead [his] breath upwards from the Base by
way of the Suṣumṇā. Having reached the abode of Brahmā he should place [his] 115
mind in the void. He should meditate thus on the perfect[387] highest reality.[388]

The very cool Ethereal Gaṅgā[389] flows from the place of Brahmā. Drinking [the Ethereal Gaṅgā], [the yogin] assuredly becomes one whose body is as hard as diamond in just one month; truly, he gets a divine body, divine speech [and] divine sight. He gets divine intellect, o goddess, and, indeed, divine hearing.

On the tip of the tongue [the yogin] should visualise the Queen of Speech shining like ten million moons [and] satiated by the *kalās* of the great *amṛta*; he instantly becomes a master poet.[390] Meditating on Lakṣmī as situated at the tip of the tongue [and] infatuated by the great *amṛta*, the yogin, o great goddess, becomes a king of yoga.[391]

[The five innate constituents]

There are said to be five innate constituents[392] in this body †which embodies the 120
supreme†.[393] When the body [of the fetus] is produced in the body of the mother through the fall of the father,[394] all [the innate constituents] arise there by the time the body [of the fetus] has reached maturity.[395] The first innate constituent is the primordial goddess Kuṇḍalinī, the second is Suṣumṇā and the third is the tongue. The fourth is the place of the palate, the fifth is the place of Brahmā. [The yogin] should raise the first innate constituent and place it in the second innate constituent. [Then] he should insert[396] the third innate constituent upwards into the fourth innate constituent. After piercing the fourth innate constituent, [the third innate constituent] should enter the fifth innate constituent.[397] This piercing that I have taught you, o Lady of the Kula,[398] is difficult to discover.

Chapter III

[Kuṇḍalinī and the flooding of the body with *amṛta*]

When she has reached the path of Suṣumṇā from the Base, the yogin should insert[399] into the uvular passage the goddess Kuṇḍalinī,[400] who has the appearance of a single thread of a spider's web [and] the splendour of ten million suns. Having broken the bolt of Śiva's door[401] with the tongue, o great goddess, he should, by holding the breath,[402] insert[403] [Kuṇḍalinī] into the abode of Brahmā, which has the splendour of ten million suns, my dear. There, in the great ocean of *amṛta* which abounds in cool waves, [the yogin] should drink the flow of nectar and rest, his mind full of ultimate bliss. He should visualise his body as satiated by the nectar of that [ocean].

By means of this divine yoga divine sight arises. Truly he becomes a Khecara,[404] and there arise the destruction of all sickness [and] the [powers of] cheating death[405] and of wandering throughout the three worlds.[406] Endowed with the [eight] powers whose first is the ability to become infinitesimal[407] [the yogin] assuredly becomes completely perfected; he becomes a ruler of yogins [and his] movement is unimpeded. [The yogin] automatically gets the strength of nine thousand elephants [and] becomes like Śiva, o goddess. Verily have I taught the truth.

Between Iḍā and Piṅgalā is the luminous[408] Suṣumṇā. There is an undecaying light there, free of the qualities of colour and shape.[409] She who looks like a sleeping serpent is the great Kuṇḍalinī. Gaṅgā and Yamunā are called Iḍā and Piṅgalā.[410] [The yogin] should insert that goddess, in the form of the supreme *amṛta*, between Gaṅgā and Yamunā, as far as the abode of Brahmā, o goddess. Truly he becomes identical with Brahmā and automatically gets an immortal body forever.[411] The goddess, having reached the abode of Śiva, the place beyond the Supreme Lord,[412] satiated by the pleasure of enjoying that place and filled with supreme bliss, sprinkling the body of the yogin from the soles of his feet to his head with the dewy, unctuous, cool nectar, o supreme goddess, proceeds again by the same path to her own home, o goddess.[413] This is the secret yoga taught [by me], o you who are honoured by the master yogins.

[Victory over death]

Shunning all sacred texts and [ritual] action such as mantra-repetition and fire-oblation, [and] freed from the notions of right and wrong, the yogin should practise yoga. He should turn the tongue upwards and insert it into the Three-peaked Mountain.[414] He should know that Three-peaked Mountain to be in the skull, below the forehead and in the region above the uvula. There is a blazing *liṅga* there, free from the process of time[415] [and] hard for even the immortals to perceive. Night is said to be in Iḍā, day in Piṅgalā. The moon and the sun, o goddess, are forever established as night and day. [The yogin] should not worship the *liṅga* by day nor by night, o goddess. He should worship the *liṅga* constantly at the place where day and night are suppressed.[416] This [existence],[417] furthermore, consists of day and night; the process of time is its true nature. By the suppression of the process of time, death is defeated.[418] [The yogin] should imagine his body as free from the process of time; he should worship [it] with the flower of thought[419] [and] he should offer it a libation of the *amṛtas* from the lotuses. By applying himself thus for six months he assuredly becomes ageless and undying. Truly, he becomes all-knowing, equal to Śiva [and] free of disease.

Inserting the tongue into the base of the palate with it pointing towards the upper mouth,[420] the yogin should drink the nectar produced there and gently suck in air with a whistling sound,[421] o goddess. Uniting the mind with the supramental state in the supportless space,[422] o goddess, he should practise natural yoga.[423] [Practising] in this way the yogin becomes ageless and undying after six months .

Placing [his] chin on the circle of sixteen vowels[424] and fixing [his] eyes between [his] eyebrows, o goddess, [the yogin] should extend [his] tongue upwards. Holding his breath by stopping Iḍā and Piṅgalā, [the yogin] should awaken Kuṇḍalinī and pierce the six lotuses. Inserting [Kuṇḍalinī], who has the appearance of a thousand lightning-bolts, into the very middle of the skull in the place that is an ocean of cool *amṛta*, he should remain there for a long time.[425]

When the yogin resides comfortably at the abode of Brahmā then [with him] at that place[426] the body appears lifeless.[427] If he should practise this yoga for a week, o goddess, then he becomes ageless and undying. With just one month's practice, he lives as long as the moon and the stars.[428] When the yogin easily breaks and enters the city of Brahmā, then he attains the state of Śiva, which consists of an eternal body,[429] o goddess. Never again does he drink at a mother's breast on the wheel of rebirth.

[Leaving the body and cheating death]

When the yogin who knows the *ātman* decides to leave this body [temporarily],[430] then, sitting up straight, he should visualise for a long time the goddess of the Base shining like ten million suns. Contracting his *jīva*, which has spread as far as the soles of his feet, he should gradually lead [it] to the place of the Base support. There he should imagine the goddess Kuṇḍalinī like the world-destroying fire devouring the *jīva*, the breath[431] and the sense-organs. Holding his breath,[432] o goddess, the yogin should raise [Kuṇḍalinī who is] radiant like a ball of lightning up from the Base and lead her to the place of Svādhiṣṭhāna.[433]

The ascetic should imagine the goddess devouring the entire *jīva* situated there. He should quickly raise [the goddess] who resembles ten million lightning bolts from there [and] having reached the place of Maṇipūra[434] practise there as before. Then, raising [her] up from there, he should lead [her] to the place of Anāhata.[435] Staying there for a moment, o goddess, he should visualise her devouring [the *jīva*] as before. Raising [her] again he should insert [her] into the sixteen-spoked lotus.[436] There too he who knows the path of yoga should visualise [Kuṇḍalinī devouring the *jīva*] as before, o goddess. Raising from there the great goddess who has devoured the *jīva* [and] has a radiance equal to that of ten million suns and leading [her] to between the eyebrows[437] [the yogin] should [by means of Kuṇḍalinī] again consume the *jīva*. The tongue, together with the mind, should break the bolt of Brahmā and duly come to rest[438] straight away in the great ocean of the supreme *amṛta*. Joining Śiva, [who is] situated there [and who is both] the supreme [and] the supreme cause, with the goddess, [the yogin] should visualise their union.[439]

If [the yogin] is keen to deceive death,[440] [then], knowing the apportionment of [the locations of] death,[441] while death[442] is approaching him he should happily remain there.[443] Below the bolt of the gateway of Brahmā is the cause of bodily death; in the region above there, o goddess, there is no opportunity for death.

When [the yogin] sees that [the time of] his death has passed, o goddess, then he should break the bolt [of the gateway] of Brahmā and lead the goddess [back] to the Base centre. [Re-]placing his *jīva*, which has been [re-]produced from the body of the goddess [Kuṇḍalinī], together with the sense-organs in their respective [places of] action, he should live happily and healthy. By this yoga, o goddess, [the yogin] can cheat an imminent death.

[Abandoning the body]

If the supremely content[444] [yogin] desires to abandon [his] mortal body then he should unite Śiva, who is in the place of Brahmā, with the goddess, pierce the void, and enter the rock of Brahmā.[445] He should place the ether element in the great ether, the air element in the great wind, the fire element in the great fire, the water element in the great ocean, the earth element in the earth, the mind in the supportless space [and] his sense-organs in the elements from ether to *prakṛti*.[446] Thus abandoning transmigratory [existence and] dependent only on the ultimate reality, untouched[447] by the five elements, the mind and the sense-organs, [the yogin] breaks the orb of the sun[448] and, absorbed in Śiva,[449] [who is] the serene abode of the ultimate reality, he becomes like Śiva.[450] Not in ten billion aeons will he return again.

If for the good of the universe he does not abandon [his] body, then he abandons it at the end of the dissolution of the universe and abides only in his own self.[451]

This is Khecarī *mudrā*, which bestows dominion over the Khecaras [and] destroys birth, death, old age, sickness, wrinkles and grey hair.

[Praise of Khecarī and devotion to Śiva][452]

There is no *vidyā*[453] like this anywhere in [any] other text. [The yogin] should not make public the very secret Khecarī *melana*,[454] o goddess, and I have proclaimed this method of the practice of [the *vidyā*] out of affection for you.

O goddess, he who does not know Khecarī, who is worshipped by all great yogins,
is in this world called a bound soul, o Pārvatī. The great yoga cannot be perfected
without my worship, even by [the yogin] who, while wandering through the three
worlds, is constantly devoted to the practice and who practises the *vidyā* obtained
from the mouth of [his] guru with his mind always focussed on Khecarī *melaka* and
60 such like. For those bound souls caught in bondage [who] do not have my grace
[and] who are intent on scorning me, yoga is a source [only] of suffering. For him
who abandons my worship, which [I], the all-knowing Śiva, have taught, [even if]
he constantly practises yoga, yoga leads to destruction.

[The yogin] should worship the universal Śiva with devotion.[455] All the gods and goddesses are pleased by him whose mind is focussed on me alone. Therefore [the yogin] should worship me and practise the yoga of Khecarī with my grace. Otherwise there will be only trouble and no *siddhi* [even] in ten million births. For him who is keen on worshipping me [and] whose mind is intent on me alone all mantras and yogas are successful, o supreme goddess.

65 Therefore, to advance in all types of yoga,[456] the yogin should worship me, o goddess, [and], delighting in Khecarī, he should practise her yoga. In [a place] free of people, animals and all disturbance,[457] [the yogin], furnished with all that is necessary for the practice[458] [and] free of all anxiety, should, in the manner described by his guru, sit on a comfortable seat and do each practice one by one, relying on the teachings of his guru.

I have taught this yoga, the best of all yogas, out of fondness for you, o great goddess. What more do you wish to hear?"

The goddess said:[459]

"O Śambhu, whose diadem is the crescent moon[460] [and] who can be attained [only] by true devotion,[461] may you be victorious. You have described well the secret [and] glorious *Khecarīvidyā*."

Chapter IV

[Drugs for *siddhi*]

"And now I shall teach you some very sacred drugs. Without drugs a yogin can never attain *siddhi*.[462]

[Having prepared] a powder of the leaves, flowers, fruits and stem, together with the root, of the plant whose name consists of the highest limb of the mendicant[463] with buttermilk and water,[464] fermented rice gruel and milk, together with honey, sugar and the like,[465] one should give[466] [to the yogin] in separate mouthfuls round essential pills [of the mixture]. †[The yogin attains]†[467] all together the loss of grey hair, great well-being, great vigour[468] and the removal of debilitating diseases. [His] ears [become like those of] a boar,[469] [his] eyes [become like those of] a bird of prey, and [his] nails [and] teeth [become] like diamonds; [he becomes] young, as fast as the wind, and lives as long as the earth, the moon and the stars.

[If the yogin] should eat powdered bulb of *vārāhī*[470] with ghee and unrefined cane-sugar, [there arise] health and growth. [If he should eat that powder] in buttermilk and water, piles are got rid of. [If he should eat it] in cow's milk, leprosy is got rid of. One should have [the yogin] drink that powder with sugar and the like and sweet water twice a day for two years. [He will become] black-haired, without grey hair or wrinkles, †[and] he gets rid of blackness on the body†.[471]

To get rid of old age and debility, the wise [yogin] should eat *guggulu*[472] with castor- 5
oil and sulphur with *triphalā*.[473]

By just one month's use of *aśvagandhā*,[474] sesame seeds, mung beans, sugar and *viśvasarpikā*,[475] there is no disease or death. With [these] five, immortality is obtained in five months, my dear.

[The yogin] should rise at dawn and eat sulphur, *triphalā* and *kuṣṭha*,[476] mixed with the three sweeteners;[477] after six months he is rid of wrinkles and grey hair.

O goddess, taking mercury, sulphur, orpiment, realgar, that which is called Rudra, namely the stem and pollen of *kunaṣṭi*,[478] and the pollen of *muṇḍikā*[479] soaked in the three sweeteners, [the yogin] becomes strong after a year.

By regularly eating powdered, dried *bhṛṅga*[480] with its root, black sesame seeds and 10
an *āmalaka* fruit in half measure, together with the three sweeteners, in one year neither diseases nor old age nor death [arise].

[The yogin] should eat one *nirguṇḍī*[481] leaf three times a day; in twelve years, o goddess, he becomes free of old age and death.

[The yogin] should use equal amounts of the pollen of *nirguṇḍī*, *amala*[482] and *muṇḍī*, anointed with sugar, ghee and honey; after a year he gets rid of grey hair and wrinkles.

In six months, sulphur, gold, orpiment, and *rudrākṣa*[483] seeds mixed with the three sweeteners bestow freedom from old age and death.

Rising at dawn, [the yogin] should eat mercury,[484] the sap of the silk-cotton tree,[485] sulphur and the three sweeteners; after six months he becomes free from old age and death."

Appendices

Appendix A: *KhV* 3.55–69 in μ and G

MATSYENDRASAṂHITĀ 16.98–17.1

अनया सदृशी विद्या क्व चिच्छास्त्रान्तरे न हि ।
खेचरीमेलनं देवि सुगुप्तं न प्रकाशयेत् ॥९८॥
तस्य चाभ्यासयोगो ऽयं तव स्नेहात्प्रकाशितः ।
मदिरा नाम या देवि सर्वयोगीन्द्रवन्दिता ॥९९॥
नैनां यो वेत्ति लोके ऽस्मिन् स पशुः प्रोच्यते शिवे ।
नित्यमभ्याशशीलस्य अटतो ऽपि जगत्त्रयम् ॥१००॥
गुरुवक्त्रोपसंलब्धां विद्यामभ्यसतो ऽपि च ।
खेचरीमेलनादिषु नित्यं सप्रेमचेतसः ॥१०१॥
न सिध्यति महायोगं मदिराराधनं विना ।
तत्प्रसादविहीनस्य तन्निन्दापरचेतसः ॥१०२॥
पशोः पाशप्रबद्धस्य योगः क्लेशाय जायते ।
सर्वज्ञेन शिवेनोक्तां पूजां संत्यज्य मादिरीम् ॥१०३॥
युञ्जतः सततं देवि योगो नाशाय जायते ।
वारुण्या तर्पयेद्देवि सर्वलोकमयं शिवम् ॥१०४॥
गौडी माध्वी च पैष्टी च तथा कादम्बरी वराः ।
कादम्बरी च द्रुमजा माध्वी मधुसमुद्भवा ॥१०५॥
पैष्टी पिष्टसमुदभूता गौडीक्षुरससंभवा ।
तासामेकतमां गृह्य तर्पयेत्सर्वदेवताः ॥१०६॥
असक्तः सुमहापूजां यदि कर्तुं च साधकः ।
कुर्याद्बिन्द्वेकदानं वा गुरुवाक्यावलम्बकः ॥१०७॥

Matsyendrasaṃhitā Witnesses: A(f. $48v^{11}$ – f. $49v^{3}$), J_6 (f. $33v^{1}$ – f. $34r^{1}$), J_7 (f. $70r^{1}$ – f. $71r^{2}$) ◇ 98–104 ≃ Ed 55–61; 105a–107b *om.* Ed; 107cd ≃ Ed 67ab; 108–109 ≃ Ed 62–63; 110 *om.* Ed; 111–112 ≃ Ed 64–65; 113ab ≃ Ed 66cd; 113c–114b *om.* Ed; 114c–115d ≃ Ed 67c, 68b–69 ◇ 98a–99b ≃ G 259a–260b; 99c–104d ≃ G 261c–266d; 105–106 *om.* G; 107 ≃ G 273; 108–110 ≃ G 267–269; 111ab *om.* G; 111c–114b ≃ G 270–272; 114c–17.1b ≃ G 260c–261b; 17.1cd ≃ G 274ab.

98c °मेलनं] °मेलन A 98d प्रकाशयेत्] प्रकारयेत् J_6J_7 99a चाभ्यासयोगो] *em.*; स्वाभ्यासयोगे A, स्वाभ्यासयोगो J_6J_7 100d अटतो] आटतो J_6 101b अभ्यसतो] अभ*श*तो A 101c °मेलनादिषु] *em.*; °मेलनादिश्च μ 101d °चेतसः] *em.*; °वेतसः μ 102c °विहीनस्य] *corr.*; °विहीनानां μ 102d °चेतसः] *corr.*; °चेतसां μ 103a °प्रबद्धस्य] *em.*; °प्रवंधस्य μ 103c °नोक्तां] J_6; °नोक्तं AJ_7 104d शिवम्] *em.*; शिवे μ 105a गौडी] गौरी A 105b वराः] A; पराः J_6J_7 105c द्रुमजा] द्रुमला A 106b गौडी°] गौरी° A ◇ °संभवा] °संभवां A 106c गृह्य] गुह्य A 106d °देवताः] °देवता A 107b कर्तुं] कर्त्तु A 107c कुर्याद्] कुयोद् J_6 107d °लम्बकः] J_6; °लम्बक AJ_7

एकबिन्दुप्रदानेन तृप्यन्ते कोटिदेवताः ।
तस्मात्संपूज्य युञ्जीत तत्प्रसादपवित्रितः ॥१०८॥
अन्यथा क्लेश एव स्यान्न सिद्धिर्जन्मकोटिषु ।
सर्वे सिध्यन्ति मन्त्राश्च योगाश्च परमेश्वरि ॥१०९॥
सम्यक्पूजाप्रयोगेन मदिरानन्दचेतसः ।
असंपूज्य पिबेद्देवि मदिरां यः स पापभाक् ॥११०॥
महाराधनशीलस्य मय्येवासक्तचेतसः ।
तस्मात्संपूजयेद्देवि सर्वयोगाभिवृद्धये ॥१११॥
मदिरानन्दितो योगी योगं युञ्जीत नित्यदा ।
विजने जन्तुरहिते सर्वोपद्रववर्जिते ॥११२॥
मृद्वासनं समास्थाय स्वगुरूक्तप्रकारतः ।
संतर्प्य शिवमीशानं देवीं देवांश्च सर्वशः ॥११३॥
तत्प्रसादेन लभते सम्यग्ज्ञानमखण्डितम् ।
एतद्योगं मयाख्यातं किं भूयः श्रोतुमिच्छसि ॥११४॥
श्रीदेव्युवाच
शम्भो सद्भावसंलभ्य जय चन्द्रार्धशेखर ।
त्वया श्रीखेचरीविद्यासाधनं गुह्यमीरितम् ॥१॥

108b तृप्यन्ते] तृप्तंते A 108c युञ्जीत] युंजीतः A 108d ॰पवित्रितः] ॰पवित्रेतः A 109a स्यान्] *em.*; श्यात् A, स्यात् J_6J_7 109b ॰कोटिषु] ॰कोदिषु A 111b मय्येवा॰] *em.*; मयैवा॰ AJ_7, मय्यैवा॰ J_6 ◇ ॰चेतसः] अचेतसः A *(unm.)* 112b योगं] योगो A 113a मृद्वासनं समास्थाय] मृद्वानसमास्थाय A *(unm.)* 113d देवांश्] देवीश् A 114c एतद] एत A

MANUSCRIPT G 259A–274B

अनया सदृशी विद्या क्व चिच्छास्त्रान्तरे न हि ।
खेचरीमेलनं देवि सुगुह्यं संप्रकाशितम् ॥२५९॥
तस्याश्चाभ्यासयोगो ऽयं तव स्नेहात्प्रकाशितः ।
एतद्योगो मयाख्यातः किं भूयः श्रोतुमिच्छसि ॥२६०॥
शम्भोः संभावनं लभ्य जयेच्चन्द्रार्कतारकं ।
खेचरी नाम या देवी सर्वयोगीन्द्रवन्दिता ॥२६१॥
एनां नो वेत्ति लोके ऽस्मिन् स पशुः प्रोच्यते शिवे ।
नित्यमभ्याशशीलस्य अटतो ऽपि जगत्त्रयम् ॥२६२॥
गुरुवक्त्रे ऽपि लब्धस्य विद्यामभ्यसतो ऽपि च ।
खेचरीमेलनाद्येषु नित्यं संसक्तचेतसः ॥२६३॥
न विद्यते महायोगो मदिदं साधनं विना ।
मत्प्रसादविहीनस्य मन्निन्दापरचेतसः ॥२६४॥
पशोः पाशविबद्धस्य योगः क्लेशाय जायते ।
सर्वमेतच्छिवेनोक्तां पूजां संत्यज्य मानवः ॥२६५॥
युज्यतः सततं देवि योगो नाशाय जायते ।
भक्त्या संतर्पयेद्देवि सर्वलोकमयं शिवे ॥२६६॥
शिवध्यानपरे पुंसि तुष्यन्ते सर्वदेवताः ।
तस्मात्संपूज्य युज्यन्तं मत्प्रसादपवित्रितम् ॥२६७॥
अन्यथा क्लेश एव स्यान्न सिद्धिर्जन्मकोटिभिः ।
सर्वे सिध्यन्ति मन्त्राश्च योगाश्च परमेश्वरि ॥२६८॥
सम्यक्पूजाप्रयोगेन मद्ध्याने मत्तमानसः ।
मामसंपूज्य योगेन पापं भवति नान्यथा ॥२६९॥
तस्मान्मां पूजयेद्देवि सर्वयोगाभिवृद्धये ।

MS G 259a–260b ≃ Ed 55a–56b; 260c–261b ≃ Ed 67c–68b; 261c–268d ≃ Ed 56c–63d; 269 *om.* Ed; 270a–271b ≃ Ed 64c–65d; 271cd ≃ Ed 66cd; 272a–273b *om.* Ed; 273cd ≃ Ed 67ab; 274ab ≃ Ed 69ab ◇ 259a–260b ≃ μ 98a–99b; 260c–261b ≃ μ 114c–115b; 261c–266d ≃ μ 99c–104d; 267–269 ≃ μ 108–110; 270–272 ≃ μ 111c–114b; 273 ≃ μ 107; 274ab ≃ μ 115cd.

260d भूयः] *corr.*; भूय G **261c** देवी] *em.*; देवि G **262a** नो] *corr.*; *न्*ो G **262d** जगत्त्रयम्] *corr.*; जगत्नयं G **263d** °सक्त°] *corr.*; °स*क्त*° G **266a** युज्यतः] *em.*; यज्यतः G **268b** जन्म°] *corr.*; ज्जन्म G **268c** सिध्यन्ति] *corr.*; सिद्धंति G **269b** मद्ध्याने] *em.*; मध्यान्हे G **270b** °वृद्धये] *em.*; °वृच्छये G

खेचर्यां नन्दितो योगी योगं युञ्जीत मन्मयम् ॥२७०॥
विजने जन्तुरहिते सर्वोपद्रववर्जिते ।
मद्वर्णं च समास्थाय स्वगुरूक्तप्रकारतः ॥२७१॥
संतर्प्य शिवमीशानं सर्वदेवोत्सवप्रदम् ।
मत्प्रसादेन महता सर्वविज्ञानवान् भवेत् ॥२७२॥
असक्तः सुमहापूजां यदि कर्तुं च साधकः ।
कुर्यादिकैकया देवि गुरुवाक्यावलम्बकः ॥२७३॥
त्वया च खेचरी विद्या सारवद्गुह्यतामियात्

272a संतर्प्य] *em.*; संतर्प G 273a असक्तः सु°] *corr.*; असक्त*स् सु*° G 273b कर्तुं] *corr.*; क*र्तुं* G 274b °वद्] *corr.*; °वत् G

Appendix B: *MaSaṃ* 17, 18 and 27

सप्तदशः पटलः

श्रीदेव्युवाच
शम्भो सद्भावं संलभ्य जयचन्द्रार्धशेखर ।
त्वया श्रीखेचरीविद्यासाधनं गुह्यमीरितम् ॥१॥
संसिद्धं केन मार्गेण खेचरीमेलनं लभेत् ।
तन्मे ब्रूहि जगन्नाथ परमानन्दनन्दित ॥२॥
श्रीभैरव उवाच
शृणु गुह्यं महादेवि सर्वतन्त्रेषु गोपितम् ।
खेचरीमेलनं लोके महायोगीन्द्रसेवितम् ॥३॥
खेचरीणामियं विद्या सद्यःप्रत्ययकारिका ।
सर्वसिद्धिप्रदा देवि जरामरणनाशिनी ॥४॥
†दार्च्छाद्† ब्रह्मकपाटस्य पशूनां दूरमार्गगा ।
असिद्धानामपि च या योगिनां परमेश्वरि ॥५॥
ब्रह्मधाम परित्यज्य आयाता नासिकापथम् ।
भित्त्वा ब्रह्मकपाटं तु यदा ध्रुवपदं व्रजेत् ॥६॥
तदा स्यात्परमानन्दं संविद्भावैककारणम् ।
ज्ञानं तथा च विज्ञानं तत्प्रसादात्स्फुरत्यपि ॥७॥
एवं योगे क्रियायां च स्थिता सकलकामदा ।
चिद्रूपा कुब्जिका नाम दुर्विज्ञेया सुरासुरैः ॥८॥
एवं कुण्डलिनीशक्तिरूर्ध्वाधोऽनेकधा गता ।
तत्स्थे योगः पदस्थे हि अणिमादिप्रसाधकः ॥९॥
तानि स्थानानि वक्ष्यामि यथा येषु च सिद्धिदा ।
मूलाधारं चतुःपत्रो बिन्दुस्त्रिवलयान्वितः ॥१०॥

μ=AJ_6J_7 ◇ A f. $49v^3$ – f. $51v^{11}$ ◇ J_6 f. $34r^1$ – f. $35v^3$ ◇ J_7 f. $71r^1$ – f. $74r^{10}$

1a ॰भावं] *em.*; ॰भाव μ 2a संसिद्धं] *corr.*; संसिद्धि A, संसिद्धिः J_6J_7 2d ॰नन्दित] J_6; ॰नंदितः AJ_7 3a श्रीभैरव उवाच] श्रीभैरवः J_6 4b सद्यः] सद्य A 5a †दार्च्छाद्†] AJ_7; दा*र्च्छा*द् J_6 ◇ ॰कपाटस्य] कपटस्य A *(unm.)* 5b पशूनां] पशुनां A ◇ ॰गा] ॰गाः A 5c या] यो A 6a परित्यज्य] *em.*; परित्य*ज्य*A, परित्य J_6J_7 *(unm.)* 6c तु] J_6; त्वु A, तु J_7 7b संविद्॰] सविद्॰ A 7d स्फुरत्य] स्पुरत्य A 9b ऽनेकधा] नकदा A 10b येषु] ॰ग्रेषु A

गमागमसमोपेत आधाराख्यः शिखिप्रभः ।
गुह्यान्तं षड्दलं दीप्तं षड्बिन्दुः परिकीर्तितम् ॥११॥
तप्तजाम्बूनदाभासं स्वाधिष्ठानं हि तद्भवेत् ।
नाभिमध्यगतं शुद्धं द्वादशारं शशिप्रभम् ॥१२॥
मणिपूरकसंज्ञानम् अर्धचन्द्रस्य मध्यगम् ।
अनाहतं दशारं तु ब्रह्मरन्ध्रान्तगं सदा ॥१३॥
शुद्धस्फटिकसंकाशं भावयेन्नादरूपकम् ।
षोडशारं महापद्मं त्रिकोणं कण्ठमाश्रितम् ॥१४॥
पूर्णचन्द्रनिभाकारं विशुद्धं मोक्षदायकम् ।
पञ्चकूटमहत्स्थानं विद्युत्कोटिसमप्रभम् ॥१५॥
मध्यदिनार्कसंकाशं भावयेद्बिन्दुरूपकम् ।
स तु नानातनोर्मध्ये शक्तिर्व्योमप्रभेदिनी ॥१६॥
ज्वालन्ती पञ्चधा रन्ध्रे सेयमाज्ञा प्रकीर्तिता ।
ब्रह्मा विष्णुश्च रुद्रश्च ईश्वरश्च सदाशिवः ॥१७॥
पृथिव्यादीनि रन्ध्राणि पञ्चपञ्चकमेव च ।
तथा च कोष्ठकाः पञ्च स्वाधिष्ठानादयः स्मृताः ॥१८॥
एतेषु स्थानभेदेषु पृथग् ध्यानं शिवोदितम् ।
तत्रैकमपि चाभ्यस्य योगी स्यादजरामरः ॥१९॥
अभ्यासेनैव नश्यन्ति पापा जन्मसहस्रजाः ।
मेलनात्शिवतां याति सुमहान् खेचराधिपः ॥२०॥
स्वतन्त्रः सर्वलोकेषु गतिरव्याहता भवेत् ।
अविज्ञाय च यः कुर्याद् गुरुवाक्यामृतं विना ॥२१॥
भक्ष्यते सोऽचिराद्देवि योगिनीभिर्न संशयः ।
य इदं परमं शास्त्रं ग्रन्थतश्चार्थतस्ततः ॥२२॥
गुरुवक्त्रात्तु लभ्येत स परां सिद्धिमाप्नुयात् ।
य इदं परमं गुह्यं खेचरीमेलकं ददेत् ॥२३॥

11a गमागम°] *em.*; गमागमौ μ ◇ समोपेत] *em.*; समोपेतौ AJ$_6$, समोयेतौ J$_7$ 11b °राख्यः] *em.*; °राख्य μ ◇ °प्रभः] *em.*; °प्रभा μ 11c गुह्यान्तं] गुह्यं तं A 12a तप्तजाम्बूनदाभासं] *em.*; सप्तजाम्बूनदाभ्यासं A, सप्तजाम्बूनदांभासं J$_6$J$_7$ 13a °संज्ञानम्] *corr.*; °विज्ञानम् μ 13d °रन्ध्रान्तगं] °रन्ध्रतिगं A 14b °रूपकम्] *em.*; °पूरकं μ 14d कण्ठम्] कठम् A 16a मध्य°] *em.*; मध्यं μ 17a ज्वालन्ती] ज्वालंति A, ज्वलंति J$_7$ 17b सेयम्] संयम् A 19b ध्यानं] धानं A 20d खेचरा°] खेभूचरा° A *(unm.)* ◇ °राधिपः] °राधिप J$_7$ 22a भक्ष्यते सोऽचिराद्देवि] भक्ष्याते सो च्चिरद्दिवि A 23b स परां सिद्धिम्] परो सिद्धिमवा° A

स एव हि गुरुर्देवि नान्यो)स्ति परमेश्वरि ।
इदं गुह्यतमं शास्त्रं पशूनां यः प्रदापयेत् ॥२४॥
अपरीक्षितवृत्तस्य स शीघ्रं नश्यति प्रिये ।
बहुधा क्लिश्यमानाय भक्तायानन्यचेतसे ॥२५॥
एकान्ते विजने स्थाने प्रवक्तव्यं विपश्चिता ।
व्याख्यानकाले कर्तव्यः पूजाविधिर्†शाढ्यतः† ॥२६॥
कुलामृतैश्च मांसैश्च कस्तूरीचन्दनादिभिः ।
रक्तवस्त्रे समाधाय विद्यापुस्तकमादरात् ॥२७॥
पूजयेत्पूर्वविधिना ततो व्याख्यानमाचरेत् ।
अथवा यद्यशक्तस्तु मानसेन कलामृतैः ॥२८॥
संतर्प्य पूज्य विजने व्याख्यानं गुप्तमाचरेत् ।
⊔⊔⊔⊔गतेनैव भावेनाराध्य पुस्तकम् ॥२९॥
शृणुयाद्विजने देशे तद्ज्ञैरयुक्तो)थवा प्रिये ।
पूर्वोक्तविधिना देवि स्वगुरूक्तप्रकारतः ॥३०॥
समभ्यस्य यथान्यायं द्वादशाब्दमतन्द्रितः ।
पर्यटेत्पृथिवीमेनां यत्र स्यान्मेलको गुरुः ॥३१॥
तं दृष्ट्वा सर्वभावेन समाराध्य प्रयत्नतः ।
आत्मनिःश्रेयसकरं तेनोक्तं सम्यगाचरेत् ॥३२॥
ज्ञानयुक्तं तु मातङ्गमपि कुर्याद्गुरुं प्रिये ।
ज्ञानविज्ञानहीनं तु षट्कर्मस्थमपि त्यजेत् ॥३३॥
यत्र यत्र विशिष्टार्थं तत्र तत्र समाश्रयेत् ।
यस्य हस्ते स्थितं दिव्यं विद्यापुस्तकमीश्वरि ॥३४॥
तस्य मूर्तिगतं देवि सकलं ज्ञानसागरम् ।
यदा यो ग्रन्थतश्चेदमर्थतश्च वदिष्यति ॥३५॥
अशेषेण जगद्धात्रि स एव परमो गुरुः ।
सर्वज्ञेन शिवेनोक्तमिदं जन्मार्बुदैरपि ॥३६॥

25d भक्तायानन्य°] भक्त्यांनन्य° A 26c कर्तव्यः] कर्त्तव्व्य A 26d †अशाढ्यतः†] AJ_7; आशाढ्यतः J_6 *(unm.)* 28b ततो] तता A 28c अथवा यद्य°] अथ वायव्य् A 28d कलामृतैः] कजामृतैः J_6 29c *omission indicated* μ 29d भावेना°] *em.*; भावना° μ 30b तद्ज्ञैर] *em.*; तत्ज्ञे A, तत्ज्ञैर् J_6J_7 31b °दशाब्दम्] दशाष्टम् A 31c पृथिवीम्] J_6; प्रथिवीम् AJ_7 32c °निःश्रेयस°] *em.*; °निश्रेयस° A, °निःश्रेय*स्व*° J_6, निःश्रेयक्य° J_7 34c हस्ते] हस्थो A 35b सकलं] A; सकुलं J_6J_7 35c यो] *द्यो* A 36d °जन्मार्बुदैर्] °जन्मार्बुदेर् A

दुर्लभं शास्त्रसारं तु दिव्यज्ञानप्रकाशकम् ।
द्वाव्‌मिौ पुरुषौ लोके सिद्धः साधक एव च ॥३७॥
अभ्यासेनैव सततं यः सर्वं परिवर्तते ।
अभीप्सुरात्मनः सिद्धिं स योगी साधकः स्मृतः ॥३८॥
सम्यगभ्यस्य विज्ञाय यः समं मेलनं चरेत् ।
सर्वसाधारणत्वेन विकल्पकुटिलोज्झितः ॥३९॥
कर्ता भर्ता च संहर्ता नित्यतृप्तो निरामयः ।
पश्यत्यात्माविभेदेन जगदेतच्चराचरम् ॥४०॥
स योगी सर्वविच्छ्रीमान् सिद्ध इत्युच्यते बुधैः ।
साधको बहुजन्मान्ते प्रयाति परमं पदम् ॥४१॥
देवैः सुदुर्लभां सिद्धिं सिद्धो याति न संशयः ।
तस्मादभ्यस्य यत्नेन खेचरीमेलनं चरेत् ॥४२॥
मेलनादप्यनभ्यासी सर्वं लभति पार्वति ।
तस्मादभ्यासहीनोऽपि मेलात्स्यादजरामरः ॥४३॥
यदा संमिलति गुरुः शिष्यं मेलनकर्मणि ।
संयोजयिष्यति शिवे तदैवं समुदाचरेत् ॥४४॥
एकान्ते विजने स्थाने पशुदृष्टेरगोचरे ।
पूजायोग्यानि वस्तूनि साधयेत्परमेश्वरि ॥४५॥
सुस्निग्धे च सुसंमृष्टे गोमयेनोपलेपिते ।
चारुवस्त्रवितानाढ्ये सर्वोपद्रववर्जिते ॥४६॥
वीरेण मदकर्पूरलघुसिन्दूररेणुभिः ।
वृत्तषट्कोण†वस्वार†वृत्तभूवलयोज्ज्वलम् ॥४७॥
कारयेन्मण्डलं देवि तत्रापि कलशं न्यसेत् ।
पूरयेद्दिव्यतोयेन रत्नगर्भं सवस्त्रकम् ॥४८॥
माल्यधूपसमायुक्तं दर्पणालंकृतं प्रिये ।
तत्र पञ्च महारत्नान् न्यसेद्विद्यां च पूर्ववत् ॥४९॥

37a °रं तु] °रत्नु A 38b यः सर्वं] *em.*; य सर्वःमुत्° μ *(unm.)* 38c अभीप्सुर] *em.*; अभीत्सुर् μ 39a अभ्यस्य विज्ञाय] *em.*; अभ्यास विज्ञात्य A, अभ्यस्य विज्ञात्य J_6, अभ्यस विज्ञात्य J_7 39d °कुटिलोज्झितः] °कुटिलोजितः A 41a °विच्छ्रीमान्] °विच्छीमान् A 43b सर्वं] *em.*; सर्वे μ 44a °मिलति] °मेलति μ 45b °दृष्टेर्] °दृष्टिर् A 46b गोमयेनोपलेपिते] गोमयेनोपःपलेंपिते A *(unm.)* 46c °नाढ्ये] °ना*र्द्ये* A 47a मद°] म° A *(unm.)* 47c °†वस्वार†°] J_6J_7; °वस्थार A 47d °वलयोज्ज्वलम्] °वल्लयोज्वंरंलम् A *(unm.)* 49b °लंकृतं] °लंच्चतं A

तदग्रे देवि साधारं पात्रं पूर्णं कलामृतैः ।
पूर्ववत्परिसंस्कृत्य पूर्वोक्तविधिनाचरेत् ॥५०॥
पूजावसाने देवेशि तत्प्रसादपवित्रितम् ।
स्नापयेत्कलशेनाङ्गं परामृतधिया गुरुः ॥५१॥
विना स्नानप्रसादाभ्यां कल्यानमयुतैरपि ।
न सिध्यति महेशानि खेचरीमेलकं प्रिये ॥५२॥
तस्मात्सर्वप्रयत्नेन तत्प्रसादं सहाभिधम् ।
सस्नानं दापयेद्विद्यां नान्यथा सिद्धिभाग् भवेत् ॥५३॥
स्नापयित्वा शिवं देवि योगस्थाने विशेषवित् ।
पञ्चाशद्वर्णमालां च स्थले वा दर्पणे ऽथवा ॥५४॥
पदे वा चन्दने दिव्ये तल्लिखेन्न तु भूतले ।
शिष्यहस्तेन देवेशि तत्र पुष्पं प्रमोचयेत् ॥५५॥
यस्मिन् वर्णे निपतितं पुष्पं तद्वरणपूर्वकम् ।
नाम चानन्दनाथान्तं दापयेद् गुरुरीश्वरि ॥५६॥
शक्तिनाम च संप्रेक्ष्य पराम्बान्तं प्रदापयेत् ।
पूर्वं प्रसादं संदग्धमहापातकसंचयः ॥५७॥
पुनश्च कलशासेकात्परामृततनुर्भवेत् ।
भूयश्च नामग्रहणात्शिवसाम्यः प्रजायते ॥५८॥
एवं कृते शिवे शिष्यो योग्यो मेलनकर्मणि ।
अन्यथा परमेशानि तदेवानर्थकृद्भवेत् ॥५९॥
इति सिद्धतनुः सिद्धो यद्यद्भावमुपासते ।
तत्तत्फलं च प्रत्यक्षं भविष्यति न संशयः ॥६०॥
इति श्रीमत्स्येन्द्रसंहितायां सप्तदशः पटलः

50a साधारं] J_6; साधारे A, साधारें J_7 50b पूरणं] पूरण° J_7 52b कल्यानं] A; कल्यानां J_6J_7 53b तत्प्रसादं] J_6; त्प्रसाद⊔ A, तत् प्रसाद J_7 55a पदे वा] यदेवा A ◇ दिव्ये] देवि A 56b पुष्पं] *em.*; पुष्प μ 56c °नाथान्तं] °नाथांतां J_6 57a शक्तिनाम च] *corr.*; शक्तिमाम चं A, शक्तिमाम च J_6J_7 57b पराम्बान्तं] *em.*; परां वा तं AJ_7, यरांवांतं J_6 59a कृते] ॠते A 59a शिष्यो] *em.*; शिष्ये μ 59d तद्] नद् A 60a °तनुः] °तनुं A 60c फलं] पलं A

अष्टादशः पटलः

श्रीभैरव उवाच
इति †सर्वज्ञपाशाद्† यस्तीर्णः संसारसागरात् ।
भुञ्जीत स्वेच्छया भोगान् स्वेच्छया योगमभ्यसेत् ॥१॥
उपादेयः प्रियो यस्मात्कौलिके प्रियमेलकः ।
अतः कुर्यादनुष्ठानं शाक्तमाणवमेव वा ॥२॥
अत्यन्तविजने स्थाने सर्वोपद्रववर्जिते ।
नितान्तं मनसो रम्ये हृद्यधूपसुगन्धिनि ॥३॥
विकीर्णपुष्पप्रकरसिन्दूरादिसुरञ्जिते ।
गुरुमण्डलकं कृत्वा भक्तिमान्योगमभ्यसेत् ॥४॥
स्थिरमासनमासीनः सकलीकृतविग्रहः ।
जितश्वासो जितमना जितकर्मा जितेन्द्रियः ॥५॥
नियोज्यं घण्टिकारन्ध्रे ␣␣␣␣␣␣␣␣ ।
अधस्ताच्चिन्तयेच्चक्रमाक्रान्ताधारमण्डलम् ॥६॥
तत्र मध्ये समोद्दीप्तां मूलशक्तिं विभावयेत् ।
प्राणान्निरुध्योर्ध्वमुखीं नयेद्भित्त्वा षडम्बुजान् ॥७॥
एकीभूता हि नादाख्या चक्रभेदक्रमेण च ।
तडिद्वलयसंकाशां स्फुरत्किरणरूपिणीम् ॥८॥
चिह्वया च निरालम्बे शून्यतेजोमये परे ।
ब्रह्मद्वारस्य गर्भे तु विसर्गाख्ये विलीयते ॥९॥
ततो रसनयोद्भेद्य प्रविशेद्ब्रह्मणः पदम् ।
तस्मिन् कुलामृतं दिव्यं पीत्वा भूयो विशेत्कुलम् ॥१०॥
तेन प्रासितमात्रेण परां सिद्धिमवाप्नुयात् ।
योगमूले स्वके स्थाने भूयस्तस्मात्समुत्थिता ॥११॥
पृथिव्याधारसंकोचादेकोच्चारक्रमेण तु ।
एतद्वागीस्वरीबीजं रहस्यं संप्रकाशितम् ॥१२॥

μ=AJ_6J_7 ◇ A f. 51v[11] – f. 54v[6] ◇ J_6 f. 35v[4] – f. 37v[3] ◇ J_7 f. 74r[10] – f. 78v[5]

2a उपादेयः प्रियो] उपदियः प्रयो A 2d शाक्तमाणवम्] J_6; शामाराण␣␣वेम् A *(unm.)*, शामाराणवम् J_7 *(unm.)* 3c नितान्तं] नितान्त॰ A 3d ॰सुगन्धिनि] ॰संुधिपिते A 4a ॰प्रकर॰] A; ॰प्रकरे J_6J_7 6b *omission indicated* μ 6d आक्रान्ताधार॰] आक्रान्तधार॰ A 7c ॰मुखीं] ॰सु␣खिं A 8a नादाख्या] नादाच्च्या A 11d समुत्थिता] समुत्थित A

व्याख्याता खेचरीमुद्रा तस्या बन्धोऽयमेव हि ।
एतस्या बन्धमात्रेण भाग्यहीनोऽपि सिध्यति ॥१३॥
मेलकं खेचरीणां च दिव्यवेषोऽभिजायते ।
अमुना संप्रदायेन यत्र यत्र विलीयते ॥१४॥
तत्र तत्र परानन्दरूपमेव प्रकाशते ।
सर्वशास्त्रार्थवेत्ता च सौभाग्यं परमं तथा ॥१५॥
काव्यं च सर्वभाषाभिः सालंकारपदोज्वलम् ।
करोति लीलया योगी रुद्रशक्तिप्रभावतः ॥१६॥
अनेनैव प्रयोगेन सर्वमात्राः स्फुरन्ति हि ।
आणवाः शाम्भवाः शाक्ता ये †केत्यु†च्चरति प्रिये ॥१७॥
मणिपूरे लयाद्वश्यं शान्तिश्रीपुष्टितुष्टयः ।
आकर्षणं पुरक्षोभो भवन्त्येव हि सिद्धयः ॥१८॥
अनाहते तु संलीनो योगी ग्रन्थिविभेदनात् ।
गिरीणां पातनं देवि कुर्यान्मृत्योश्च वञ्चनम् ॥१९॥
विशुद्धेऽप्यमृताधारे योगस्तु स्यादसंशयः ।
क्षुत्तृषादाहनिर्मुक्तो जरारोगविवर्जितः ॥२०॥
आज्ञास्थानगतो योगी त्रैलोक्यमपि पश्यति ।
त्रिकालज्ञः स्वयं कर्त्ता स एव परमेश्वरः ॥२१॥
अतीतं वेत्ति नाभिस्थो वर्त्तमानं हृदि स्थितः ।
आज्ञास्थानगतो योगी सर्वं जानाति सर्वदा ॥२२॥
अधुना चोन्मनीभावः परतत्त्वोपलब्धये ।
पारम्पर्यक्रमायातो ब्रह्माण्डोदरमध्यगः ॥२३॥
यल्लिङ्गाधारमध्यस्थं मध्ये शक्त्यङ्कुरान्वितम् ।
यवमात्रप्रमाणं तु त्रिकोणाकृतिमुत्तमम् ॥२४॥
निष्कलं यत्परं तेजः परस्य परसंस्थितम् ।
जवमणीन्द्रियं यद्वद्विस्फुरश्चैव दृश्यते ॥२५॥
तथाकृतिर्भवेत्तस्य मीलनोन्मीलनानि च ।
प्रथमं भेदयेच्चक्रं नाभिजं नाडिभिर्युतम् ॥२६॥

15a परानन्द°] A; परानन्दा° J_6J_7 16b °ज्वलं] *em.*; °ज्वलां μ 19d मृत्योश्] मृत्युश् A ◇ वञ्चनम्] *em.*; वंचनां μ 20a ऽप्य°] *em.*; त्य° μ 22b स्थितः] *em.*; स्थितं μ 23a चोन्मनी°] वोन्मनी° A   24c यव°] यत्र A   25b परस्य परसंस्थितम्] परस्परसंस्थित A *(unm.)*   25c जव°] जवा° J_7 25d विस्फुरश्] *em.*; विस्फुराश् AJ_7, वि*ुराश् J_6

तदूर्ध्वे हृदयावस्थं चक्रं वै कुलसंज्ञकम् ।
हृच्चक्रं भेदयेत्पश्चात्कण्ठचक्रं ततः शनैः ॥२७॥
तदूर्ध्वे लम्बिकां भेद्य नासाग्रं तु ततो नयेत् ।
नासाग्रात् श्वाससंभिन्नं भ्रूमध्ये संनिवेशयेत् ॥२८॥
श्वासेन सहितं बीजं तेजोरूपं ललाटके ।
गत्वा लक्षं ललाटस्थं प्रविशेत्सूर्यसंनिभम् ॥२९॥
कुञ्चिकाढ्यं ततः सूक्ष्मा ⊔⊔⊔णु च सूक्ष्मकम् ।
उद्घाटयेत्ततो द्वारं शिवद्वारार्गलं महत् ॥३०॥
बिन्दुद्वारार्गलं भित्त्वा दुर्भेद्यं त्रिदशैरपि ।
ब्रह्माण्डोदरमित्युक्तं योगिनीसिद्धसेवितम् ॥३१॥
तदेतदङ्गुलोत्सेधं कपाले संव्यवस्थितम् ।
प्रवेशात्स्पर्शनं तत्र बालानामिव जायते ॥३२॥
शक्तितत्त्वावबोधो हि विज्ञानं सिद्धसाधनम् ।
परतत्त्वावबोधश्च ज्ञानं मोहप्रसाधनम् ॥३३॥
भुक्तिमुक्त्योर्द्वयोर्हेतुः परमानन्दतां गतः ।
जीवन्मुक्तिमवाप्नोति वत्सरार्धान्न संशयः ॥३४॥
प्राप्तद्वादशकेनैव शिवसाम्यबलः प्रिये।
सर्वार्थकृत्यं सूक्ष्मत्वं सर्वज्ञत्वं विशुद्धता ॥३५॥
नित्यानन्दस्वभावत्वं सर्वव्यापित्वमेव च ।
अणिमा लघिमा प्राप्तिः प्राकाम्यं गरिमा तथा ॥३६॥
ईशित्वं च वशित्वं च यच्च कामावसायिता ।
स्यान्महासिद्धयस्त्वेता अष्टौ विज्ञानयोनयः ॥३७॥
योगिनः संप्रवर्तन्ते वत्सरात्परमेश्वरि ।
अथापरं प्रवक्ष्यामि साधनं परमं प्रिये ॥३८॥
विधिनानुत्थितं पूर्वं मया च वरवर्णिनि ।
अन्येषां देवदेवानां ब्रह्मादीनां च दुर्लभम् ॥३९॥
बिन्दुजीवजलाक्रान्तं वर्तुलं चन्द्रमण्डलम् ।
बिन्दुप्राणानिलाक्रान्तं त्रिकोणं वह्निमण्डलम् ॥४०॥

27d कण्ठचक्रं] *em.*; कण्ठं वक्त्रं μ 28c नासाग्रात्] *em.*; नासाग्रे μ 30b *omission indicated* μ
32b कपाले] J_6; कलाये A, कयाले J_7 33a ∘बोधो] ∘बोधे J_6^{ac} 35c ∘कृत्यं] A; ∘कृत्वं J_6J_7
36b ∘व्यापित्वम्] *em.*; ∘व्याप्तित्वे A, ∘व्याप्तित्वं J_6J_7 38c अथापरं] अथातः सं∘ A

आपूर्य वामया नाड्या मुञ्चेद्दक्षिणया बहिः ।
पुनर्दक्षिणयापूर्य बहुशो वामया त्यजेत् ॥४१॥
एवं विशुद्धनाडीकः कुम्भकानां शतं शतम् ।
कुर्याद्बहिश्च हंसेन सहजेनान्तरस्थितम् ॥४२॥
स पश्यति जगत्कीर्णं तेजसः परमाणुभिः ।
दृष्टेति प्रत्ययं कुर्यात्प्रत्येकमयुतं यदा ॥४३॥
तदा पश्यति नासाग्रे हृदयेन्दूज्ज्वलमहः ।
तयोः संचिन्तयेदैक्यं तत्रात्मानं स पश्यति ॥४४॥
अतिमग्नं मनः कुर्यात्तस्मिन् पुर्यष्टकात्मके ।
ततः स प्रियसाङ्गत्यादुद्रतामाप्य दीप्यति ॥४५॥
शक्तिबन्धप्रयोगेण सप्तरात्रं निरोधकः ।
कोदण्डद्वयमध्यस्थं बिन्दुनादेन भेदयेत् ॥४६॥
एवमभ्यसतस्तस्य प्रत्ययः संप्रजायते ।
याममात्रादधृुवं त्यक्त्वा गगने भवति स्थितः ॥४७॥
द्वादशान्ते दिनार्धेन दृष्ट्वा साक्षान्महेश्वरम् ।
संप्राप्य प्रियसाङ्गत्यं शिवसायुज्यमाप्नुयात् ॥४८॥
सुखमासनमासीनः सकलीकृतविग्रहः ।
किंचिदभ्युन्नतोरस्को मयूराञ्चितमस्तकः ॥४९॥
विस्रस्तांसः स्थिरो भूत्वा रसनां घण्टिकाबिले ।
संयोज्य परमेशानि ध्यानं कुर्याज्जितेन्द्रियः ॥५०॥
अत्यन्तनिपुणं कुर्यात्सुषुम्णान्तर्गतं मनः ।
शक्तिक्षोभात्ततस्तस्य परोऽभिव्यज्यते ध्वनिः ॥५१॥
तदेव सहजं बीजं तत्र संयोजयेन्मनः ।
क्षणात्क्षोणीं परित्यज्य गगने भवति स्थिरः ॥५२॥
मुहूर्ताद्वीक्षते सर्वं तेजोमयमिदं जगत् ।
याममात्रं तदा तेजस्तदेव परिपश्यति ॥५३॥

42a °कः] °क° A 42c बहिश्च] *em.*; बहिछ μ 43d प्रत्येकमयुतं] *em.*; प्रत्येकंमयुतं μ 44b °येन्दूज्ज्वलमहः] *em.*; °यैंदोज्वलंमहः A, °येदोज्वलंमहः J_6J_7 45d आप्य दीप्यति] J_6; अप्यदीप्यति A, आय्पदीप्यति J_7 47c °मात्राद] °मात्रा μ 47d गगने भवति स्थितः] J_6; गमने भव⌴स्थित A, गमने भवस्थितः J_7 48b दृष्ट्वा] *em.*; दृष्टा μ 49a सुखमासनमासीनः] J_6; सुखासासनमासिन A, सुखमासनमासीन J_7 51c °क्षोभात्ततस्] J_6; °क्षोभां ततस् A, °क्षोभा ततस् J_7 52a सहजं] सहसं A 52c क्षोणीं] J_6; क्षोणी AJ_7

तदा तस्य निवर्तन्ते निखिलाश्चित्तवृत्तयः ।
†यामलं† यमसंकल्पो यदा स्थाणुवदास्थितः ॥५४॥
यदा ब्रह्माण्डभाण्डस्थं सर्वं प्रत्यक्षमीक्षते ।
अहोरात्रेण सर्वाणि साक्षात्तत्त्वानि पश्यति ॥५५॥
तद्रूपश्चेत् †परिषतस्† तदासौ जायते शिवः ।
नियोज्य घण्टिकारन्ध्रे रसनां निश्चलात्मिकाम् ॥५६॥
भ्रूमध्ये चक्षुषी न्यस्य स्थिरं कृत्वा मनो हृदि ।
क्षीरोदार्णवनिर्मग्नं पद्मद्वयपुटीकृतम् ॥५७॥
पिबन्तं ब्रह्मरन्ध्रेण क्षीरधारामृतं हिमम् ।
रोमकूपैर्विनिर्गत्य कोटिशः क्षीरबिन्दुभिः ॥५८॥
अभेद्यपाण्डुरान्तस्थमिवात्मानं विचिन्तयेत् ।
अजरामरतामेति मासमात्रं न संशयः ॥५९॥
मासावधि महेशानि योगमेकं शिवोदितम् ।
दिने दिने द्वियामान्तं यामान्तं वा समुच्चरेत् ॥६०॥
एकेनैव तु योगेन भुवनान्तमनुव्रजेत् ।
द्वितीयेन तु योगेन सप्तद्वीपावधिं व्रजेत् ॥६१॥
तृतीयेन तु योगेन शिवलोके महीयते ।
अतीत्य सकलान्लोकान्पृथग्भोगान्प्रभुज्य च ॥६१॥
शरीराय महायोगी चन्द्रद्वीपे सुखं वसेत् ।
श्रीदेव्युवाच
अक्षयं नाथ कं लोकं वद देव महेश्वर ॥६३॥
[श्रीभैरव उवाच]
सर्वं पूर्वं मयाख्यातं किं न बुध्यसि पार्वति ।
त्रैलोक्यं क्षयते सर्वं सहस्रयुगपर्यये ॥६४॥
कल्पाख्यं ब्रह्मणः स्थानं वैकुण्ठं चैव वैष्णवम् ।
कैलाशं रुद्रसंस्थानं क्षीयते च महाक्षये ॥६५॥
अक्षयं चन्द्रद्वीपं तु यत्र देवी कुलाम्बिका ।
तिष्ठते च मया सार्धं सत्यं सत्यं महातपे ॥६६॥

55b ◦मीक्षते] ◦मीक्षसे A 56a †परिषतस†] AJ_7; परिखतस् J_6 59a अभेद्य] J_6; अमेघ◦ A, अमेद्य◦ J_7 ◇ ◦स्थम्] *em.*; ◦स्थाम् μ 61d ◦वधिं] ◦वलिं A 62d प्रभुज्य] यः भुज्य A 63d महेश्वर] *em.*; महेश्वरं μ 64a ◇ सर्वं] *corr.*; शिव μ 64c क्षयते] A; क्षायते J_6J_7 65a ब्रह्मणः] J_6; ब्रह्मण AJ_7 66b कुलाम्बिका] A; कुजांविका J_6J_7

योगिन्यस्तत्र या देवि सिद्धाश्च वरवर्णिनि ।
इच्छारूपधराः सर्वे सर्वे चामोघशक्तयः ॥६७॥
स्वतन्त्राश्च स्वरूपाश्च सर्वे कुब्जेश्वरप्रभाः ।
किमत्र बहुनोक्तेन जल्पितेन पुनः पुनः ॥६८॥
क्षयपातविहीनं तु चन्द्रद्वीपं वरानने ।
तत्क्षये यौवनानन्दः क्रीडते स्वेच्छया प्रिये ॥६९॥
कल्पकोटिशतैस्तस्य क्षयो नैव प्रजायते ।
न च सांसारिका व्याप्तिस्तस्य भूयः प्रवर्तते ॥७०॥
पशुमार्गस्थितो नित्यं योनियोन्यन्तरं व्रजेत् ।
तस्मात्सर्वप्रयत्नेन गुरुं तोष्य महेश्वरि ॥७१॥
प्रबोद्धव्यमिदं शास्त्रं संसारं तर्तुमिच्छता ।
येन सिद्धिमवाप्नोति सत्यं सत्यं न संशयः ॥७२॥

इति श्रीमत्स्येन्द्रसंहितायामष्टादशः पटलः

69a क्षयपात°] *em.*; क्षपयात° μ **70c** व्याप्तिस्] *em.*; व्याप्ति° μ **70d** तस्य] *em.*; °त्वस्य AJ_6, स्वस्य J_7 **72b** तर्तुम्] *em.*; वर्तुम् AJ_6, वर्त्तुम् J_7

सप्तविंशः पटलः

ईश्वर उवाच
क्षेत्रज्ञानविहीनस्तु बाह्यचक्रमनाः क्षमः ।
सर्वतीर्थाधिकं स्नानं योगी देवि समाचरेत् ॥१॥
लोकेशः केशवो रुद्रः ईशश्चैव सदेश्वरः ।
निगद्यन्ते च विड्मूत्ररजोरेचकसारकाः ॥२॥
दृढलावण्यशौक्ल्यघ्नदेहस्थैर्यगद†क्षमः† ।
क्रमादमी प्रणश्यन्ति क्रियते विधिना यदि ॥३॥
दिव्यानुजः सुरश्रेष्ठः सूतो यज्ञो हरिः स्वयम् ।
अतिदुष्टः स्वयं रुद्रो लेभे ईशः सुरद्रवम् ॥४॥
सदाशिवो वरो ज्ञेयस्तेषां क्रममिमं शृणु ।
विजने जन्तुरहिते सुपात्रे चामरीरसम् ॥५॥
तत्र मेहनजं सारं कृत्वा चैवादिपुष्पकम् ।
पिङ्गलीवालुकं वारि सम्यगोंकारसंभवम् ॥६॥
तथा मथनजं दिव्यं ब्रह्मरन्ध्रविनिर्गतम् ।
एकीकृत्य धरातोयैः संस्कृत्य च यथाविधि ॥७॥
कर्पूरकुंकुमादीनि तस्मिन्विन्यस्य मेलयेत् ।
तेन प्रमर्दयेद्देहमापादतलमस्तकम् ॥८॥
नासजं †नास्त्यकं† कुर्यादजरामरफलाप्तये ।
मासेन देवदेवेशि नित्यमन्तः प्रदर्शयेत् ॥९॥
वलीपलितनाशश्च दृढलावण्यमेव च ।
भविष्यति महेशानि नाडीशुद्धिर्गदक्षयः ॥१०॥
अनेन विधिना देवि निर्विकल्पेन चेतसा ।
यश्चरेत्तस्य संसिद्धिर्जायते ह्यजरामरः ॥११॥

μ=AJ_6J_7 ◇ A f. 68v[7] – f. 69v[10] ◇ J_6 f. 47v[8] – f. 48v[1] ◇ J_7 f. 100r[7] – f. 102r[1]

1b बाह्य°] वाघ्र° A ◇ °मनाः] *conj.*; °मना μ 1c सर्व°] सर्वं A 1d योगी देवि समाचरेत्] *em.*; योग देंवी समं चरेत् A, योगं देवी समं चरेत् J_6J_7 2b ईशश्चैव] *em.*; ईशः सैव μ 2c निगद्यन्ते] निमद्यंते A 3a °शौक्ल्य°] °शौक्ल° A 4b सूतो] सूनो A 4c अतिदुष्टः] अनिद्रुष्टः A 4c रुद्रो] *em.*; रुद्रे μ 4d ईशः सुरद्रवम्] *em.*; द्रशः सुरद्रवः A, ईशः सुरुद्रवः J_6J_7 5c जन्तु°] नंतु° A 6c पिङ्गलीवालुकं] पिगजीवालुजं J_6J_7 6c वारि] सारि A 7a मथनजं] मथनलं A 8b तस्मिन्] *em.*; तस्य μ 8c °मर्दयेद] *em.*; °मर्दये μ 9d नित्यम्] J_6; नित्यंम् AJ_7 ◇ प्रदर्शयेत्] A; प्रदर्शनात् J_6J_7

क्षेत्रतीर्थमये देहे यत्तीर्थं शिवनिर्गतम् ।
सर्वपापक्षयकरं वलीपलितनाशनम् ॥१२॥
करोति नात्र संदेहस्त्रिकालाभ्यङ्गयोगतः ।
षण्मासाल्लभते सत्यमजरामरतां प्रिये ॥१३॥
त्रिकालोद्वर्तनाद्वर्षाद्वलीपलितहा भवेत् ।
एककालप्रयोगेन त्रिवर्षादजरामरः ॥१४॥
विकल्पो नात्र कर्तव्यस्तर्हि सिद्धिर्न जायते ।
अविकल्पप्रवृत्तस्य योगिनः सिद्धिरुत्तमा ॥१५॥
सर्वपापक्षयश्चैव सौकुमार्यं प्रजायते ।
दिव्यं शिवमयं तीर्थं तीर्थकोटिफलप्रदम् ॥१६॥
रात्रौ पात्रान्तरे सर्वं कुर्याद्योगी समाहिताम् ।
चन्दनं कुङ्कुमं कुष्ठं हारिद्रं गोमयं तिलम् ॥१७॥
कर्पूरमगुरुं चन्द्रं गुग्गुलं कङ्गुकाघृतम् ।
गन्धकं च समालोड्य प्रातर्देहं प्रमर्दयेत् ॥१८॥
अनेन विधिना मासात्सूर्यकल्पो भवेन्नरः ।
वलीपलितनिर्मुक्तो जायते ह्यजरामरः ॥१९॥
रात्रौ कृत्वा महेशानि पात्रे सर्वामरीसुधाम् ।
तालकं कनकं गन्धं रुद्राक्षं च मनःशिलाम् ॥२०॥
पिष्ट्वा संलोड्य स्वदेहं मर्दयेत्प्रातरुत्थितः ।
मासाद्भवति देवेशि सत्यं पावकसंनिभः ॥२१॥
वलीपलितनिर्मुक्तः सिद्धिः स्यादजरामरा ।
दिवा संक्षिप्य पात्रान्तः सायं मर्दनमाचरेत् ॥२२॥
घृष्ट्वा गुग्गुलुना धूपं वस्त्रावृततनौ ददेत् ।
संदग्धगोमयं भस्म मेलयित्वामरीरसे ॥२३॥
संमिश्रोन्मत्तकरसं तेन देहं प्रमर्दयेत् ।
मर्दनादेव षण्मासाज्जायते ह्यजरामरः ॥२४॥

12a चेत्रतीर्थमये] *em.*; चेत्रं तीर्थमया AJ_7, चेत्रं तीर्थं मया J_6 14a त्रि°] द्वि° J_6 17c कुष्ठं] *em.*; कुष्टं μ 17d हारिद्रं] दारिद्रं A 18a कर्पूरमगुरुं चन्द्रं] J_6; कर्पूरुगुरुं चंद्रं च A *(unm.)*, कर्पूरगरुं चंद्रं J_7 *(unm.)* 18c गन्धकं] ⌈रो⌉धकं A 20c तालकं कनकं] J_6; तलकं कंनकं A, तलकं कनकं J_7 21a स्व°] *em.*; सं° μ 21d °निभः] °निभं A 22b °मरा] J_6; °मराः AJ_7 23a घृष्ट्वा गुग्गुलुना] J_7; घृष्टा गुग्गुलना A, घृष्ट्या गुग्गुलुना J_6 23b °तनौ ददेत्] °ननौ दवेत् A 23c °दग्ध°] *em.*; °दग्धा° A, °दग्ध्वा J_6J_7

सर्वतो विषनाशश्च भविष्यति न संशयः ।
यो नित्यं मर्दयेदेनं द्वादशान्तमखण्डितम् ॥२५॥
सर्वपापविनिर्मुक्तः सर्वव्याधिविवर्जितः ।
अजरश्चामरो भूत्वा जीवेदाचन्द्रतारकम् ॥२६॥
अविकल्पमतिर्देवि यः सदा मर्दयेत्तनुम् ।
तस्य न व्याधिजा भीतिर्न जरामृत्युतो ऽपि च ॥२७॥
अनेन देवि स्नानेन सर्वतीर्थफलोदयः ।
भवति नात्र संदेहः सत्यं सत्यं मयोदितम् ॥२८॥
पशुपाशप्रबद्धाश्च शिवज्ञानपराङ्मुखाः ।
दिव्यामरीसुधास्नानं न विन्दन्ति बहिर्मुखाः ॥२९॥
अप्रकाश्यतमं चेदं रहस्यं ते प्रकाशितम् ।
शिवेनोदाहृतं देवि नापरीक्ष्य प्रदापयेत् ॥३०॥

इति श्रीमत्स्येन्द्रसंहितायां सप्तविंशः पटलः

27c °भीतिर] °भितिर् A 28c भवति] *em.*; लभति AJ_6, लभते J_7 29b °मुखाः] J_6; °मुख्य A, °मुखा J_7 29d °मुखाः] मुखा A 30b ते प्रकाशितम्] तं प्रकाशिते A

---

26 *om.* A

Appendix C: works cited in the *Bṛhatkhecarīprakāśa*

In the following list the names of cited works are followed by the location (if I have found it) of the citation(s) in the published edition (if one is available) of the work and then the location of the beginning of the citation in the manuscript. In general, I have sought to identify only those citations that are from haṭhayogic works. I have not listed unattributed citations that I have been unable to identify. The sign "≃" indicates that the citation is found in a slightly different form in the edition that I have consulted. Where I am uncertain of the identity of the text being referred to, its name or its author's name is given in single inverted commas.

'Aṃjane': f: 42(3)v^{mg}

Atharvaśira[upaniṣad]: f. 86(1)v^{5}

Amarakośa: f. 29r^{10}, f: 70v^{mg}, f. 110v^{2}

Amṛtabindūpaniṣad: f. 90r^{9}

Aṣṭādhyāyī: 1.4.82 at f. 59v^{9} (*"iti sūtrāt"*)

Uttaragītā: f. 59r^{mg}

Kapilatantra:[486] f. 14r^{9}

Kālāgnirudropaniṣad: f. 86(1)v^{8}

'Kālidāsa': f. 42(1)r^{8}, f. 110r^{9}

Kulaprakāśatantra: f. 42(1)v^{5}, f. 88v^{mg}

Kulārṇavādau: f. 45v^{10}

Kaurmagītā: f. 89v^{3}

Kaurme Śivagītā: f. 66v^{4}, f. 85r^{5}, f. 85r^{10}, f. 89v^{mg}, f. 101r^{8}

Gāruḍa[purāṇa]: f. 63v^{7}, f. 67r^{9}, f. 67v^{5}, f. 68v^{5}

Gītāsāra: "ekonaviṃśādhyāye" f. 16v^{6}

'Gorakṣa': f. 25r^{mg},[487] f. 42(3)v^{4}, f. 45r^{mg}[488]

Gorakṣaśataka$_{N}$: 67 at f. 11v^{8}; 64 at f. 12r^{1}, 133–134 at f. 26r^{5} (attributed to *Haṭhapradīpikā*), 43 at f. 99r^{7}, 25–28 at f. 99v^{7}, 142 at f. 100r^{mg}, 24cd at f. 100r^{3}, 72c–76d at f. 103v^{mg}, 11 at f. 108v^{1} (=*HP* 1.35), 12 at f. 108v^{5} (=*HP* 1.44)

Carakasaṃhitā: f. 78v^{8}

Jābala[upaniṣad]: f. 86(2)r^{9}

Jaiminyaśvamedhagālava: f. 74r^{4}, f. 74r^{10}, f. 74v^{7}, f. 75r^{mg}, f. 75v^{1}

Tattvakaumudī: f. 57r^{mg}

Tattvapradīpikā: f. 69v^{mg}, f. 107v^{mg}

Tantrarāja: f. 27v^{2}, f. 42(1)v^{2}, f. 42(1)v^{9}, f. 42(2)r^{5} (=citation at f. 42(1)v^{2}), f. 42(2)r^{6} (=citation at f. 42(1)v^{9}), f. 64r^{2}, f. 73v^{3}, f. 74r^{1}, f. 78r^{1}, f. 78r^{9}, f. 78v^{5}, f. 82v^{2}, f. 90v^{8}, f. 105r^{mg}, f. 106v^{mg}

[*Taittirīya*] *śruti:* f. 42(1)r^{8}

Dakṣiṇamūrtisaṃhitā: f. 105r^{6}

Dattātreyayogaśāstra: see *Sāṃkṛtidattātreyasaṃvādaprakaraṇa*

'Devalaḥ': f. 91v^{7}

Dhātupāṭha: f. 102v^{8}

Nandipurāṇa: f. 92r^{5}

Nārāyaṇīyayogasūtravṛtti: f. 57v^{2}, f. 90v^{2}

Nārāyaṇīyavṛtti: f. 93r^{2}

Nārāyaṇīyasūtravṛtti (ad Kṣurikopaniṣad): f. 90r^{11}

Niruktaśeṣa: f. 11r^{6}.

Padmapurāṇa: f. 84v^{3}

Pādmagītā: f. 90r^{mg}

Pādmaśivagītā: f. 76r^{mg}

Pādme Kapilagītā: f. 25r^{7}, f. 68r^{1}, f. 89r^{10}

Pārthiveśvaracintāmaṇi: f. 84v^{4}

Pauṣkaraprādurbhāva: 17th *adhyāya* (of *Gāruḍapurāṇa*?) with Nīlakaṇṭha's *vyākhyā*, the *Yogacintāmaṇi*: f. 67v^{1}, f. 83r^{mg}

Prabodhacandrodaya: f. 110r^{9}

Brahmayāmala: f. 42(1)v^{1}, f. 42(2)r^{1} (=previous citation)

Bhāgavata: f. 55r^{3}, *"ekādaśe skandhe"* f. 16v^{2}, f. 95v^{8}, *"paṃcame"* f. 69v^{6}, *"śrīdhara-vākyāyām"* f. 78r^{7}, *"dvitīyaskande"* f. 82v^{6}

Bhagavadgītā: 8.13ab at f. 17v^{1}, f. 65v^{11}, f. 66r^{mg}, 6.13 at f. 98v^{10}, 6.44a at f. 101r^{12}, f. 104r^{2}, 6.17 at f. 107v^{1}, 6.11d at f. 107v^{10}

Bhojavṛtti: f. 90r^{7}

'Mahākapilapañcarātre': f. 42(1)v^{8}, f. 42(2)v^{4}

Mahāhārakatantra: f. 88v^{mg}

Mahābhārata: "puṣkaraprādurbhāve saptadaśādhyāye" f. 24v$^{8-10}$, *"bhārate yājñaval-kyaḥ":* f. 73r^{mg}, f. 74r^{3}, f. 75r^{2}, f. 75v^{3}, *"bhārate":* f. 75r^{8}, *"bhārate kaśyapastutau":* f. 85v^{7}, *"mokṣadharme bhārate":* f. 92v^{11}, *"śāntau bhīṣmena":* f. 93r^{9}, *"bhārate pau-ṣkare saptadaśādhyāye nīlakaṃṭhena"* f. 97r^{6}

Mahābhāṣya: f. 57r^{5}

Mantramahodadhi: f. 105^{mg}

Mālatīmādhava: 5.1a at f. 68r^{mg}

'Yājñavalkya': f. 43r^{9}, f. 66v^{mg}, f. 76r^{3}, f. 77v^{2}, f. 80v^{1}, f. 82r^{6}, f. 86(2)r^{3}, f. 97r^{5}, f. 98v^{6}, f. 108v^{6}

Yājñavalkyagītā: f. 85v^{7}, f. 97r^{10}

Yājñavalkyasaṃhitā: f. 92r^{1}, f. 96r^{3}, f. 96r^{11}

Rudrahṛdaya: f. 85v^{10}

Yogacintāmaṇi: f. 25r^{2}

Yogataraṅginī: f. 73v^{6}

Yogatārāvalī: f. 89r^{4}

Yogapradīpikā:[489] f. 37r^{7}

Yogabīja: 183ab at f. 8v^{6}; 91–98 at f. 19v^{4}, 141cd at f. 26v^{7}, 131 at f. 37r^{2}, 125–127 at f. 37r^{5}, ≃73 at f. 45r^{mg}, f. 45r^{11}, ≃179, 182a–183b, 173c–176b and ≃177cd at f. 64r^{3}, 146–147 at f. 88r^{5}, 148–149 at f. 88v^{2}, 150–152b at f. 88v^{6}, 135c–136b at f. 90r^{4}, 102 at f. 91r^{2}, 104 at f. 91r^{4}, 106cd at f. 91r^{7}, 108a–110b at f. 91v^{11}, 15c–17d at f. 93r^{8}, 153 and 157–159 at f. 101r^{10}, ≃159a–160b at f. 101v^{1}, 113cd at f. 102v^{4}, 116–117 at f. 102v^{5} (=*DYŚ* 286–289), 120cd at f. 102v^{9}, 121c–122b at f. 103r^{2}, 123c–124b at f. 103r^{4}, 94a at f. 104r^{11}

Yogaratnakārikā:[490] f. 89v^{9}

Yogavāsiṣṭha: f. 64r^{9}

Yogasāra: f. 12r^{2}

Yogasiddhāntacandrikā: f. 93r^{2}

Yogasūtra with Vyāsa's *Bhāṣya:*[491] 3.50 at f. 12r^{7}–f. 12v^{3}; f. 15r^{4}; f. 16r^{8}; f. 16v^{4}; f. 16v^{8}; 3.29 at fol.21r^{mg}, 3.25 at f. 41v^{4}, 4.1 at f. 64r^{mg}, f. 64r^{10}, 3.21 at f. 73r^{11}, f. 76v^{mg}, 3.37 at f. 77v^{9}, 3.38 at f. 78r^{4}, f. 81r^{4}, f. 82v^{7}, 2.1–2 at f. 85v$^{4-6}$, 1.2 at f. 87v^{4}, 89a–90b at f. 87v^{4}, 2.29 at f. 89v^{5}, 3.28 at f. 96v^{11}, 1.33 at f. 109v^{2}

'Ratnāvalī': f. 86(1)v^{7}

Rāmāyaṇa: f. 97v^{mg} *("vālmīkīye")*

Liṅga[purāṇa]: f. 109r^{8}

'Vāmadevarṣi': f. 98v^{10}

Vāyavīyasaṃhitā: f. 88v^{mg}

Vāyupurāṇa:[492] f. 15r^{6}, f. 88r^{1}, f. 88r^{3}, f. 88v^{2}, f. 88v^{6}, f. 89v^{5}, f. 90r^{7}, f. 95r^{1}1, f. 97v^{8}, f. 107r^{7}

Vāyusaṃhitā: f. 86(1)v^{11}, f. 92r^{4}

Vāsiṣṭhasaṃhitā: 1.50 at f. 59r^{9} (without attribution)

Viśvāmitrakalpa: f. 92v^{1}

Viśvāmitrasaṃhitā: f. 90r^{10}, f. 90v^{2}

'Vyākaraṇagraṃthe': f. 25r^{4}

'Vyāsaḥ': f. 84v^{7}

Śatarudriya: f. 84v^{6}

'Śākaloktamaṃtra': f. 24r^{11}

Śāradātilakatantra:[493] f. 42(1)v^{7}, f. 42(2)v^{1} (=previous citation)

'śāstram':[494] f. 26v

'śiva':[495] f. 95v^{7}, f. 95v^{11}

Śivagītā: f. 107v^{11}

Śivatāṇḍava: f. 105v^{6}

Śivapaṃjaramārkaṇḍeyastotra:[496] f. 84v^{5}

Śivapurāṇa: f. 86(2)r^{9}

Śivarahasya: f. 86(2)r^{4}, f. 86(2)r^{9}

Śivasaṃhitā:[497] 4.13 at f. 8v^{8}, 4.6ab at f. 8v^{10}, 3.11–15 at f. 11r^{1}; 5.2c–9b at f. 14v^{9}; 3.52c–54 at f. 16r^{10}; 5.167cd, 5.169ab, 5.170–171 at f. 24v^{5}, 5.132 at f. 25r^{3}, ≃ 5.158-159d at f. 44v^{4}, 1.17 and 1.18cd at f. 45r^{10}, 3.30ab and 3.30ef at f. 46v^{10}, f. 61r^{mg}, f. 66r^{11}, 2.4ab, 2.1–3 at f. 67r^{7}, 2.6ab and 2.10 at f. 67v^{3}, 5.29–30, 5.34 at f. 74v^{mg}, 4.13 at f. 87r^{7}, 5.15 at f. 88r^{2}, 3.27c–f at f. 93r^{3}, 3.35b–37b at f. 93r^{6}, 5.10–13 at f. 93v^{2}, 3.39–41 at f. 93v^{5}, ≃ 3.51c–52 at f. 95v^{3}, 3.64 at f. 96r^{2} (*"śive-na"*), 3.65ab at f. 96r^{3} (attributed to *"datta"*), 3.68–70 at f. 96v^{5} (*"śivena"*), ≃ 3.72–74 at f. 97r^{4}, 5.159a–d at f. 100v^{4}, 5.209–210 at f. 100v^{7}, 5.214cd and 211cda at f. 100v^{8}, 4.101 at f. 103v^{5}, 4.105cd at f. 104r^{9}, 5.234abc and 235ac at f. 104v^{4}, 3.22–23 at f. 107v^{12}

Śivārādhanadīpikā: f. 86(1)r^{8}

Śulbasūtra: f. 21v^{1}

'Śaivavratadaśake madīyaḥ saṃgrahaḥ': f. 86(1)r^{4}

Śaivāgama: f. 86(3)v^{9}

'Śrīdharā': f. 82v^{mg}

Śrīsūkta: f. 46r^{4}

Sāṃkṛtidattātreyasaṃvādaprakaraṇa:[498] 76–99 at f. 8r^{5}; 201–207 at f. 10r^{5}; 32–38 at f. 11r^{10}; 92 at f. 15v^{6}; 173–175 f. 16v^{1}; 158–161 at f. 47r^{1}, 157 at f. 59r^{9} (without attribution), 43 at f. 80v^{8}, 23–24 at f. 88r^{4}, 40–51 at f. 88v^{8}, 64 at f. 89v^{7}, f. 90r^{1}, 138–140 at f. 93r^{5}, 162–164 at f. 95v^{3}, 173 at f. 95v^{8}, 182–3 at f. 95v^{11}, 243–245 at f. 97r^{11}, 250 at f. 101r^{2}, 257–8 at f. 101r^{7} (unattributed), 259 at f. 101r^{9}, 260–261 at f. 101v^{3}, 263–267 at f. 101v^{7}, 268–269 at f. 101v^{11}, 270 at f. 102r^{5}, 286–289 at f. 102v^{5} (=*YB* 116–117 and attributed to *YB*), 285 at f. 102v^{6}, 283 at f. 102v^{9}, 274 at f. 103r^{3}, 295–296 and 293 at f. 103r^{8}, 107–113 at f. 107r^{5}

Siṃhasiddhānta: f. 42(1)v^{2}, f. 42(2)r^{7} (=previous citation)

'siddhāntāt': f. 100r^{4}

Siddhāntāgama: f. 86(1)v^{1}

Sudarśanasaṃhitā: f. 86(3)v^{mg}

Saundaryalaharī (saṭīkā): f. 98r^{7}

Skandapurāṇa: f. 26v^{8} (*"kedārakhaṇḍa adhyāya 65 tad uktaṃ... saṃgītaprastāvane nāradaṃ prati śivena"*), f. 42(1)r^{1}, f. 86(1)v^{2}, f. 107v^{2} (*"kedārakhaṃḍe"*)

Svarodaya: f. 42(1)v^{mg}, f. 42(2)r^{3} (=previous citation), f. 68r^{11}, f. 69r^{3}, f. 73v^{11}, f. 74v^{mg}, f. 75r^{4}

Haṃsopaniṣad: 16–17 at f. 26v^{5}

Haṭhapradīpikā: 1.11 at f. 10r^{4}, 3.32 at f. 20r^{7}, 4.3–5 at f. 23v^{1}, 3.46ab, 3.47–48 at f. 26r^{3}, 3.50bc, 3.51 at f. 26r^{7}, 4.68ab at f. 26v^{10}, 4.23–24 at f. 33v^{8}, 4.10 at f. 37v^{4}, f. 44r^{7}, 3.46ab at f. 44v^{9}, 4.37 at f. 72r^{2} (attributed to Gorakṣa), 2.44 at f. 90v^{9}, 3.6–7d at f. 90v^{10}, f. 91r^{3}, ≃2.51a–52b at f. 91r^{5}, 2.57a–58b at f. 91r^{8}, ≃2.60a–62b at f. 91r^{9}, 2.68–69 at f. 91v^{2}, 2.72 at f. 91v^{4}, 1.59 at f. 93r^{11}, 1.62a–d at f. 93v (attributed to Gorakṣa), 1.20 at f. 93v^{7} (unattributed), 1.62e–63d at f. 94v^{6}, 3.18c–19d at f. 101v^{12}, 3.25–27 at f. 102r^{5}, ≃3.24 at f. 102r^{9}, 3.51cd at f. 102r^{11}, 3.110 at f. 102v^{10}, 3.70 at f. 103r^{3}, ≃3.79ef at f. 103r^{10}, 3.90abefgh and 3.91ab at f. 103v^{1}, 4.10 at f. 104r^{10}, 1.12 at f. 107v^{1}, 1.13 at f. 107v^{3}, 1.36 at f. 108v^{3}, 1.48e–h at f. 108v^{7}

The following works are mentioned but not cited at the indicated places in the commentary:

Karaṅkinītantra: f. 28r^{1}

'kārikā': f. 99r^{1}

Gurugītā: f. 11r^{7}

Caraka[saṃhitā]: f. 18r^{10}, f. 97r^{2}, f. 110r^{mg}

Tattvakaumudī: f. 37r^{mg}

Tantrarāja: f. 35v^{9}, f. 38v^{2}

Dattātreyatantra: f. 27v^{mg}, f. 27v^{3}, f. 28r^{1}

Nāgārjunataṃtra: f. 27v^{1}, f. 27v^{3}, f. 28r^{1}

Pādmaśivagītā: f. 5v^{1}, f. 86(1)v^{10}

Prabodhacandrodaya: f. 46r^{1}

Bhāvaprakāśa: f. 18r^{10}, f. 97r^{2}

Bhiṣakśāstra: f. 18r^{10}, f. 110r^{5}

Mārttaṃḍagītā: fol. 18r^{mg}

'Mohanadāsa': f. 20r^{2}

Yājñavalkyasaṃhitā f. 47r^{2}

'Yājñavalkya': f. 34r^{mg}, f. 94v^{2}

Yogatārāvalī: f. 32r^{4}, f. 38r^{2}

Rudrayāmala: f. 13v^{6}, f. 28v^{5}

Liṅgapurāṇa: f. 86(3)v^{4}

Vāgbhaṭṭa: f. $18r^{10}$

Vāyupurāṇa: f. $99r^{3}$ *("upamanyu")*

Viśvālayatantra: f. $106r^{3}$

Śivakavaca: f. $86(3)r^{8}$

Śivapurāṇa: f. $86(2)r^{5}$, f. $86(3)v^{4}$

Śivamatsyeṃdrasaṃhitā: fol. $5r^{mg}$

Śivarahasya: f. $85v^{3}$, f. $86(3)v^{4}$

Śivasaṃhitā: f. $6v^{1}$, f. $34r^{mg}$

Śivārcanacaṃdrikā: f. $37v^{mg}$

Suśruta[saṃhitā]: f. $18r^{10}$

Saṃgītadarpaṇa: f. $49r^{mg}$

Saṃgītaratnākara: f. $49r^{mg}$

Saundaryalaharīvyākhyā of Lakṣmīdhara: f. $6v^{1}$, f. $9v^{2}$

Svarodaya: f. $38v^{2}$

Skandapurāṇa: f. $85r^{2}$ *("Brahmottarakhaṃḍa")*, f. $86(2)r^{5}$, f. $86(3)v^{4}$

Abbreviations

Primary sources

ATU	*Advayatārakopaniṣad*
AM	*Abhaṅgamālā*
AY	*Amanaskayoga*
AP	*Amaraughaprabodha*
AŚ	*Amaraughaśāsana*
KSS	*Kathāsaritsāgara*
KT	*Kiraṇatantra*
KMT	*Kubjikāmatatantra*
KRU	*Kularatnoddyota*
KAT	*Kulārṇavatantra*
KJN	*Kaulajñānanirṇaya*
KU	*Kṣurikopaniṣad*
GŚ$_{\mathrm{N}}$	*Gorakṣaśataka*$_{\mathrm{N}}$
GSS	*Gorakṣasiddhāntasaṃgraha*
GBP	*Gorakhbāṇī pad*
GBS	*Gorakhbāṇī sākhī*
GhS	*Gheraṇḍasaṃhitā*
JRY	*Jayadrathayāmala*
TĀ	*Tantrāloka*
TŚBM	*Triśikhībrāhmaṇopaniṣad, mantrabhāga*
DYŚ	*Dattātreyayogaśāstra*
DU	*Darśanopaniṣad*
DhBU	*Dhyānabindūpaniṣad*
NBU	*Nādabindūpaniṣad*
NSA	*Nityāṣoḍaśikārṇava*
NT	*Netratantra*
NTU	*Netratantroddyota*
BKhP	*Bṛhatkhecarīprakāśa*
BVU	*Brahmavidyopaniṣad*
MaSaṃ	*Matsyendrasaṃhitā*
MKS	*Mahākālasaṃhitā*

MBh	*Mahābhārata*
MKSK	*Mahākālasaṃhitā, Kāmakalākhaṇḍa*
MKSG	*Mahākālasaṃhitā, Guhyakālīkhaṇḍa*
MVUT	*Mālinīvijayottaratantra*
YKU	*Yogakuṇḍalyupaniṣad*
YCU	*Yogacūḍāmaṇyupaniṣad*
YTU	*Yogatattvopaniṣad*
YB	*Yogabīja*
YV	*Yogaviṣaya*
YŚU	*Yogaśikhopaniṣad*
YS	*Yogasūtra*
RAK	*Rasārṇavakalpa*
VU	*Varāhopaniṣad*
VS	*Vasiṣṭhasaṃhitā*
VD	*Vivekadarpaṇ*
VM	*Vivekamārtaṇḍa*
ŚP	*Śārṅgadharapaddhati*
ŚS	*Śivasaṃhitā*
ṢCN	*Ṣaṭcakranirūpaṇa*
SYM	*Siddhayogeśvarīmata*
SSP	*Siddhasiddhāntapaddhati*
HP	*Haṭhapradīpikā*
HPJ	*Haṭhayogapradīpikājyotsnā*
HR	*Haṭharatnāvalī*
HT	*Hevajratantra*

Other abbreviations

ĀSS	Ānandāśrama Sanskrit Series
IFP	Institut français de Pondichéry
KSTS	Kashmir Series of Texts and Studies
MMSL	Maharaja Man Singh Library
NAK	National Archives Kathmandu
NCC	New Catalogus Catalogorum
NGMPP	Nepal-German Manuscript Preservation Project

Notes

1 See verse 1.16.

2 See e.g. *Haṭhapradīpikājyotsnā* 1.1.

3 The compound *khecarīmudrā* is in fact used at just two places in the *Khecarīvidyā*: 2.82a and 3.54a. At the first occurrence it refers to the physical practice, while at the second it seems to refer to the result of the sum of the practices described in the text. Elsewhere the physical practice is called simply *abhyāsa*, "the practice".

4 On these different recensions of the *Haṭhapradīpikā* see the descriptions of witnesses H2 and *H3* on pp. 55–6.

5 At vv. 955–7, Jayatarāma lists eleven texts which he has consulted in order to compose his work but the *Khecarīvidyā* is not among them. Much of the *Jogpradīpakā*'s description of *khecarīmudrā* is clearly derived from the *Khecarīvidyā* (see for example vv. 665–670 which is very similar to the *Khecarīvidyā*'s fourth *paṭala*) and cannot be found in Jayatarāma's main source, the long recension of the *Haṭhapradīpikā*, so it seems certain that either Jayatarāma did consult the *Khecarīvidyā* or that one of the texts he lists was the *Khecarīvidyā* by another name or contained large parts of it.

6 This association with the Nātha order is almost certainly a retroactive attribution. There is little in the text that connects it with any specific tradition, apart from general evidence of roots in Kaula tantrism. It does not contain a systematic description of its yoga, nor does it call its yoga *ṣaḍaṅga*, "having six ancillaries", or *aṣṭāṅga*, "having eight ancillaries". It contains no statements of its ontological standpoint. Other than the manuscript colophons there is nothing to link it with Ādinātha. The four tantras mentioned in the text (see note 8) help little in locating it within a specific tradition. The *Vivekamārtaṇḍa* was itself probably attributed to Gorakṣanātha some time after its composition (see note 9). The mention of a *Jālasambaratantra* in the *Kularatnoddyotatantra* (see note 205) and the *Khecarīvidyā*'s use of the system of six *cakra*s found in texts of the Paścimāmnāya cult of Kubjikā suggest a possible link with the latter. *Matsyendrasaṃhitā* 44.27 declares *etat te paramāmnāyam auttaraṃ paścimānvayam*: "this [that I have taught] you is the supreme higher tradition, consonant with/following the western [tradition]", and *Matsyendrasaṃhitā* 18.67a–68b describes all Yoginīs and Siddhas as *kubjeśvaraprabhāḥ*, "resembling Kubjeśvara". Members of the cults connected with the *Matsyendrasaṃhitā* and

the *Mahākālasaṃhitā*, the two works with which the *Khecarīvidyā* is most closely linked, add the suffix *-ānandanātha* to their initiatory names (*MaSaṃ* 17.57; JHA 1976:5). This suffix is rarely found in the names of Nātha yogins but is added to the names of Kaula initiates. See *Tantrālokaviveka* 29.42 and, for the cult of Śrīvidyā, *Nityotsava* p.37, ll. 1–3. The names by which the goddess is addressed in the *Khecarīvidyā* are common in Kaula and Vidyāpīṭha Śaiva texts. Thus *vīravandite* (*KhV* 2.18, 2.110) is found at *Mālinīvijayottaratantra* 3.28, 3.58, 7.4, *Tantrasadbhāva* (NAK 5-445) 9.199, *Picumata* (NAK 3-370) 56.87, 56.89, 85.54, *Jayadrathayāmala* 4.2.463, *Kubjikāmatatantra* 6.48 etc.; *kuleśvari* (*KhV* 2.124) occurs many times in the *Kubjikāmatatantra*. I am grateful to Alexis SANDERSON for providing me with these references.

7 MEULENBELD (1999: vol. IIA pp. 749–50) gives a description of the text which is derived from that of WHITE *(loc. cit.)*.

8 Four other works are mentioned at 1.14c–15b. Because of variants among the witnesses and a lack of manuscripts of the works mentioned, establishing their identities is difficult, and establishing their dates even more so. See the notes to the translation for further details.

9 BOUY (1994:18) lists the names by which this text has been called: *Gorakṣapaddhati*, *Gorakṣasaṃhitā*, *Gorakṣaśata*, *Gorakṣaśataka*, *Gorakṣayogaśāstra*, *Haṭhayoga*, *Haṭhayogagorakṣaśataka*, *Jñānaprakāśaśataka*, *Jñānaśataka*, *Muktisopāna*, *Vivekamārtaṇḍa*, and *Yogamārtaṇḍa*. (I have not included the following titles from his list: *Haṭhagrantha*, *Haṭhayogacintāmaṇi*, *Yogacintāmaṇi* and *Yogasāgara*. These are reported by BRIGGS (1938:256) as names by which the *Gorakṣaśataka* is referred to in its commentary in his manuscript P, but are probably no more than honorific ways of referring to the *mūla*.)

A text called *Vivekamārtāṇḍa* and attributed to Viśvarūpadeva has been edited and published in the Trivandrum Sanskrit Series (No. 119). It is a work in six *prabodhas*, the last of which, entitled *Yogasādhana*, closely matches the text of the *Gorakṣaśataka* as edited by Nowotny. This sixth chapter has also been edited, as the *Vivekamārttaṇḍa*, in the *Gorakṣagranthamālā* series (GGM 75) from a copy of a manuscript in Jodhpur (MMSL No. 2027) which consists of the sixth chapter alone. Only in this chapter is the practice of *khecarīmudrā* described, so the reference in the *Khecarīvidyā* cannot be to any of the other five *prabodhas*. In the present state of research, it cannot be definitively stated whether the first five *prabodhas* were composed (or compiled) and prefixed to the already extant sixth, or whether they were all composed together, with the sixth becoming more popular and attaining a life of its own. I concur with BOUY (1994:21) and KUVALAYĀNANDA & SHUKLA (1958:14–15) in preferring the former hypothesis.

Nowotny has edited the *Gorakṣaśataka* from four manuscripts, the oldest of which is dated *samvat* 1791 (1733–34 CE). There is a manuscript in the Oriental Institute Library, Baroda (accession number 4110) whose colophon reads *iti śrīgorakṣadevaviracito vivekamārttaṃḍaḥ samāptaḥ* // ❀ // *saṃvat* 1534 (1476–77 CE). The text of this manuscript corresponds closely to Nowotny's edition of the *Gorakṣaśataka*, although it omits 24 verses found in the edition, including verse four, in which the work calls itself *Gorakṣaśataka*. Another manuscript of the *Vivekamārtaṇḍa* in

the Oriental Institute Library, Baroda (accession number 2081), which is undated but appears to be old, also transmits a work that closely matches Nowotny's edition of the *Gorakṣaśataka*. In GHAROTE & BEDEKAR's *Descriptive Catalogue of Yoga Manuscripts* (1989:356–357) the "Additional Particulars" section for MS No. 8047 in the Jodhpur Oriental Research Institute, entitled *Vivekamārtaṇḍa* and dated *samvat* 1879, reads "It is Gorakṣaśatakam". In the *Gorakṣasiddhāntasaṃgraha*, which can be dated to the seventeenth century (BOUY 1994:19), there are four quotations from a text called *Vivekamārtaṇḍa* all of which can be found in Nowotny's edition of the *Gorakṣaśataka*. A commentary on the *Siddhasiddhāntapaddhati* entitled *Nāthanirvāṇa* cites at least 55 verses which can be found in Nowotny's edition of the *Gorakṣaśataka*, attributing them to the *Vivekamārtaṇḍa* (BOUY 1994:23).
In GHAROTE & BEDEKAR's catalogue (1989:44–59), of 62 manuscripts called *Gorakṣaśataka* and 5 called *Gorakṣasaṃhitā*, the oldest dated manuscript (Varanasi Sanskrit College MS No. 3759) was written in *samvat* 1696 (1638–9 CE).
This evidence indicates that the work now generally called the *Gorakṣaśataka* was known as the *Vivekamārtaṇḍa* before the seventeenth century. This seems a more fitting name for a text which in its shortest available complete form consists of 157 verses (KUVALAYĀNANDA & SHUKLA 1958:7) and a verse of which ($GŚ_N$ 200) ascribes it to Ādinātha. Recensions of the text consisting of a hundred or so verses do exist, but are either incomplete (e.g. BRIGGS 1938:284–304, which names the six ancillaries of yoga at verse 7 but stops half-way through the description of the second ancillary, *prāṇāyāma*, at verse 101) or are attempts by commentators to produce a coherent *śataka* (KUVALAYĀNANDA & SHUKLA's 1958 edition). There is a different text called *Gorakṣaśataka* which is complete in 101 verses. This unedited work was used to compile the first chapter of the *Yogakuṇḍalyupaniṣad*; see BOUY 1994:40. It is perhaps through confusion with this work that the *Vivekamārtaṇḍa* came to be known as the *Gorakṣaśataka*. BOUY (1994:20–24) notes in detail other concordances between the *Vivekamārtaṇḍa* and the different recensions of the longer *Gorakṣaśataka*, and suggests that the *Gorakṣaśataka* may "sometimes" *(parfois)* have been known as the *Vivekamārtaṇḍa*, but does not remark on the diachronic nature of the change of name. A new edition of the *Vivekamārtaṇḍa*, drawing on the large number of variously named manuscripts of the text that exist, would make an important contribution to the study of the historical development of *haṭhayoga*.

10 *ŚP* 4374 = *VM* 7, *ŚP* 4418 = *VM* 59. *ŚP* 4372–4419 contains verses from various works on yoga (the edition has *ete yogaśāstrebhyaḥ* after verse 4419) and describes the first of two types of *haṭhayoga*, which is said to have been practised by Gorakṣa, as opposed to the second type, which was practised by the sons of Mṛkaṇḍa (*ŚP* 4372). Over half of the other verses of this passage are from the *Dattātreyayogaśāstra*.

11 BOUY (1994:82) has shown that the *HP* borrows from the following texts: the *Vivekamārtaṇḍa*, the original *Gorakṣaśataka*, the *Vasiṣṭhasaṃhitā* (*Yogakāṇḍa*), the *Dattātreyayogaśāstra*, the *Amaraughaprabodha*, the *Khecarīvidyā*, the *Yogabīja*, the *Amanaskayoga*, the *Candrāvalokana*, the *Uttaragītā*, the *Laghuyogavāsiṣṭha* and possibly also the *Śivasaṃhitā*. To these can be added the *Kaulajñānanirṇaya* (*KJN* 3.2c–3b ≃ *HP* 4.33) and possibly the *Kulacūḍāmaṇitantra* (a half-verse from which

is cited in Kṣemarāja's *Śivasūtravimarśinī ad* II.5 and found at *HP* 3.53ab). The absence of a source text or textual parallels for *HP* 3.22–36 suggests that this passage on the haṭhayogic *ṣaṭkarmas* may have been composed by the compiler of the text. I have been unable to find references to similar practices in tantric works. These cleansing techniques, which may have been developed from medical practices, are thus probably a unique feature of *haṭhayoga*.

12 Bouy *(loc. cit.)* identifies at least eleven of the works from which the *Haṭhapradīpikā* borrows but this does not help him since none of these works have themselves been satisfactorily dated. He sees the lack of a reference to the *Haṭhapradīpikā* in Mādhava's *Sarvadarśanasaṅgraha* as strong enough evidence to claim that the date of composition of that work (the second half of the fourteenth century) is the *terminus a quo* of the *Haṭhapradīpikā*. (This evidence is not conclusive. The *Sarvadarśanasaṅgraha* often relies on only a limited number of texts of a given discipline. I am grateful to Dominic Goodall and Harunaga Isaacson for pointing this out to me.) The *terminus ad quem* of the *Haṭhapradīpikā* is established by a manuscript of Mummaḍideva Vidvadācārya's *Saṃsārataraṇi* in the collection of the Maṭha of the Śaṅkarācārya of Purī. The manuscript is described by Mitra (1886:301) and the work, which is a commentary on the *Laghuyogavāsiṣṭha*, has been edited by V.S. Panasikara. In it the *Haṭhapradīpikā* is cited seven times and mentioned by name at five of the citations. The Purī manuscript is dated *samvat* 1581 (1524 CE) and is described as "incorrect" and "corrupt" by Mitra which leads Bouy to infer that the *Haṭhapradīpikā* "ne saurait être postérieure au xve siècle". Gharote & Bedekar (1989:438–9) list a manuscript of the *HP* in the collection of the Sanskrit University Library, Varanasi (No. 30109) which is dated 1553. Bouy (1994:84 n.357) understands this to mean *Saṃvat* 1553 which is odd since elsewhere Gharote & Bedekar indicate when a date is *Saṃvat*. Perhaps Bouy has seen the university catalogue, which I have not. He concludes that if the date is correct "on pourrait fixer le *terminus ad quem* de la HP en 1496".

13 We can also perhaps discount the possibility of the *Khecarīvidyā* having been composed in the modern Marāṭhī-speaking region, on account of the absence of any of the esoteric physiological terminology characteristic of the texts composed in that region at about the same time as the composition of the *Khecarīvidyā*, i.e. Jñāndev's *Abhaṅgamālā* and *Lākhoṭā*, and the *Siddhasiddhāntapaddhati*. See note 259 for more details.

14 Detailed descriptions of the individual sources consulted to establish the critical edition of the *Khecarīvidyā* (including its citations in other works) can be found on pp. 35–57.

15 It is of course only through shared errors that one can confidently establish that witnesses share a hyparchetype (Vasudeva 2004:xxxii). The many such errors that support the division of the witnesses of the *KhV* are not listed here. A full collation of all the witnesses of the *KhV* can be found at http://www.khecari.com

16 On the evidence of this contamination see page 14.

17 See page 40 for a detailed discussion of the *Bṛhatkhecarīprakāśa* and its author Ballāla.

18 The abbreviation *MaSaṃ* has been used in order to avoid confusion with the abbre-

viation MS in its usual sense of "manuscript".

19 I am grateful to Csaba Kiss for passing on to me the fruits of his research on the *Matsyendrasaṃhitā* and his forthcoming edition of the text will no doubt shed much more light on this fascinating work. In a preliminary paper, he writes "[The *Matsyendrasaṃhitā*] seems to be a remarkable text, or collection of texts, of a relatively late phase of the Śaiva tradition, particularly of its yogic teachings. It is long, detailed and mostly rather well-preserved. It might provide some clues for, among other things, the understanding of the transition from the early Indian yoga traditions (Pātañjala and Śaiva) to the late and fully developed haṭha-yogic teachings as well as perhaps of the transition from the early Kula traditions to the later Kaula teachings associated with the figure of Matsyendra. It might also throw some light on the connection between the Kaula traditions of the Paścimāmnāya and Dakṣiṇāmnāya, and the Nātha tradition of haṭha-yogins. The [*Matsyendrasaṃhitā*] is an encyclopaedic compilation of yogic techniques: from *āsana*s and *prāṇāyāma* to visualisation and *mudrā*s, from mantra techniques to *maṇḍala*s, the text describes a whole world of religio-psychological practices and rites... its Kaula layer might not be the central or earliest one. It might contain some material from other, e.g. Saiddhāntika, sources. No doubt, the [*Matsyendrasaṃhitā*] also incorporates later haṭha-yogic material." (Csaba Kiss 2004:5–6). Later in the same paper (p. 12) he examines the *dhyāna* of Parameśāna and Caṇḍikā described in *paṭala* 7 and concludes that the *MaSaṃ*'s Caṇḍikā may be a variant of the goddess Kubjikā, adding "The concealment of Kubjikā's name and this unusual, or to put it in another way, forced and arbitrary juxtaposition of Śiva and Kubjikā could be seen as a tendency to de-Śāktaize the cult of Kubjikā and to conceal all its sectarian marks. It might indicate that the text in fact belongs to a Kaula yoga tradition originating from a masculinised version of Kubjikā's cult."

20 See e.g. *Haṭhapradīpikā* 1.5.

21 On this affiliation see note 6. It seems likely that the teachings of the text have not always been associated with Matsyendranātha. The text shows clear signs of accretion and his name is found only in the frame story told in the first and last *paṭala*s.

22 A *Śivamatsyendrasaṃhitā* is mentioned in the margin of f. 5r of the *Bṛhatkhecarīprakāśa* (witness S).

23 I am grateful to Alexis Sanderson for reproducing for me part of a letter on this subject that he wrote to Professor Wezler in 1994. He concludes "The literature of the bhang-drinking Kaulas appears to be from eastern India. As to its date, I know no evidence that it predates the establishment of Islam in that region". In a later paper (2003:n. 43) Sanderson writes "It is probable that the use of cannabis for spiritual intoxication was adopted following the example of Muslim ascetics in India such as those of the Madāriyya order, founded by Badīʿ ad-dīn Shāh Madārī, an immigrant who settled in Jaunpur, where he died c. 1440 (Trimingham 1973:97), an order notorious for its use of hashish". See also Meulenbeld 1989.

24 Personal communication from Alexis Sanderson 2005.

25 On Śāstṛ, see Fuller 1992:53, 54, 89, 214 and the following passages from south Indian Śaivasiddhānta works: *Rauravāgama* vol. 3, *paṭala* 49, which describes the

worship of five village deities, including Śāstṛ; *Ajitāgama* vol. 3, *paṭala* 83 and *Īśānaśivagurudevapaddhati*, *Kriyāpāda paṭala* 58, which describe the installation of Śāstṛ.

26 See SANDERSON 1988:687.

27 Devī's request is found at 2.5–11b. The following is an edition of witness A f. $7r^{3-8}$:

> *dehaśuddhiḥ kathaṃ deva kathaṃ syād āsanakramaḥ* |
> *prāṇāyāma⟨ḥ⟩ kathaṃ proktaḥ pratyāhāra⟨ḥ⟩ kathaṃ bhavet* ||5||
> *kathaṃ sā dhāraṇā yoge dhyānayogaś ca kīdṛśaḥ* |
> *kathaṃ śrīkuṇḍalinīyogaṃ triliṅgārcāpi kīdṛśī* ||6||
> *kāni kṣetrāṇi dehe 'smin kāni tīrthāni śaṅkara* |
> *sarvasnānādhikasnānaḥ kaḥ paraḥ parameśvara* ||7||
> *kāny auṣadhaprayogāṇi kiṃ ca deva rasāyanam* |
> *kathaṃ syāt pādukāsiddhi⟨r⟩ dehasiddhiḥ kathaṃ bhavet* ||8||
> *vetālasiddhiś ca kathaṃ kapālasya ca sādhanam* |
> *katham añjanasiddhi⟨ḥ⟩ syād yakṣiṇīsiddhir eva ca* ||9||
> *aṇimādi kathaṃ deva yoginīmelanaṃ katham* |
> *etāny eva tathānyāni bhavatā sūcitāni ca* ||10||
> *tāni sarvāṇi me brūhi vistareṇa maheśvara* |

7c °snānaḥ] *em.*; °stāna *cod.* 7d parameśvara] *em.*; parameśvaraḥ *cod.* 8a kāny] *em.*; kāy *cod.* ◇ °prayogāṇi] *em.*; °prayogāni *cod.* 8b ca deva] *em.*; cid eva *cod.* 10c etāny] *em.*; etany *cod.* 10d bhavatā] *em.*; bhavantā *cod.*

Dehaśuddhi, *āsanakrama*, *prāṇāyāma*, *pratyāhāra*, *dhāraṇā* and *dhyāna* yoga are described in *paṭala*s 2–7 respectively. *Kuṇḍalinīyoga* and the *liṅgatraya* are described in *paṭala*s 22 and 23. *Paṭala*s 26 and 27 describe *tīrtha*s and *kṣetra*s in the body. *Auṣadhaprayoga*s and *rasāyana* are described in *paṭala*s 28 (=*KhV paṭala* 4) and 29. *Pādukāsiddhi* is described in *paṭala* 30. *Paṭala* 31 covers *vajrasiddhi*—the *dehasiddhiḥ* in 2.8d is probably a corruption of *vajrasiddhiḥ*. *Vetālasiddhi*, *kapālasādhana*, *añjanasiddhi*, *yakṣiṇīsiddhi*, *aṇimādi* and *yoginīmelana* are described in *paṭala*s 32, 33, 35, 34, 36 and 37 respectively. Thus it seems likely that *MaSaṃ paṭala*s 8–21, 24–25 and 39–54 were not part of the text when Pārvatī's questions were posed.

28 11.1–3 (A f. $30r^{3-5}$):

> *atha naivedyam utsṛjya mukhavāsādi dāpayet* |
> *mudrāś ca darśayet paścāt pūjānte sarvasiddhaye* ||1||
> *dakṣavyāṃśau bhujau devi parivartya tathāṅgulīḥ* |
> *tarjanībhyāṃ samākrānte †sarvārdhamadhyame†* ||2||
> *aṅguṣṭhau tu maheśāni kārayet saralāv api* |
> *eṣā hi khecarīmudrā sarvasiddhipradāyinī* ||3||

1a utsṛjya] *em.*; utsṛjyaḥ *cod.* 3a aṅguṣṭhau] *em.*; aṅguṣṭau *cod.*

29 In note 27 it was observed how *MaSaṃ paṭalas* 28 and 29 correspond to Devī's request to hear about *auṣadhaprayogāṇi*. All the other subjects she lists correspond to single *paṭalas*, so it is likely that either *paṭala* 28 or *paṭala* 29 is a later addition to an earlier recension of the text. *Paṭala* 28 lists various herbal preparations while *paṭala* 29 begins *śrīdevy uvāca | sarvauṣadhamayī (em.; sarvoṣadhamayīṃ* A*) śambho yā parā siddhimūlikā....* This appears to be capping the previous *paṭala* and suggests that *paṭala* 28 (=*KhV paṭala* 4) might be part of an earlier layer of the text and thus the *MaSaṃ* may be the source of *KhV paṭala* 4. The superiority of μ's readings in *KhV paṭala* 4 adds weight to this theory. However, the fact that the various different metres in *paṭala* 28 are not used elsewhere in the earlier parts of the *MaSaṃ* argues in favour of *paṭala* 29 being part of the earlier layer.

30 Critical editions of *MaSaṃ paṭalas* 17, 18 and 27 are included in the appendices.

31 The readings without *na* may be attempts by redactors to reject Kaula ritual.

32 Critical editions of this passage as it is found in μ and G are included in the appendices because the number of variants, additions and omissions, and the reordering of the verses make it difficult to compare the different passages by referring only to the apparatus of the critical edition.

33 Most of this passage is obscured in R_2 as a result of attempts to paste together the damaged manuscript, but at the few places where it is legible it shares readings with the *KhV* manuscripts.

34 A similar attempt at expunging a reference to Kaula practices involving alcohol can be seen at *Siddhasiddhāntapaddhati* 5.14, where the Lonavla edition has *jñāna-bhairavamūrtes tu tatpūjā ca yathāvidhi*. All the manuscript witnesses read *surādibhiḥ* for *yathāvidhi*. The editors of the text also collated four printed editions and presumably at least one of them reads *yathāvidhi* (the apparatus is negative so one cannot be sure). MALLIK adopts *surādibhiḥ* in her 1954 edition; her witness Ha reads *yathāvidhiḥ*.

35 Some of μ's *aiśa* forms are listed on pp. 15–16.

36 However, *KhV* 3.69ab (≃*MaSaṃ* 17.115ab) suggests that the topic of Khecarī is not finished until then. Perhaps the *madirā* passage was an early interpolation in the text. G seems to have attempted to resolve the problem of context by shifting *MaSaṃ* 17.114cd to before *MaSaṃ* 17.99c but this only results in further confusion over who is talking to whom.

37 The half-verse at μ's 17.111ab has nothing with which to connect it syntactically but it fits well at *KhV* 3.64ab. I can only guess that the redactor of the *KhV* version inserted this half-verse in order to make sense of a passage rendered nonsensical due to the omission of μ's 17.110 and that this half-verse found its way into μ due to conflation of the sources.

38 Evidence supporting this analysis (which is probably a simplification of a contaminated transmission—more details will be found in the forthcoming edition of the *MaSaṃ* by KISS) can be seen at the following places:
J_6 to J_7 and A: e.g. 1.40d, 2.30b, 3.20a, 3.61a, 3.64d; *MaSaṃ* 18.20c.
J_6 to J_7 to A: e.g. 1.42c; *MaSaṃ* 18.32b, 18.47d, 18.59a, 27.18a, 27.29b.
J_6 and J_7 to A: e.g. 2.20b, 3.56b, 3.56c, 3.62c; *MaSaṃ* 27.4d, 27.7a, 27.1b, 27.2c, 27.3a. The identical omissions found in all three witnesses at *KhV* 2.103d and

MaSaṃ 17.29c, 18.6b and 18.30b indicate that they share a hyparchetype.

39 The reading *kaulikatarpaṇāt* was evidently too much for the redactors in the tradition of β's K_5, which has *śaṅkarapūjanāt.*

40 For readings shared by R_2 with μ alone, see e.g. 2.31d, 97d, 98b, 108d, 121b, 3.47b; with μ and G, 2.29c, 50d, 3.36c; with G alone, 2.69c, 3.27d; with the *Khecarīvidyā* manuscripts alone, e.g. 2.33d, 96c, 111d, 3.9a, 66cd; with *D* alone, 3.39ab, 40d, 41a, 44a.

41 *U* does, however, keep 9a's *granthataḥ*.

42 Bouy (1994:102) has demonstrated how the compiler of the *upaniṣad* borrowed from an unedited work called *Gorakṣaśataka* (entirely different from the well-known *Gorakṣaśataka* edited by Nowotny—see note 9) to compile the first chapter.

43 The colophon at the end of *paṭala* 2 of the *Bṛhatkhecarīprakāśa* (witness S) reads: *iti śrīādināthanirūpite mahākālataṃtrāntargatayogaśāstre umāmaheśvarasaṃvāde dvitīyaḥ paṭalaḥ pūrṇaḥ*, suggesting that the *Khecarīvidyā* is part of a *Mahākālatantra.* However, this is hard to reconcile with 1.14c where a *Mahākālatantra* is distinguished from the *Khecarīvidyā.*

44 *Haṭhapradīpikājyotsnā* 1.1: *ādināthakṛto haṭhavidyopadeśo mahākālayogaśāstrādau prasiddhaḥ*. White (1996:169) says that Nārāyaṇa, the commentator on Atharvan *upaniṣad*s, refers to a *Mahākālayogaśāstra* as a treatise on *haṭhayoga.* I have been unable to locate this reference.

45 I am grateful to Dominic Goodall for suggesting this possibility.

46 Goudriaan *(loc. cit.)* also identifies the *Mahākālasaṃhitā* with the *Mahākālayogaśāstra.* His reasons for this are not clear. It may be due to a mistake in the NCC (Raghavan 1969b:188) where a manuscript of the *Mahākālasaṃhitā* in the collection of the Asiatic Society of Bengal is wrongly said to be of the *Khecarīvidyā/Mahākālayogaśāstra* (from the description by Shastri (1905:11) it appears to consist of the first eight *paṭala*s of the *Mahākālasaṃhitā Guhyakālīkhaṇḍa*).

47 It is likely that at least some of the *Mahākālasaṃhitā* postdates the *KhV. MKSG* 11.698–1065 teaches two types of yoga, gradual *(krāmika)* and subitist *(haṭha). Haṭhayoga* is said to be very dangerous: many Brahmarṣis have died from it, so it should not be practised (11.702–3). The *krāmika* yoga has eight ancillaries and instructions for it are taken directly from the *Vasiṣṭhasaṃhitā* (dated by Bouy to pre-1250 CE (1994:118)) with a few minor doctrinal alterations, including at *MKSG* 11.939a–954b a visualisation of Guhyakālī substituted for that of Hari found at *VS* 4.33b–64d. Thus *MKSG* 11.707a–964b and 11.1020c–1057 match closely *VS* 1.19–4.73 and 6.8–53. Somewhat surprisingly in the light of vv. 702–3 mentioned above, instructions for *haṭhayoga* are included at *MKSG* 11.966a–1020b. The only practice described is the haṭhayogic *khecarīmudrā* and the instructions seem to be a précis of the *KhV.* Although no verses are taken directly from the *KhV*, the instructions to cut and lengthen the tongue, and the descriptions of the tongue's attainment of successively higher places in the head in three year stages, correspond to those taught in the *KhV.* The many rewards described almost all have direct parallels in the *KhV* and the ascription of the ability to prevent *doṣa*s found at 11.985 is suggestive of *KhV* 2.82a–101b. Such parallels cannot be found in other texts that describe the technique. The main aim of the technique as described in the *MKS* and

Khecarīvidyā is *amṛtaplāvana*, flooding the body with *amṛta*, not *bindudhāraṇa*, retention of the *bindu*, the aim of the practice in most other works (on these two aims, see page 28). The one glaring difference between the *MKS* passage and the *KhV* is that the *MKS* nowhere mentions Khecarī, calling the practice *rasanāyoga*, "tongue yoga". Why this should be so is unclear. The *Vasiṣṭhasaṃhitā*, while retaining tantric features such as visualisations of Kuṇḍalinī and *amṛtaplāvana*, does not call any of its yogic techniques *mudrā*s and it may be that the writer of the passage on *rasanāyoga* was remaining faithful to this tradition.

Jhā (1976:5–9) does not ascribe any great age to the *MKS*, suggesting the twelfth century CE as the earliest possible date of its composition. He believes it was composed (or compiled) to establish a tantric *saṃpradāya* that was not anti-vedic. Thus at *MKSG* 4.196 the Veda is praised above all tantric works. The earliest external evidence for the *MKS* are citations in the seventeenth-century *Tārābhaktisudhārṇava*.

48 See e.g. *Yoginītantra paṭala* 7.1–27 which contains descriptions of the *svapnavatī*, *mṛtasañjīvanī*, *madhumatī* and *padmāvatī vidyā*s. Cf. *Tantrarājatantra paṭala* 34.

49 The practice was already called *khecarīmudrā*—the *Vivekamārtāṇḍa* mentioned at *KhV* 1.14d calls it thus (*GŚ*$_N$ 64). Cf. *Kularatnoddyota* 3.105–108, which is cited in note 96.

50 *Matsyendrasaṃhitā* 17.1cd (≃ *KhV* 3.69cd): *tvayā śrīkhecarīvidyāsādhanaṃ guhyam īritam* // 1 //.

51 In verse 9 the reading found in μ and K3 has been adopted, in which it is said that the yogin will become a Khecara from eating a particular herbal preparation.

52 μ does include the fourth *paṭala* but it is found ten *paṭala*s after those that correspond to the first three of the *Khecarīvidyā*.

53 On the likelihood of *MaSaṃ paṭala* 28 being the source of the *KhV*'s fourth *paṭala* see note 29.

It is on the strength of the *KhV*'s fourth *paṭala*, in which 8c–9b describes a preparation containing mercury, sulphur, orpiment and realgar and verse 14 describes a preparation containing mercury, that White (1996:169) has called the entire *KhV* "a paradigmatic text of the Siddha alchemical tradition". In the first three *paṭala*s there are two verses where it is said that alchemical *siddhi*s arise as a result of perfection of the practice (1.68 and 1.75), but other than that, there is nothing that could be described as specifically alchemical. The bizarre practices described at 2.72–79 suggest an attempt to render external alchemical practice redundant by effecting similar techniques within the realm of the body (see the notes to the translation). The thesis of White's work is that Rasa Siddhas (alchemists) and Nāth Siddhas (*haṭhayogins*) "if they were not one and the same people, were at least closely linked in their practice" (ibid.:10). It seems that they were not "one and the same people" but that many of the similarities in the terminology of their practices are due to the texts of both schools being couched in the language and theory of earlier tantric works. White himself suggests (ibid.:97–101) that Gorakhnāth brought together several disparate schools when he established the Nātha *saṃpradāya* "as a great medieval changing house of Śaiva and Siddha sectarianism" (ibid.:100). None of the textual descriptions of the trainee *haṭhayogin*'s abode suggests that it might be used as a laboratory (e.g. *DYŚ* 107–111, *HP* 12–13) while the peripatetic lifestyle of the perfected *haṭha* adept is incompatible with the encumbrances of alchemical experimentation. During my fieldwork, the *haṭhayogin*s with whom I travelled would buy beads of fixed mercury to wear in their *jaṭā* from Brahmin *rasavādin*s who lived at the *tīrtha*s through which the ascetics passed on their annual pilgrimage cycle.

54 The section from 3.55 to the end of *paṭala* 3 would have been as it is found in the *MaSaṃ* manuscripts.
The original chapter describing the *vidyā* of Khecarī was probably the first chapter in the text from which it was taken. *Khecarīvidyā* 1.1–44 contains several verses that emphasise the importance of the text and the worship of the book in which it was written, giving the passage an introductory flavour. These verses could themselves be later additions but they contain references to *melaka*, a goal of the practice of the *vidyā* that is mentioned only in the earliest layer of the text. One problem with this theory is the inclusion of the *Vivekamārtaṇḍa* among the tantras listed at 1.14c–15b. This work does not contain a description of a Khecarī mantra but does describe the tongue practice. Perhaps the list originally included the name of a different work and this was changed to *Vivekamārtaṇḍa* when the instructions for the practice were added to the text.

55 It is likely that at this stage the text was not divided into three *paṭala*s in the same way that it is in the edition. Witness G has no chapter divisions, while the *MaSaṃ* manuscripts divide the *paṭala*s at different places from the *KhV* manuscripts.

56 The verses describing the practice have some internal contradictions and are unlikely all to have been composed together. See, for example: *paṭala* 3, in which vv. 1–14, 15–22, 23–25b, 25c–32b and 32c–55b are different descriptions of similar practices; 2.101c–102b, which mentions *cālana* as one of the four stages of the practice even though it is not mentioned in *paṭala* 1 (see also note 366); 2.107–115 and 3.23–25b, which use phrases common in other, more explicitly haṭhayogic texts (e.g. *ūrdhvaretas*, *unmanī*, *śūnya*, *sahaja yoga*) but conspicuous by their absence elsewhere in the *KhV*; 1.55, where the tongue ready for the practice is said to be able to reach the top of the head, having passed the eyebrows several years earlier, while at 1.73 the *siddhi*s effected by the practice are said to arise between the eyebrows (cf. note 245).

57 Only G shows no clear evidence of contamination.

58 Where there are two or more equally acceptable readings it is usually that found in the greatest number of witnesses which has been adopted.

59 Nowhere in the edition has a reading found only in R_2 or T been adopted.

60 In compiling this list of *aiśa* peculiarities I have used that given by GOODALL (1995: xxiv), which he in turn drew from a list compiled by Alexis SANDERSON.

61 This reading is corrected to *abhyāsaḥ* in MFB and I have adopted the corrected form in the edition.

62 This reading is found corrected to *asmiṃs tantravare* in N.

63 This reading is found in $S\beta\gamma$ and is an attempt to alter *vikhyātā vīravandite*, the reading found in $\mu\alpha_3$ which has been adopted in the edition.

64 This anacoluthon is found repaired in G.

65 This survey of texts is of course by no means exhaustive. There is undoubtedly more

material to be unearthed. The most fertile area for research is likely to be the texts of tantric Śaivism.

66 *tassa mayhaṃ Aggivessana etad ahosi | yan nūnāhaṃ dantehi dantam ādhāya jivhāya tāluṃ āhacca cetasā cittaṃ abhiniggaṇheyyaṃ abhinippīḷeyyaṃ abhisantāpeyyan ti | so kho ahaṃ Aggivessana dantehi dantam ādhāya jivhāya tāluṃ āhacca cetasā cittaṃ abhiniggaṇhāmi abhinippīḷemi abhisantāpemi | tassa mayhaṃ Aggivessana dantehi dantam ādhāya jivhāya tāluṃ āhacca cetasā cittaṃ abhiniggaṇhato abhinippīḷayato abhisantāpayato kacchehi sedā muccanti | seyyathā pi aggivessana balavā puriso dubbalataraṃ purisaṃ sīse vā gahetvā khandhe vā gahetvā abhiniggaṇheyya abhinipīḷeyya abhisantāpeyya evam eva kho me aggivessana dantehi dantam ādhāya jivhāya tāluṃ āhacca cetasā cittaṃ abhiniggaṇhato abhinippīḷayato abhisantāpayato kacchehi sedā muccanti | āraddhaṃ kho pana me Aggivessana viriyaṃ hoti asallīnaṃ upaṭṭhitā sati asammuṭṭhā sāraddho ca pana me kāyo hoti appaṭippasaddho ten'eva dukkhappadhānena padhānābhitunnassa sato | evaṃrūpā pi kho me Aggivessana uppannā dukkhā vedanā cittaṃ na pariyādāya tiṭṭhati | tassa mayham Aggivessana etad ahosi | yan nūnāhaṃ appānakaṃ jhānaṃ jhāyeyyan ti...* (p.242 l.23–p.243 l.5).

67 *tassa mayhaṃ Aggivessana etad ahosi | ye kho keci atītaṃ addhānaṃ samaṇā vā brāhmaṇā vā opakkamikā dukkhā tippā kaṭukā vedanā vedayiṃsu etāvaparamaṃ nayito bhiyyo | ye pi hi keci anāgatam addhānaṃ samaṇā vā brāhmaṇā vā opakkamikā dukkhā tippā kaṭukā vedanā vedayissanti etāvaparamaṃ nayito bhiyyo | ye pi hi keci etarahi samaṇā vā brāhmaṇā vā opakkamikā dukkhā tippā kaṭukā vedanā vediyanti etāvaparamaṃ nayito bhiyyo | na kho panāhaṃ imayā kaṭukāya dukkarakārikāya adhigacchāmi uttariṃ manussadhammā alamariyañāṇadassanavisesaṃ | siyā nu kho añño maggo bodhāyāti |* (p.246 ll.20–30).

68 *tassa ce bhikkave bhikkuno tesaṃ pi vitakkānaṃ vitakkasaṅkhārasanthānaṃ manasikaroto uppajjant'eva pāpakā akusalā vitakkā chandūpasaṃhitā pi dosūpasaṃhitā pi mohūpasaṃhitā pi tena bhikkhave bhikkhunā dantehi dantam ādhāya jivhāya tāluṃ āhacca cetasā cittaṃ abhiniggaṇhitabbaṃ abhinippīḷetabbaṃ abhisantāpetabbaṃ | tassa dantehi dantam ādhāya jivhāya tāluṃ āhacca cetasā cittaṃ abhiniggaṇhato abhinippīḷayato abhisantāpayato ye pāpakā akusalā vitakkā chandūpasaṃhitā pi dosūpasaṃhitā pi mohūpasaṃhitā pi te pahīyanti te abbhatthaṃ gacchanti | tesaṃ pahānā ajjhatam eva cittaṃ santiṭṭhati sannisīdati ekodihoti samādhiyati |.*

69 *...khuradhārūpamo bhave |*
jivhāya tāluṃ āhacca udare saññato siyā |
alānacitto ca siyā na cāpi bahu cintaye |
nirāmagandho asito brahmacariyaparāyano |
ekāsanassa sikkhetha samaṇopāsanassa ca |
ekattaṃ monam akkhātaṃ eko ve 'bhiramissasi |
atha bhāsihi dasa disā |.

70 E.g. *GŚ*$_N$ 65, *ŚS* 3.93. See also *KhV* 2.107 and note 377.

71 The earliest date for the composition of the Pali canon that we can confidently assert is the last quarter of the first century BCE. See e.g. SCHOPEN 1997:23–25.

72 *ūrusthottānacaraṇaḥ savye kare karam itaraṃ nyasya tālusthācalajihvo dantair dantān asaṃspṛśan svaṃ nāsikāgraṃ paśyan diśaś cānavalokayan vibhīḥ praśāntātmā caturviṃśatyā tattvair vyatītaṃ cintayet ||1||...*

...*dhyānaniratasya ca saṃvatsareṇa yogāvirbhāvo bhavati* //6//.

73 *athānyatrāpy uktaṃ / atha parāsya dhāraṇā / tālurasanāgra(°āgra°*] *em.* ISAACSON & GOODALL; *°āgre* Ed.)*nipīḍanād vāṅmanaḥprāṇanirodhanād brahma tarkeṇa paśyati / yadātmanātmānam aṇor aṇīyāṃsaṃ dyotamānaṃ manaḥkṣayāt paśyati tadātmanātmānaṃ dṛṣṭvā nirātmā bhavati / nirātmakatvād asaṃkhyo 'yoniś cintyo mokṣalakṣaṇam iti / tat paraṃ rahasyam iti / evaṃ hy āha*

> *cittasya hi prasādena hanti karma śubhāśubham /*
> *prasannātmātmani sthitvā sukham avyayam aśnuta iti* //20//
> (*aśnuta*] *corr.*; *aśnutā* Ed.)

athānyatrāpy uktam / ūrdhvagā naḍī suṣumṇākhyā prāṇasaṃcāriṇī tālv antar vicchinnā / tayā prāṇa (prāṇa] *em.*; *prāṇā* Ed.) *oṃkāramanoyuktayordhvam utkramet / tālv adhy agraṃ parivartya cendriyāṇi saṃyojya mahimā mahimānaṃ nirīkṣeta / tato nirātmakatvam eti / nirātmakatvān na sukhaduḥkhabhāg bhavati kevalatvaṃ labhate (labhata*] *corr.*; *labhata* Ed.) *iti* /.

74 The absence of a fixed lower limit for the date of the *Khecarīvidyā* makes it impossible to prove that these Śaiva works predate it. However, it is a chronology of ideas that is important here. The *khecarīmudrā* of the *Khecarīvidyā* combines elements of the tantric Śaiva physical practices described in this section with the non-physical tantric *khecarīmudrā* described in the following section in a way that is not found in these tantric works. The *khecarīmudrā* of the *Khecarīvidyā* must postdate its individual elements as found in these texts. It seems very likely that the *Khecarīvidyā* itself also postdates these works: the latest of them (see note 101) are the *Kubjikāmatatantra* and the *Kularatnoddyota*, early works of the Paścimāmnāya in which the system of six *cakra*s is found for the first time (see *KMT paṭala*s 11–13 and note 433). This system is found well developed in the *Vivekamārtaṇḍa*, a work mentioned at *KhV* 1.16.

75 *KT* 59.34c–35b:

> *kumbhakaṃ tu tataḥ kṛtvā kaṇṭham āpīḍya sasphuram* //34//
> *jihvātālusamāyogāt tatkṣaṇotkramaṇaṃ bhavet* /

The verse is as found in the Mysore codex (University of Mysore, Oriental Research Institute MS P 285/10). At 34d, the Nepalese MS of c. 924 CE (NAK 5-893; NGMPP Reel No. A 40/3) has *kṛtam āviśya tatpuṭam*.

76 E.g. *Brahmavidyopaniṣad* 73–74. See also note 236.

77 References to these other passages can be found later in this chapter where the corporealisation of subtle visualisation techniques into gross physical practices is explored in detail.

78 The tantric Śaiva *karaṇa*s become known as *mudrā*s in the texts of *haṭhayoga*. *HP* 1.56 describes the stages of *haṭha*[*-yoga*] and has *mudrākhyaṃ karaṇam* as the third stage. Ballāla (*BKhP* f. 37v[7]), explaining *HP* 4.10, glosses *karaṇaṃ* with *mudrā*. SINGH (1979:33) quotes (without reference) a definition of *karaṇa*: *karaṇaṃ dehasanniveśaviśeṣātmā mudrādivyāpāraḥ* and translates it with "disposition of the limbs of the body in a particular way, usually known as *mudrā* i.e. control of certain organs and senses that helps in concentration". Similarly, *AY* 1.20 uses *karaṇa* as

a synonym of *mudrā*. The headstand (or shoulderstand) is known as *viparītaṃ karaṇam* or *viparītakaraṇī* in haṭhayogic texts: see e.g. *GŚ*$_N$ 135, *HP* 3.6, 3.76–78.

79 *JRY Bhairavānanavidhi Bhūmikāpaṭala* 153c–162b (f.193v–f.194r):

> *pibed dhārāmṛtaṃ tac ca yad dugdhaṃ gostanair iva //153//*
> *tenāmṛtena tṛptas tu valīpalitavarjitaḥ /*
>
> *viṣṇumastakasaṃprāptā rasanā śūnyasaṃgame //156//*
> *īṣat sparśavivarjā tu tālurandhragatā tathā /*
> *dvijacañcupuṭaprakhyaṃ vaktraṃ kṛtvā tathā dvija //157//*
> *uddhṛtya tad anu sparśaṃ yāvad bhāvaṃ sthirīgatam /*
> (**194r**) *dṛḍhabhāvagato yogī svasthaṃ plavam avāpnuyāt //158//*
> *tatrasthasya ca viśrāmād gandhadvayavicāraṇāt /*
> *parāmṛtaṃ prasravati śūnyendurasanāhatam //159//*
> *tadāsvāditacidrūpam ūrdhvaṃ gacchaty aśaṅkitam /*
> *kauñcikotpāṭanaṃ hy eṣa śivaśaktisamāgamaḥ //160//*
> *†śivavyāptikṛtodyānaṃ plutoccārordhvadṛkkriyaḥ† /*
> *lalanātāluke yojya spandaśaktiyutaṃ dadet //161//*
> *kaṇṭhotthatāluvivaraṃ yāvad dvādaśabhūmikāḥ /*

153c dhārā°] *conj.* SANDERSON; vāra° *cod.* 153d dugdhaṃ] *em.* SANDERSON; ugdhaṃ *cod.* 156c °saṃprāptā] *em.*; °saṃprāpta *cod.* 157a īṣat] *em.* SANDERSON; īṣa *cod.* 157c dvijacañcupuṭa°] *em.* SANDERSON; dvikacuṃcupuṭa *cod.* 160c kauñciko°] *em.* SANDERSON; krauñciko° *cod.* 160d °samāgamaḥ] *em.* SANDERSON; °samāgama *cod.*

80 SANDERSON has made the conjectural emendation of *krauñciko°* to *kauñciko°* on semantic grounds, with the support of *KMT* 8.73d *kuñcikodghāṭayed bilam* and parallel metaphors found in the *Śrīpīṭhadvādaśikā* (NAK 5.358 ff.93v–95r: v. 5) and the *Kālīkulakramasadbhāva* (NAK 1-76: 2.87ab). (SANDERSON has similarly emended *JRY* 1.45.184b *kruñcikodghāṭamatratam* to *kuñcikodghāṭamātrataḥ* and *Yoginīsaṃcāraprakaraṇa* (part of the *JRY*'s third *ṣaṭka*) 1.31b *kruñcikodghāṭam* to *kuñcikodghāṭam*. The *JRY* passage describes the Alaṃgrāsa stage in the yoga of the *vāmasrotas* while the *Yoginīsaṃcāraprakaraṇa* passage lists names of works with titles echoing the names of the phases of the *JRY*'s *vāmasrotas* yogas.) At *MaSaṃ* 17.8c Kuṇḍalinī is called both *cidrūpā* (cf. *JRY Bhairavānanavidhi Bhūmikāpaṭala* 160a) and *kuñcikā*. Cf. *MaSaṃ* 18.30a.

81 This passage has verbal parallels in the *KhV*. Compare *JRY* 2.157cd with *KhV* 1.74ab: *kākacañcupuṭaṃ vaktraṃ kṛtvā tadamṛtaṃ pibet*, "making the mouth like the open beak of a crow, [the yogin] should drink the *amṛta* therein" (see also note 267) and 2.159a with *KhV* 3.42ab: *parāmṛtamahāmbhodhau viśrāmaṃ samyag ācaret*, "[The tongue] should duly relax in the great ocean of the supreme *amṛta*."

82 *MVUT* 21.1–8:

> *athātaḥ paramaṃ guhyaṃ śivajñānāmṛtottamam /*

vyādhimṛtyuvināśāya yogināṃ upavarṇyate //1//
ṣoḍaśāre khage cakre candrakalpitakarṇike /
svarūpeṇa parāṃ tatra sravantīm amṛtaṃ smaret //2//
pūrvanyāsena saṃnaddhaḥ kṣaṇam ekaṃ vicakṣaṇaḥ /
tatas tu rasanāṃ nītvā lambake viniyojayet //3//
sravantam amṛtaṃ divyaṃ candrabimbāt sitaṃ smaret /
mukham āpūryate tasya kiṃ cil lavaṇavāriṇā //4//
lohagandhena tac cātra na pibet kiṃ tu nikṣipet /
evaṃ samabhyaset tāvad yāvat tat svādu jāyate //5//
jarāvyādhivinirmukto jāyate tat pibaṃs tataḥ /
ṣaḍbhir māsair anāyāsād vatsarān mṛtyujid bhavet //6//
tatra svāduni saṃjāte tadāprabhṛti tatragam /
yad eva cintayed dravyaṃ tenāsyāpūryate mukham //7//
rudhiraṃ madirāṃ vātha vasāṃ vā kṣīram eva vā /
ghṛtatailādikaṃ vātha dravad dravyam ananyadhīḥ //8//

Codices: K_{ED}=The KSTS edition, with selective *variae lectiones* from K_1, K_2, K_3 and K_1; V=Benares Hindu University c 4106, paper, Śāradā; J=Śrī Raghunātha Temple Library, Jammu, MS No. 1524/ka, paper, Devanāgarī; P=Deccan College, Poona MS No. 488, Collection of 1875–6, paper, Devanāgarī. Somdev VASUDEVA kindly provided me with the variant readings of witnesses V, J and P.

2b °kalpitakarṇike] K_{ED}; °kalpitakalpitam VJ, °kalpitam P *(unm.)* 3c rasanāṃ] K_{ED}VJ; rasatāṃ K_3P 3d viniyojayet] VJP; viniyojayat K_{ED} 4b °bimbāt sitaṃ] K_1VJP; °bimbasitaṃ K_{ED} 5d svādu] K^{pc}_{ED}V; sādu K^{ac}_{ED}, sādhu J, sādhv a° P 6a jarā°] K_{ED}P; jaya° J 7a tatra] K_{ED}VP; tac ca J ◇ svāduni] K^{pc}_{ED}VJ; sāduni K^{ac}_{ED}, sādhuni P 8b vasāṃ] K_{ED}VJ; ⌈vaṃ⌉saṃ P 8d dravad] K_{ED}VJ; dravyād P

83 *MVUT* 14.11-15 describes a similar (but subtler) practice, "the introspection of taste" *(rasarūpā dhāraṇā)*: "Now I will teach the taste-introspection, which is revered by Yogins, whereby the attainment of all flavours arises for the Yogin. One should contemplate, with a focussed internal faculty, the Sensory Medium of taste as resembling a water-bubble on the tip of the tongue. It is located at the end of [the] royal nerve *(rājanāḍī)*, it is cool, six-flavoured and smooth. Then, within a month one savours flavours. Rejecting the salty [flavours] etc., when he reaches sweetness, the Yogin, swallowing that, becomes the vanquisher of death after six months. [He is] freed from aging and disease, black-haired, undiminished is [the splendour of] his complexion. He lives as long as the moon, the stars and the sun, practising now and again." (translation VASUDEVA 2004:333).

MVUT 15.16–19 teaches the "introspection of the tongue" *(jihvādhāraṇā)*: "The yogin should contemplate his own tongue as having the colour of the moon. Within ten days he will achieve the sensation of the absence of his own tongue, as it were. After six months the single-minded [practitioner] can taste what is far away. Within three years he directly savours the supreme nectar, whereby the Yogin is freed from old age and death. Even if he is addicted to forbidden drinks he commits no sin..." (ibid.:264).

KMT 9.19–20 teaches a visualisation of the mouth filling with *amṛta* that has arisen at the uvula, in which the *amṛta* seems to be equated with the Aghora mantra.

84 See *JRY* 4.2.157b *tālurandhragatā*; *KJN* 14.50c *ūrdhvakām* (cf. *KhV* 2.80a); *KJN* 6.18b *brahmavilaṃ gataḥ* (cf. *KhV* 1.55d); *KJN* 6.26d *svavaktreṇa saṃyutām* (cf. *KhV* 2.64d); *KMT* 23.159d *lambakaṃ tu vidārayet*.

85 *KJN* 14.50–54b:

ata ūrdhvaṃ paraṃ guhyaṃ sarvavyādhivimardakam /
rasanām ūrdhvakāṃ kṛtvā manas tasmin niveśayet //50//
satatābhyāsayogena maraṇaṃ nāśayet priye /
kṣaṇena mucyate rogair vyādhimṛtyujarādibhiḥ //51//
naśyate vyādhisaṃghātaṃ siṃhasyaiva yathā mṛgāḥ /
kṣaṇena naśyate vyādhiḥ kaṭukakuṣṭhanāśanam //52//
susvādena mahādevi valīpalitanāśanam /
kṣīrasvādena medhāvi amaro jāyate naraḥ //53//
ghṛtasvādopamaṃ devi svātantryaṃ tu tathā bhavet /

50a ūrdhvaṃ paraṃ] *em.* Griffiths; ūrdhveśvaraṃ Ed. 50c rasanām ūrdhvakāṃ] *em.*; rasanā ūrddhakaṃ Ed. 51ab °ābhyāsayogena maraṇaṃ] *conj.*; °ābhyāsayet tat tu muhūrttaṃ Ed. 52d kaṭuka°] *conj.*; kaṭuke Ed. 54a °opamaṃ] *em.*; °opamanaṃ Ed. *(unm.)* 54b svātantryaṃ tu tathā] *em.*; svātantran tu yathā Ed.

Both *MVUT* 21.1–8 (see note 82) and *KJN* 14.50–54b are followed by passages on *mṛtakotthāpana*, reanimating corpses, and *paradehapraveśana*, entering another's body.

86 Govind Dās Yogīrāj said that the liquid tasted fishy at first, then salty, then like butter, then like ghee and finally had a taste that could not be described. Bernard (1982:68) reported "At first it was thick, heavy, and slimy; eventually, it became thick, clear, and smooth".

87 *KJN* 6.18–19:

prasārya dantarāyaṃ tu yāvad brahmabilaṃ gataḥ /
amṛtāgraṃ rasāgreṇa duhyamānaḥ sudhīr api //18//
māsena jinayen mṛtyuṃ satyaṃ satyaṃ mahātape /
rasanāṃ tālumūle tu kṛtvā vāyuṃ pibec chanaiḥ //19//
ṣaṇmāsam abhyased devi mahārogaiḥ pramucyate /

18a dantarāyaṃ] *em.*; danturāyān Ed. 18d duhyamānaḥ] *conj.* Sanderson; dahyamāna Ed. 19a jinayen] *em.* Sanderson; jitayen Ed. 19c rasanāṃ] *em.*; rasanā Ed. 20a °māsam] *em.*; °māsād Ed.

88 The *dantarāya* is the *rājadanta*, on which see note 258; *brahmabila* is a synonym of *brahmarandhra*, on which see note 240.

89 *KJN* 6.23–26:

yad rājadantamadhyastham bindurūpaṃ vyavasthitam /
amṛtaṃ tad vijānīyād valīpalitanāśanam //23//
śītalasparśasaṃsthāne rasanāṃ yujya buddhimān /
valīpalitanirmmuktaḥ sarvavyādhivivarjitaḥ //24//
na tasya bhavate mṛtyur yogayānaparaḥ sadā /
rasanāṃ tālumūle tu vyādhināśāya yojayet //25//
tiṣṭhañ jāgran svapaṅ gacchan bhuñjāno maithune rataḥ /
rasanāṃ kuñcayen nityaṃ svavaktreṇa tu saṃyutām //26//

23a yad] *conj.*; dvau Ed. ◇ rājadanta°] *em.*; rājada*° Ed. 23c tad] *em.*; taṃ Ed. 24a śītala°] *em.*; śītalaṃ Ed. 24b yujya] *conj.* GRIFFITHS; kṛtvā tu Ed. *(unm.)* 25c rasanāṃ] *em.*; rasanā Ed. 26b bhuñjāno] *em.* GOODALL (26ab =*KMT* 8.78cd); bhuñjan Ed. *(unm.)* 26c rasanāṃ] *em.* GRIFFITHS; rasanaṃ Ed. 26d saṃyutām] *em.* GRIFFITHS; saṃyutam Ed.

90 This "mouth" probably refers to the opening above the uvula. See note 322.

91 *KMT* 23.158–162:

athānyaṃ api vakṣyāmi prayogaṃ mṛtyunāśanam /
saṅkocya mūlacakraṃ tu janmasthaṃ dhārayet kṣaṇāt //158//
saṅghaṭṭaṃ pīḍanaṃ kṛtvā lambakaṃ tu vidārayet /
lambakāmṛtasantṛpto jayen mṛtyuṃ na saṃśayaḥ //159//
dāhaṃ śoṣaṃ tu santāpaṃ vaivarṇaṃ vā mahādbhutam /
nāśayeta varārohe anenābhyāsayogataḥ //160//
rasanāṃ śūnyamadhyasthāṃ kṛtvā caiva nirāśrayām /
na dantair daśanān spṛṣṭvā oṣṭhau naiva parasparam //161//
tyajya sparśanam eteṣāṃ jinen mṛtyuṃ na saṃśayaḥ /
eṣa mṛtyuñjayo yogo na bhūto na bhaviṣyati //162//

159a saṃghaṭṭaṃ] *em.*; saṃghaṭṭe Ed. 160a dāhaṃ śoṣaṃ tu santāpaṃ] *em.*; dāhaśoṣas tu santāpo Ed. 160b mahādbhutam] *em.* GRIFFITHS; mahadbhutam Ed. 161b nirāśrayām] *em.*; nirāśrayam Ed.

92 Cf. *KhV* 2.82c–88d.

93 This has happened to Dr. Ṭhākur when practising *prāṇāyāma* for long periods and to his son when holding his breath while swimming. Satyānanda SARASVATĪ (1993:280) reports "when prana is awakened in the body, the tongue will move into [the *khecarīmudrā*] position spontaneously". I have been introduced to a man who had no knowledge of yogic techniques but whose tongue assumed the *khecarīmudrā* position while he was under the influence of LSD.

Praṇavānand SARASVATĪ (1984:203–4) says that before birth a baby's tongue is in the *khecarīmudrā* position and has to be flicked out after parturition. This breaks the baby's *yoganidrā* ("yogic sleep"), it starts to breathe, experiences hunger and thirst, and beholds *saṃsāra*. An aside attributed to "the haṭhayogic tradition" *(haṭhayogasaṃpradāyaḥ)* is found in the *Haṭharatnāvalī* between vv. 2.135 and 2.136. This corrupt passage appears to say that a fetus practises *lambikāyoga* while in the womb but that at birth the tongue falls down and is bound by the frenum. In a private communication, Dr. Lucy Colfox has told me that babies are in fact born with their tongues in their mouths.

94 Cf. VASUDEVA's definition of *mudrā* cited on page 26.

95 The *Kularatnoddyota* can be dated to approximately the twelfth century CE at the latest. See note 101.

96 The eight *mudrās* correspond to the eight *mātṛs* listed at *KMT* 15.6–7. *Kularatnoddyota* 3.105–108 (I am grateful to Somdev VASUDEVA for providing me with his unpublished edition of *KRU* 3.95a–129b, to which I have added the variants from witness V):

> *sarvadvārāṇi saṃrudhya mārutaṃ saṃniyamya ca /*
> *lalanā ghaṇṭikāntasthā antaḥsrotonirodhikā //105//*
> *ākuñcya karapādau tu muṣṭibandhena suvrate /*
> *ūrdhvonnataṃ mukhaṃ kṛtvā khastham ardhaprasāritam //106//*
> *stabdhe ca tārake kṛtvā ākuñcyādhāramaṇḍalam /*
> *vyomamārgagatāṃ dṛṣṭiṃ manaḥ kṛtvā tadāśrayam //107//*
> *catvarasthaṃ varārohe karaṇaivaṃvidhaṃ matam /*
> *mudreyaṃ khecarī proktā sarvamudreśvareśvarī //108//*
>
> Q=NAK 5427 (NGMPP A 40/21), palm-leaf, Kuṭila, ca. 12th cent. CE; R=NAK 116 (NGMPP A 206/10), paper, Nevārī, dated *saṃvat* 754 (= 1634 CE); S=NAK 55142 (NGMPP A147/10), paper, Devanāgarī; T=NAK 55151 (NGMPP 149/1), paper, Nevārī; U=NAK 42454 (NGMPP A 146/6), paper, Nevārī; V=Chandra Shum Shere c.348, paper, Nevārī.
>
> 105a saṃrudhya] QSTU; saṃrudhyāṃ R, saṃrundhya V 105c lalanā] QSTUV; lalanāṃ R 105d °sroto°] *em.* VASUDEVA; °śroṇi° R, °srota° SV, °śrota° QTU 106a ākuñcya karapādau ca] RSV; ākuñcya karapādau tu Q, ākuñcya karapādo tu T, ākutra kalapādo tu U 106b °bandhena] QST; °bandhana R, °vānūna U, °vāndhana V 106d khasthaṃ] QRSUV; khasthāṃ T 107a stabdhe ca] QTV; tathaiva R, sokṣava° S, stāva U 107c °gatāṃ] QSUV; °gatā R, °gataṃ T 107d manaḥ] QRSTU; mama V ◇ madāśrayam] *conj.* GRIFFITHS; mamāśrayam V, samāśrayam *cett.* 108a catvarasthaṃ] *em.* SANDERSON; tvaccārasthaṃ QRV, catvārasthaṃ STU 108b karaṇaivaṃvidhaṃ] R; karaṇevaṃvidhaṃ QSTUV

97 The "crossroads" *(catvara/catuṣpatha/catuṣkikā)* is in the region of the *brahmarandhra*. See *TĀ* 15.94 and Jayaratha *ad loc.*, *Tantrālokaviveka ad* 5.55a and *NTU* p.147, l.18. I am grateful to Alexis SANDERSON for providing me with these references.

98 *JRY Bhairavānanavidhi Bhūmikāpaṭala* 159a.

99 *KJN* 6.19d.

100 *KRU* 3.110a–112b (for details of the witnesses see note 96):

> *svādhiṣṭhānasya vāmāṅge datvā cittaṃ sureśvari |*
> *paramāmṛtasaṃpūrṇaṃ smarec cakram anāmayam ||110||*
> *sahasrāraṃ mahāmāye vidyāyoginisaṃyutam |*
> *plāvayann amṛtaughena sarvaṃ dehaṃ vicintayet ||111||*
> *mudreyaṃ śaśinī proktā sarvakāryārthasādhanī |*
>
> 111a sahasrāraṃ] QRSV; sahastāraṃ T, sahasrāya U 111b yogini] *short final* i *metri causa* 111c plāvayann] QRSV; plāvayenn TU 111d sarvaṃ dehaṃ] Q; sarvāṃ dehāṃ R; sarvadehaṃ ST, sarvadeha° U, sarvā dehaṃ V 112a śaśinī] QRSTV; śakhinī U

101 The *Kularatnoddyota* must postdate the *Kubjikāmatatantra* since much of it is derived from that work. The *Kubjikāmatatantra* itself postdates the root tantras of Trika Śaivism (Sanderson 1986:163–164). The earliest witness of the *Kularatnoddyota* is a Nepalese palm-leaf manuscript from about the twelfth century CE (manuscript Q in the apparatus in note 96).

102 For detailed studies of *mudrā* in tantric Śaivism see Vasudeva 1997 and Padoux 1990b.

103 *KMT* 6.81c–82b gives a *nirvacana* derivation of the name Khecarī: *khagatir hy ūrdhvabhāvena khagamārgeṇa nityaśaḥ | carate sarvajantūnāṃ khecarī tena sā smṛtā ||* "Motion in the ether arises through the higher existence [?]. Of all creatures, she who always goes *(carate)* by way of the ether *(khagamārgeṇa)* is known as Khecarī." In the *Siddhayogeśvarīmata* (which is devoted to the Yoginī cult—see *paṭalas* 13, 22 and 29 for detailed descriptions of Yoginīs), Khecarī seems to be used as a synonym of Yoginī at 29.20. Sanderson (1987:15) describes Yoginīs as "both supernatural apparitions and human females considered to be permanently possessed by the mother goddesses [cf. *SYM* 22.5ab]. They were to be invoked and/or placated with offerings of blood, flesh, wine and sexual fluids by power-seeking adepts..."

104 See *JRY mudrāṣaṭka* 2.636a, 644d (f.32r), 648d (f.32v); *Parātrīśikā* 1; *Yoginīhṛdaya cakrasaṅketa* 5d etc. The Bhairavāgama is the entire corpus of Tantras of the Mantramārga, excepting those of the Śaiva Siddhānta. For an explanation of the different categories of texts in tantric Śaivism see Sanderson 1988.

105 *KJN* 9.2ab: *sarvasiddhiyoginīnāṃ khecarīṃ sarvamātarīm |*. Cf. *KMT* 15.10, where the eight *mātṛs* are said to be born from the bodies of the Khecarīs: *khecarītanusaṃbhūtāś cāṣṭau mātryaḥ*. In the Buddhist *Hevajratantra*, Khecarī is located at the top of the circle of Yoginīs (*HT* 1.8.15, 1.9.12).

106 At *KJN* 14.93 *paramāmṛta* is located at the *khecarīcakra*. *KMT* 14.65–67 and 15.82 say that the Dūtīs and Yoginīs flood the world with *amṛta* when disturbed *(kṣubdhāḥ)* but this is not said in the description of the Khecarīs in *paṭala* 16.

107 cf. *KMT* 25.214.

108 *TĀ* 32.4ab: *tatra pradhānabhūtā śrīkhecarī devatātmikā |*.

109 *TĀ* 32.64:

> *ekaṃ sṛṣṭimayaṃ bījaṃ yadvīryaṃ sarvamantragam |*
> *ekā mudrā khecarī ca mudraughaḥ prāṇito yayā ||64||*.

110 At *TĀ* 32.26 the *karaṅkinī* variant of the *khecarīmudrā* is described. As well as adopting other physical gestures, the yogin is to touch his palate with his tongue—*jihvayā tālukaṃ spṛśet*. This brings to mind the meditational techniques described in the passages cited above from the Pali canon, the *Viṣṇusmṛti* and the *Maitrāyaṇīyopaniṣad* and is one of the first instances of such practices being linked with the name *khecarīmudrā*. However this should not be seen as significant in the development of the haṭhayogic *khecarīmudrā*. It adds nothing to what is found in the pre-āgamic passages cited above and appears to be simply an instruction on what should be done with the tongue during *sādhana* on the same lines as, say, instructions to gaze at the tip of the nose. Instructions to press the tongue to the palate in the manner of those pre-āgamic passages are found elsewhere in the texts of tantric Śaivism and *haṭhayoga* (see e.g. *Skandapurāṇa* 179.40, *Mṛgendratantra yogapāda* 18c–19b, *Mataṅgapārameśvarāgama yogapāda* 2.27, *KMT* 7.85a, *Bṛhadyogiyājñavalkyasmṛti* 190, *Yājnavalkyasmṛti* 3.199, *HP* 1.45–46 and *DYŚ* 70) and the occurrence of such an instruction in the *Tantrāloka*'s description of a variant of *khecarīmudrā* is probably coincidental.

111 *JRY* 4.2.597d.

112 *Netratantroddyota* 7.32.

113 Perhaps surprisingly, no specific mention is made of flying in the *KhV*. *Khecaratva*, "being a Khecara", is often said to be a reward of the practice but is never specifically said to entail the ability to fly. *Khecaratva* and flying are distinguished in many other texts: a list of *siddhi*s at *KJN* 14.16–19 has both *bhūmityāga*, "leaving the ground", at 17a, and *khecaratva* at 19b; *SSP* 5.34–41 contains a list of *siddhi*s attained after different durations of practice: in the seventh year the yogin becomes *kṣitityāgī* and in the ninth he becomes a Khecara; *AŚ* p.4 ll.11–12 gives a list of *siddhi*s starting with *bhūmityāga* and culminating in *khecaratvapratiṣṭhā*. In his translation of *Vātulanāthasūtra* 1, ŚĀSTRĪ adds "Khecara denotes the man who has made a remarkable progress in the spiritual realm and has, as a result thereof, occupied that state in which one always lives and moves in the ether of consciousness" (translation p.1 n.2).

Explicit mentions of flying are common in the Bhairavāgama. Many of the *JRY*'s *mudrā*s result in the *sādhaka* rising into the air: at 4.2.592d in the description of the *daṃṣṭriṇī mudrā* we read *trisaptāhāt kham utpatet*, "after three weeks he rises up into the air"; at 4.2.632a the result of *karaṅkinī mudrā* is *praharārdhāt plaved vyomni*, "after ninety minutes he floats in the void". The Kashmiri exegetes did not take such passages literally: commenting on *TĀ* 32.16c, where Abhinavagupta has quoted a description of the *triśūlinī mudrā* from the *Yogasaṃcāra* by which "[the yogin] leaves the ground" *(tyajati medinīṃ)*, Jayaratha writes *medinīṃ tyajatīti dehādyahantāpahastanena parabodhākāśacārī bhaved ity arthaḥ*, "when the text says that he leaves the ground it means that he will move in the sky of absolute consciousness by throwing off identification with the body, [the mind, the vital energy] and [the void]" (SANDERSON's unpublished translation). Perhaps the composer(s) of the *KhV* also took this position. We know that folk tales of flying yogins were current at the time of its composition (DIGBY 1970:11–15) and other haṭhayogic texts do mention *bhūmityāga* but not in the context of *khecarīmudrā* (see e.g. *DYŚ* 155,

GhS 5.56; but cf. *MaSaṃ* 18.52 which mentions *kṣitityāga* as the result of a *dhyāna* in which, among other physical attitudes, the tongue is to be placed above the palate). The absence of any mention of *khecarīmudrā* in Ballāla's explanation of *trailokyabhramaṇa ad KhV* 3.6 is telling: *antarikṣamārgeṇa guṭikāvat*, "going by way of the atmosphere like [when one consumes] a pill". Similarly, the *Jogpradīpakā* makes no mention of flying in its lengthy description of *khecarīmudrā*, nor in its description of the *ākāśadhāraṇā*, but does say that *vāyudhāraṇā* results in *gaganagamana* (MS *bhāṃ*; MS *nāṃ* and the edition read *gaganamagana*). Today *khecarīmudrā* is often said by yogins to bestow the power of flight (see note 153). It is perhaps this association which led WHITE (1996:169) to translate the title of the *KhV* with "The Aviator's Science; or The Arcane Science of Flight".

114 See *ŚS* 4.22 (=*HP* 3.5).

115 Not everywhere in the texts of *haṭhayoga* is the practice called *khecarīmudrā*. In the descriptions at *GŚ*$_N$ 131–152, *ŚS* 3.80–95 and *SSP* 6.84 it is not named. In *AŚ* pp.1–3 it is said to be a *sāraṇā*. *MKSG* 11.966a–1020b calls the technique simply *rasanāyoga*, "tongue yoga". *GŚ*$_N$ 70 and *HP* 3.36 give alternative names for *khecarīmudrā*: *nabho mudrā* and *vyomacakra* respectively. *GhS* 3.7 also calls the practice *nabho mudrā*.

116 Although I distinguish between tantric Śaivism and *haṭhayoga*, and between the texts of both, it should be stressed that there is no clear-cut division between the two. The *Śivasaṃhitā*, an archetypal haṭhayogic manual, calls itself a tantra (4.7, 4.25). The *Khecarīvidyā* does the same (1.16) and itself exemplifies the futility of trying to differentiate too strictly between tantric and haṭhayogic works. The origins of many of the practices that are considered quintessentially haṭhayogic can be traced to tantric works (e.g. the haṭhayogic *khecarīmudrā* and the *mūlabandha*, on which see note 299). Similarly, haṭhayogic works contain references to aspects of tantrism that might be thought to have no place in such texts. Thus the yogin who has perfected *sītkārī prāṇāyāma* is said to be "esteemed by the circle of yoginīs" *(yoginīcakrasammānyaḥ)* at *HP* 2.55. In the absence of any yardstick by which to evaluate a text's contents and classify it as haṭhayogic or not, the best method is perhaps to see whether the text considers itself as teaching *haṭhayoga*. However, for the period prior to the composition of the *HP*, this would limit us to the *Dattātreyayogaśastra*, the *Yogabīja*, the *Śārṅgadharapaddhati*, the *Amaraughaprabodha* and the *Śivasaṃhitā*. After the *HP*, the number of explicitly haṭhayogic works increases considerably but these are for the most part commentaries and derivative texts, such as the so-called Yoga Upaniṣads. Exceptions include the *Haṭharatnāvalī* and the *Gheraṇḍasaṃhitā*. At the risk of opening myself to accusations of *ativyāpti*, I include all of the works identified by BOUY (see my note 11) as being used to compile the *HP*, as well as the *Śārṅgadharapaddhati*, the *Amaraughaśāsana* and post-*HP* works which teach *haṭhayoga*, when I talk of "haṭhayogic texts".

117 On this *tattva* see e.g. *Yonitantra* 2.10 and its introduction, p. 27.

118 On which see HEESTERMAN 1964:22–27 and BODEWITZ 1973:213–318.

119 *HP* 3.53ab: *ekaṃ sṛṣṭimayaṃ bījam ekā mudrā ca khecarī* /. This half-verse is also cited by Kṣemarāja in his *Śivasūtravimarśinī* (II.5) where he attributes it to the *Kulacūḍāmaṇitantra*.

120 Although I refer to corporealisation as a "process", the traffic was not all one-way. Thus the transformation by some tantric exegetes of the sex act, or of yogic practices, into mental techniques is the opposite of corporealisation.

121 *TĀ* 5.22a–23b:

> *somasūryāgnisaṃghaṭṭaṃ tatra dhyāyed ananyadhīḥ |*
> *taddhyānāraṇisaṃkṣobhān mahābhairavahavyabhuk ||22||*
> *hṛdayākhye mahākuṇḍe jājvalan sphītatāṃ vrajet |*

122 Textual parallels are described in detail in the notes to the translation.

123 See *SYM paṭala* 11; *MVUT* 16.53–54; *KJN* 5.5–13; *NT paṭala* 7, in which the second of the two techniques taught is called *khecarīmudrā*; *ṢCN* 41–46. Cf. *SYM paṭala* 12 and *MVUT* 14.11-15, 15.16–19 (on which see note 83).
It might be argued that just because the physical *khecarīmudrā* is not mentioned in these texts, that does not mean that it was not practised: many tantric works allude to sexual rites without describing their practical details. Perhaps it was for the guru to instruct the *sādhaka* in the physical practice. However Kṣemarāja's commentary on *NT* 7.16–22 (p. 158 ll. 10–17) describes the technique whereby *śakti* enters the central channel: the *mattagandhasthāna* (i.e. the anus—see *Tantrālokaviveka ad* 6.185c–186b) is to be contracted and relaxed (the passage is cited in full in note 299). Kṣemarāja's mentioning here of a physical practice not alluded to in the *mūla* argues against his having any knowledge of the physical *khecarīmudrā*. The subtle physiology necessary for it is in place: commenting on 7.1–5 (p.147 l.14) he cites a passage describing the sixteen *ādhāras* including the *sudhādhāra*, "the nectar *ādhāra*", which is *lambhikasya* [sic] *sthitaś cordhve*, "situated above the uvula", and *sudhātmakaḥ*, "consisting of nectar" (cf. *Svacchandatantroddyota* 7.218a–226b and *Tantrālokaviveka* 5.55).
The idea of a subtle *khecarīmudrā* persists in the texts of *haṭhayoga*. Thus *HP* 4.43-53, in a section on *rājayoga*, describes *khecarīmudrā* and the flooding of the body with *amṛta* but makes no mention of tongues. Cf. *VS* 4.41–46, 6.23–41 and *Jñāneśvarī* 6.247–260 (Kiehnle 1997:138–9), which describe similar processes but do not call them *khecarīmudrā*.

124 *HP* 3.46–48 (cf. *KhV* 2.68ab and *GBS* 137):

> *gomāṃsaṃ bhakṣayen nityaṃ pibed amaravāruṇīm |*
> *kulīnaṃ tam ahaṃ manye itare kulaghātakāḥ ||46||*
> *gośabdenoditā jihvā tatpraveśo hi tāluni |*
> *gomāṃsabhakṣaṇaṃ tat tu mahāpātakanāśanam ||47||*
> *jihvāpraveśasambhūtavahninotpāditaḥ khalu |*
> *candrāt sravati yaḥ sāraḥ sā syād amaravāruṇī ||48||*

125 Cf. the *JRY* passage cited in note 79 where the tongue, when "at the aperture of the palate" *(tālurandhragatā)*, is described as "in contact with the void" *(śūnyasaṃgame)*, and "free from the slightest touch" *(īṣatsparśavivarjā)*.

126 *GŚ$_N$* 69:

> *cittaṃ carati khe yasmāj jihvā carati khe gatā |*
> *teneyaṃ khecarīmudrā sarvasiddhair namaskṛtā ||69||*

127 On the Kashmiri exegetes' interpretation see Kṣemarāja ad *NT* 7.32 cited on page 26.

128 By "early texts" here I mean those texts which probably or definitely predate the c.1450 CE *HP*. The works which have been used to compile the *HP* are listed in note 11. Besides the *Khecarīvidyā*, three of those texts include descriptions of the haṭhayogic *khecarīmudrā*: the *Gorakṣaśataka* (64–70, 131–152), the *Dattātreyayogaśāstra* (272–273) and the *Śivasaṃhitā* (3.80–95, 4.51–59). The *Siddhasiddhāntapaddhati* probably predates the pre-1363 CE *Śārṅgadharapaddhati* (the description of nine *cakras* at *ŚP* 4351–4363 paraphrases that at *SSP* 2.1–9) and describes an unnamed *khecarīmudrā* at 6.84. The *Amaraughaśāsana* describes an unnamed *khecarīmudrā* on pages 1–2. The composition of this last work, whose authorship is ascribed to Gorakṣanātha, can be dated to before 1525 CE, the date of the manuscript from which it has been edited. It is quite different in style from other haṭhayogic works and, uniquely among such texts, calls the haṭhayogic practices described in its first few verses *sāraṇās*. *Sāraṇā* is one of eighteen processes in the alchemical refinement of mercury described in a quotation in the *Sarvadarśanasaṅgraha*'s ninth chapter (p.205, l.11).

129 These two approaches are later manifestations of the structural poles of Śaivism as identified by SANDERSON (1993:57): "Śaivism in its great internal diversity is the result of the interplay of two fundamental orientations, a liberation-seeking asceticism embodied in the Atimārga and a power-seeking asceticism of Kāpālika character within the Mantramārga." The distinction between liberation-seekers and power-seekers is blurred in haṭhayogic texts but this division into two poles is still helpful in understanding the different approaches to the practice of *haṭhayoga*.

The ideological tensions within the Nātha order are explained by the Nāthas themselves with a legend that is first found in a fourteenth-century Bengali and Sanskrit work, the *Gorakṣavijaya*, and which spread throughout North India. Matsyendranātha, the first human guru of the Nāthas, has become ensnared in the ways of wine, women and song. He is at the palace of the queen of Kadalīdeśa, "Banana country", and passes his time intoxicated, enjoying the company of the sixteen hundred dancing girls who live in the palace. The queen of Kadalīdeśa, fearing that attempts might be made to rescue her new lover, has banned men from the palace. Gorakṣanātha, Matsyendra's disciple, learns of his downfall and sets out to rescue him. He disguises himself as a dancing girl, gains entry to the palace and brings his guru back to his senses by instructing him through song and dance. Gorakṣa then turns all the women into bats and the two of them leave Kadalīdeśa.

This is the basic structure of the legend, which is now found in many different versions. It is interpreted as describing a reformation by Gorakṣa of the Kaula practices taught by Matsyendra. Matsyendra is often described as the originator of kaulism or the *yoginīkaula* tradition: he is the author of the *Kaulajñānanirṇaya* and Jayaratha (*ad TĀ* 1.7) says that 'Macchanda' is famous for being the propagator of the entire *kulaśāstra*. Gorakṣanātha, on the other hand, is portrayed in legend as a more austere and ascetic figure and this is borne out in the Sanskrit texts attributed to him. The original *Gorakṣaśataka* bears little trace of any Kaula inheritance. The interpretation of this legend shows that the contradictions within the Nāthas' texts were apparent to the Nāthas themselves but is a simplification of a more complicated situation in which, for example, the haṭhayogic texts attributed to Dattātreya show less tantric influence than those of Gorakṣa.

130 *ŚP* 4365a–4371b:

> *pūrvābhyastau manovātau mūlādhāranikuñcanāt |*
> *paścime daṇḍamārge tu śaṅkhinyantaḥ praveśayet* ||4365||
> *granthitrayaṃ bhedayitvā nītvā bhramarakandaram |*
> *tatas tu nādajo bindus tataḥ śūnye layaṃ vrajet* ||4366||
> *abhyāsāt tu sthirasvānta ūrdhvaretāś ca jāyate |*
> *parānandamayo yogī jarāmaraṇavarjitaḥ* ||4367||
>
> *atha vā mūlasaṃsthānām udghātais tu prabodhayet |*
> *suptāṃ kuṇḍalinīṃ śaktiṃ bisatantunibhākṛtim* ||4368
> *suṣumṇāntaḥ praveśyaiva pañca cakrāṇi bhedayet |*
> *tataḥ śive śaśāṅkābhe sphurannirmalatejasi* ||4369
> *sahasradalapadmāntaḥsthite śaktiṃ niyojayet |*
> *atha tatsudhayā sarvāṃ sabāhyābhyantarāṃ tanum* ||4370||
> *plāvayitvā tato yogī na kiṃ cid api cintayet |*

131 In the *SSP* (1.66, 2.6, 6.84), *AŚ* (p.1, p.10) and *BVU* (73–76), we find descriptions of the subtle physiology underlying *khecarīmudrā* not referred to in other Sanskrit manuals of *haṭhayoga* in which *amṛta* is secreted at the *daśamadvāra*, "the tenth door", at the end of the *śaṅkhinīnāḍī*, which is located at the *rājadanta* (on which see note 258). *ŚP* 4591–4612 teaches techniques for *videhamukti*, "bodiless [i.e. final] liberation", and *kālavañcana*, "cheating death", similar to those described at *Khecarīvidyā* 3.43c–53b. In the *ŚP* passage, the yogin shuts the nine doors of the body but leaves the tenth open if he wants to abandon his body; if he wants to enter a trance in which death cannot take him but from which he can return, he should shut the tenth door. The tenth door is "frequently referred to in old and medieval Bengali literature" (Dasgupta 1976:240), such as the *Gorakṣavijaya*, and also in the Hindī poems of Gorakhnāth: see *GBS* 135 and *GBP* 11.3. Cf. *AM* 51.1. For analyses of the workings of the *śaṅkhinī nāḍī* see Dasgupta 1976:239-243 and White 1996:254–255.

132 On *nāda* and *bindu* see notes 138 and 325.

133 On *udghāta*, "eruption [of the breath]", see Vasudeva 2004:402–409.

134 See note 9. I have not consulted manuscripts of this unedited text but have relied on the first *adhyāya* of the *Yogakuṇḍalyupaniṣad*, which Bouy (1994:102) has shown to contain eighty of the *Gorakṣaśataka*'s one hundred verses.

135 On *śakticālana* see note 366.

136 *DYŚ* 278–280.

137 *GŚ*$_N$ 69a–70b (a more detailed description is given at *GŚ*$_N$ 131–148):

> *khecaryā mudritaṃ yena vivaraṃ lambikordhvataḥ |*
> *na tasya kṣarate binduḥ kāminyāśleṣitasya ca* ||69||
> *yāvad binduḥ sthito dehe tāvan mṛtyubhayaṃ kutaḥ |*

138 *Bindu* is used more often than *amṛta* when describing the fluid that is to be stored in the head. However the two do seem to be interchangeable: at *KJN* 5.23 in a description of flooding the body we find *bindudhārānipātaiś*, "with the descent of the flow of *bindu*", while at $GŚ_N$ 141b the yogin is instructed to hold the *somakalāmṛtam* in the *viśuddhicakra* and keep it from the mouth of the sun.

139 While the theory of *bindudhāraṇa* is simple enough, there are problems with it in practice. When the tongue is placed in the hollow above the palate the throat is sealed off and saliva gradually accumulates in the mouth (see *MVUT* 21.4, cited in note 82). Eventually the mouth fills up with this fluid and something has to be done with it. Bernard (1982:68) would at first return his tongue to its normal position so that he could swallow it. After some time he was able keep his tongue above the palate while swallowing small amounts. Svoboda (1986:279) was taught to practise *khecarīmudrā* while performing the headstand. He says "Your guru will warn you that whenever you feel something dripping onto your tongue you should not swallow but instead come down out of the posture and let the secretion flow from your mouth into your hand. This is Amrita, which should be taken to your guru, who will put it into a special paan and only then make you eat it." The passage describing *khecarīmudrā* at $GŚ_N$ 138–152 comes after instructions for *viparītakaraṇa*, the headstand, and 144c could be understood as instructing the yogin to come out of the posture to drink the *amṛta* that has accumulated.

The headstand, the chin-lock and *khecarīmudrā* are the three techniques useful for *bindudhāraṇa*. No root text of *haṭhayoga* groups them together but Ballāla does so in the *BKhP* (f. 100v[2]): *khecaryā viparītakaraṇyā jālaṃdharabaṃdhena caṃdrasya bandhanena sūrye hutavahe* (*huta°] em.* Sanderson; *hata°* S) *vāmṛtabiṃdvapatanād dehasya jīvanaṃ sidhyatīti tattvaṃ* |

140 References to the drying up of the juices of the body as an aim of haṭhayogic practice also conflict with the idea of *amṛtaplāvana*: at $GŚ_N$ 77 *mahāmudrā* is said to result in *rasānāṃ śoṣaṇam*, "drying up of fluids"; in a description of *kumbhaka*, breath-retention, *YB* 135cd reads *recake kṣīnatāṃ yāti* (*em.*; *yāte* Ed.) *pūrakaṃ śoṣayet sadā*, "on exhalation [the yogin] becomes weak; inhalation always dries out [the body]"; Kiehnle (1997:136) reports that according to the *Jñāneśvarī* (no reference is given), "the liquids of the body are dried up" by the heat of rising Kuṇḍalinī. The Rāmānandī ascetics with whom I lived during my fieldwork are intent on the drying out and mortification of the body, to which end they perform *dhūnītap*, the austerity of sitting surrounded by smouldering cow-dung fires in the midday sun.

141 It is perhaps possible to reconcile *bindudhāraṇa* with *amṛtaplāvana* by understanding *khecarīmudrā* as sealing one aperture but opening another, thereby diverting the *amṛta* away from the fire in the stomach and into the *nāḍī*s of the body. White (1996:253–255) hints at this and at $GŚ_N$ 141 *amṛta* is said to go *unmārgeṇa*, "by the wrong path", having cheated the mouth of the sun. However the two aims are never described together in the texts. The long version of the *Haṭhapradīpikā* (H_2 5.301 at f. 114v[6–7]) does describe *bindudhāraṇa* as a reward of two to three years of *amṛtaplāvana* but does not suggest that *khecarīmudrā* results in both simultaneously: *amṛtāpūrṇadehasya yogino dvitrivatsarāt | ūrdhvaṃ pravarttate reto aṇimādiguṇodayaḥ ||*.

142 The earliest layer of the *KhV* mentions *melaka* and *khecaratva* as rewards of the practice, and includes a passage on the worship of *madirā*, alcohol, thus suggesting roots in Kaulism. However the passages on the physical practice that were inserted into this earliest layer show fewer Kaula features. The absence of sexual symbolism or allusions to tantric rites involving the consumption of bodily power-substances (see note 333) is striking. The insertion of the tongue into the hollow above the palate and the drinking of the resultant fluid has obvious parallels with such Kaula practices (see e.g. *TĀ* 4.131, *MaSaṃ* 18.11; cf. *HT* 2.4.38–39). This suggests that the compilers of the *Khecarīvidyā* came from a more ascetic or yogic tradition than the Kaula text which they used as the framework for their compilation.

143 White (1996:99) lists the following groups as coming under the aegis of the Nātha order in the twelfth to thirteenth centuries: Pāśupatas, Kāpālikas, Śāktas, Maheśvara Siddhas, Rasa Siddhas, and Buddhist Siddhācāryas.
While containing some internal contradictions as a result of its inclusivism, the *HP* also seems deliberately to avoid mentioning issues that could cause division among rival groups. Thus, while Kuṇḍalinī and the *nāḍī*s are described, the *cakra*s are mentioned just once (under the name *padmāni*, "lotuses"), at 3.2 (=*ŚS* 4.21), where it is said that they are pierced by Kuṇḍalinī when she is awakened. Descriptions or lists of individual *cakra*s do not appear. Different schools of yogins had different systems of *cakra*s and by avoiding a specific description of such a system the *HP* avoids alienating any schools. At *HP* 1.3 Svātmarāma says that he has composed the text for those who do not know *rājayoga* because of their being confused in the darkness of many doctrines *(bhrāntyā bahumatadhvānte)*.

144 A glance through Gharote & Bedekar's *Descriptive Catalogue of Yoga Manuscripts* (1989) quickly reveals the extent of this growth.

145 On their patronage, see for example the account of the relationship of Mahārājā Mān Siṅh of Jodhpur (fl. 1783–1841 CE) with Ayas Dev Nāth in Gold 1995. Callewaert & Beeck's word-index of devotional Hindī literature (1991:q.q.v.) gives many more instances of the vernacular appellation of the Nāthas, *jogī*, than of those of ascetics of other orders, e.g. *vairāgī* and *saṃnyāsī*, suggesting their dominance of the ascetic milieu in the medieval period.

146 In the vernacular texts of the Nāthas composed during this period, the dominant yogic paradigm is that of *ulṭā sādhanā*, "the regressive process", which "involves yogic processes which give a regressive or upward motion to the whole biological as well as psychological systems which in their ordinary nature possess a downward tendency" (Dasgupta 1976:229). *Bindudhāraṇa* is a key part of this process.

147 See *YŚU* 5.39c–42d, of which the first of the two lines not found in the $GŚ_N$ describes the yogin as *samāhitaḥ* while the second has been redacted to avoid $GŚ_N$ 69d's *kāminyāśleṣitasya ca*, "and of [the yogin] embraced by an amorous woman". *DhBU* 79a-86b and *YCU* 52–59 are almost identical to $GŚ_N$ 64–71. Upaniṣadbrahmayogin's commentary to *DU* 6.37–38 (which does not describe *khecarīmudrā*) mentions *amṛtaplāvana* but only of a *liṅga* in the forehead.

148 The *GhS* can be dated to approximately 1700 CE. See the introduction to my edition of the text, pp. xiii–xiv.

149 As *haṭhayoga* entered the Vedāntic mainstream it was slowly stripped of its tantric

heritage. The *GhS* turns *vajrolīmudrā*, the practice of urethral suction, into a simple physical posture (*GhS* 3.39). (The original *vajrolīmudrā*, which was first used to draw up combined sexual fluids, is described at *DYŚ* 299–314.) This process of suppression of tantric elements was given a boost by the Hindu Renaissance of the British period when Hindu apologists felt a need for a monolithic homogeneous Hinduism with which to enter into a dialogue with Christianity. A generous helping of Victorian prudery was thrown into the mix and since then all but the most broad-minded commentators on *haṭhayoga* have dismissed or ignored practices that have left-hand tantric origins. VASU's 1914 edition of the *Śivasaṃhitā* omits entirely the description of the original *vajrolīmudrā* "as it is an obscene practice indulged in by low class Tantrists" (p.51). RIEKER's commentary on the *HP* written in 1972 under the guidance of B.K.S. Iyengar, a well-known *haṭhayoga* teacher from Pune, describes the *vajrolī-*, *sahajolī-* and *amarolī- mudrās* as "a few obscure and repugnant practices... a yoga that has nothing but its name in common with the yoga of a Patanjali or a Ramakrishna" (1992:127).

150 In *Yoga in Modern India* (2004), ALTER shows how modern yoga practice in India has been shaped by western ideas of fitness, physiology and nature cure. The traditional practice of *haṭhayoga* continues, albeit chiefly among ascetics who do not speak English and are thus relatively uninfluenced by modern scientific paradigms. These traditional yogins are not mentioned in ALTER's work. DE MICHELIS (2004) examines the history of modern yoga, concentrating on its philosophical and theoretical underpinnings as promulgated by the Brahmo Samaj, Swami Vivekananda and B.K.S.Iyengar.

151 The now commonplace identification of *rājayoga* with the yoga of Patañjali's *Yogasūtras* dates from the late nineteenth century CE (see DE MICHELIS 2004:178–180). The phrase *rājayoga* is not found in any Sanskrit texts other than those of *haṭhayoga*, in which it is usually the goal of practice rather than the method and is equated with *samādhi* (see *HP* 4.3 and *GhS* 7.17). *DYŚ* 160ab says that *rājayoga* arises through *bindudhāraṇa*. *GhS* 7.3–6 teaches that *rājayoga* encompasses six types of *samādhi: dhyāna, nāda, rasānanda, laya* (these four are produced by *śāmbhavī, khecarī, bhrāmarī* and *yoni mudrā*s respectively), *bhakti* and *manomūrcchā* ('trance'). *HR* 2.105 says that the successful practitioner of *vajrolīmudrā* becomes a *rājayogī*. Some texts teach yogas beyond *rājayoga*: *YB* 143 describes *mahāyoga*, of which *mantra, haṭha, laya* and *rāja* are but levels; after *rājayoga*, *ŚS* 5.208 teaches *rājādhirājayoga*, "the king of kings amongst yogas".

Lāl Jī Bhāī added an interesting slant to the modern idea of *haṭhayoga* being a preliminary practice for *rājayoga*. He told me that *rājayoga* is itself merely a preliminary for *khecarīmudrā*, which in turn leads to the awakening of Kuṇḍalinī.

152 On this long-term *samādhi* see note 425. Ascetics who have practised such *samādhi* (often interring themselves for days or weeks) earn the honorific Hindī title *samādhiṣṭh*, "in *samādhi*".

Since *khecarīmudrā* is a part of yogic practice, it is not surprising that it should be seen as a means to *samādhi*, the *summum bonum* of all yogas. However the trend for subordinating all yogic practice to the goal of *samādhi* is sometimes taken to extremes. See for example SHUKLA (1966:6–7), who analyses the six cleaning practices of *haṭhayoga*, following the interpretation of the *GhS*. *Neti*, the cleansing of the nasal and oral passages, facilitates *khecarīmudrā*, which leads to *rājayoga*. *Karṇadhauti*, ear-cleaning, facilitates the hearing of the internal *nāda*, which again leads to *samādhi*. *Trāṭaka*, staring without blinking, cleans the eyes, facilitating *śāmbhavīmudrā*, the knower of which "becomes one with Brahman". Thus, for SHUKLA, the authors of the haṭhayogic texts "have all along kept the goal of Advaita in view".

153 On the absence of textual evidence linking *khecarīmudrā* with flying see note 113. Praṇavānand SARASVATĪ (1984:204), while acknowledging that *khecarīmudrā* can make the body so light that it rises into the air, explains flying by means of *khecarīmudrā* as the upward movement of breath. For him, the aim of yoga is the cleansing of the *antaḥkaraṇa*. Lāl Jī Bhāī of Rishikesh told me two reasons why he believed flying was possible through *khecarīmudrā*. Firstly, he once sneaked into a Nātha yogin's meditation room, seeking initiation, and found him floating above the ground. Secondly, he had had to remove the fan and lamp from his own meditation room because on more than one occasion he had come out of his meditation to find himself on the other side of the room, having fallen onto the lamp or with his hair caught in the fan. He took this to be evidence that he had flown across the room.

154 As well as emphasising the ineffableness of the fruits of the practice, my informants were adamant that, contrary to instructions found in haṭhayogic texts, guarantees along the lines of "if you do x for y months, z will happen" cannot be made. Each individual's experience is unique.

155 *KJN* 12.3–9 includes descriptions of the *vratin* as *unmattākṛti*, "resembling a madman", *kaśmala*, "dirty", and *nagna*, "naked". *MaSaṃ* 44.2 describes the *sādhaka*: *avadhūto jaṭābhasmanarāsthikṛtabhūṣaṇaḥ* (*em.*; °āḥ A) / *maunī karāśanī bhūtvā paryaṭan pṛthivīm imām* // "Having cast off worldly concerns, wearing matted hair, ashes and human bones, silent, using his hand as a plate [?], wandering the earth".

156 H2 5.331 (f. 117v[6]).

157 H2 5.255 (f. 110r[1–2]): *apavitra pavitro vā sarvāvasthāṃ gato pi vā* / *khecarīṃ* (*em.*; *khecarī cod.*) *kurute yas tu sa siddho nātra saṃśayaḥ* //; H2 5.258 (f. 110r[6–7]): *sahasāpi bhaven mokṣaḥ* (*em.*; *mokṣa cod.*) *saha cāṇḍālapaṇḍitaiḥ* (*em.*; °*paṃḍitaḥ cod.*).

158 The two numerically strongest ascetic orders in India today are the Vaiṣṇava Rāmānandīs and the Śaiva Dasnāmī Saṃnyāsīs. It is notoriously difficult to obtain accurate estimates of ascetic numbers (see e.g. GROSS 1992:118–125). VAN DER VEER (1989:xiii) says that "the Ramanandis have become probably the largest monastic order of North India". CLARK (2004:172) calculates the number of Dasnāmīs to be about 100,000. At the Hardwar Kumbh Melā in 1998 a Rāmānandī Tyāgī *mahant* claimed that the Rāmānandīs numbered about 2,000,000 and the Saṃnyāsīs 1,500,000. The next largest order is that of the Udāsīs who trace their origin to Śrīcand, the eldest son of Guru Nānak. The Rāmānandī Tyāgīs and the Nāgās of both the Saṃnyāsīs and Udāsīs closely resemble the Nāthas in both appearance and lifestyle. The number of Nāthas at the Hardwar Kumbh Melā was less than five hundred and they did not have their own procession *(julūs)* on the main bathing

days.

159 My ethnographic informants are described on pages 60–61.

160 This is only a guiding principle and does not apply to the subgroups. Thus the order of, for example, the witnesses in β (other than those of β_1 which are grouped together because of their similarity) is the order in which they were collated.

161 In this description of the sources of the text of the *Khecarīvidyā*, *paṭala* and verse numbers refer to those of the edition unless stated otherwise.

162 The Asiatic Society of Bengal lost its majesty many years ago but the siglum A was already taken when R_1 and R_2 were collated.

163 Because of the bad condition of the manuscript and the way in which its fragments have been pasted together, I cannot be certain from my microfilm printout that the verso of the last folio really ends with chapter 3, but it seems likely. The left side of 11v is obscured, but there is enough room for the final one and a half *pāda*s of the last verse as finished on 11a.

164 This verse is attributed to Bhartṛhari (*Śatakatrayādisubhāṣitasaṃgraha* v. 697).

165 F. 42(2) is an expansion (introduced with *"prasaṃgāt"*), in a later hand, of the commentary found on f. 42(1)v.

166 Only one side of f. 42(3) is written on.

167 Samvat and Śaka dates corresponding to 1840 CE are found in the final colophon, but these probably refer to a date when the manuscript changed hands. The inserted lines are written in a different hand from the rest of the codex.

168 On these manuscript groups, see page 5.

169 See for example his description of the coprophagic *ajarī kriyā* at f. $47v^{2-4}$, quoted in my notes to the translation of 2.76c–77b, or his detailed description of the preparation for and technique of *vajrolī mudrā* at f. $103v^{1}$–f. $104r^{6}$, which goes into more detail than any other haṭhayogic text and suggests at least close acquaintance with a practitioner of the technique, if not mastery by the commentator himself.

170 PETERSON (1883:117) lists a manuscript entitled *Mahākālayogaśāstre Khecarīvidyā*. It is ascribed to Ādinātha, is dated Samvat 1805 and consists of 300 verses in 15 folios. I have assumed this to be MS P and have not listed it among the unconsulted manuscripts.

171 The readings of R_1 are very similar to those of J_1, more so in fact than those of J_5 which is paired with J_1 to make the subgroup γ_2. The large number of minor errors in R_1 has, however, meant that J_1 and J_5 match one another more often than do J_1 and R_1. To keep the apparatus as concise as possible J_1 and J_5 have been dealt with as a subgroup.

172 Three other manuscripts entitled *Khecarīvidyā* were described in the Institute's catalogue but could not be found by the library staff (No. 187 on p.164 of Part 2c of the catalogue, dated Samvat 1867, 7 folios; No. 5321 in part 21, 20th century, 2 folios, incomplete; No. 18376 on p.236 of part 4, 20th century, 14 folios). By their descriptions it would appear that they contain the work found in MS O rather than that found in the other *KhV* manuscripts.

173 BOUY (1994:82) has shown how the *Haṭhapradīpikā* is for the most part an anthology of passages from other works.

174 There may be more verses from the *Khecarīvidyā* elsewhere in the text: I have not gone through all of the manuscript in detail.
175 Another MS of the *Matsyendrasaṃhitā* in the MMSL (No. 1785), reported as complete by Vyas & Kshirsagar (*ibid.: loc.cit.*) is in fact incomplete. It ends during the 13th *paṭala*, before the *paṭala*s which contain the *Khecarīvidyā*.
176 This is very likely to be MS V.
177 "...*facere Çivam deae Umae exponentem magicam per aerem incedendi scientiam*" (loc.cit.).
178 This could be J2. The date and number of folios correspond but J2 has 8 rather than 9 lines to a side.
179 The majority of my informants are Vaiṣṇava Rāmānandī Tyāgīs. This is because I have spent more time in their company than that of other orders, but also reflects their being the numerically strongest ascetic order in India today (on this point see note 158).
I discuss in detail the practice of yoga by Rāmānandī Tyāgīs in Mallinson 2005.
180 When additions are reported in the bottom register of the apparatus of the critical edition, they are always to be found after the *pāda* under whose verse number and letter they are reported.
181 E.g. 1.17d where μ has *devi* for the *prītyā* found in all the other witnesses and I report it.
182 E.g. 2.45c where K2 has °*jyād* for the readings *syād*, °*khyā* and °*sthād* found in the other witnesses and I do not report it.
183 E.g. 2.68b where K3 has *yogaṃ na* for the other witnesses' *yogena* and I do not report it (*-aṃ* and *-e* are easily confused in Devanāgarī).
184 I have used small asterisks to indicate when an *akṣara* is legible (to me) only with external help (usually the readings of the other witnesses).
185 E.g. *kāryya* for *kārya* and *tatva* for *tattva*.
186 E.g. *ūrdhva* written as *ūrdha*, *ūrddha* and *ūrdva* at 3.26b.
187 E.g. *cintayed vratī* at 3.37b where I report *ca tāṃ* and *priye* as variants of *vratī* but do not report the corresponding forms *cintayec* and *cintayet*.
188 E.g. 2.58a where J3 has the unmetrical *guṇītaḥ* but I report that β has *guṇayutaḥ*.
189 E.g. 1.22c where I have reported that J2 and K2 agree with VPC in reading *nārpayed* when in fact they read *nāryayed* and *nāryayad* respectively.
190 *BKhP* f. $1v^{6-8}$: *atha—atha kadā cid ādināthaḥ priyāvinodena lokopakārāya sarvataṃtrāṇi samāmnāya paścād devyā teṣāṃ jarāmaraṇanāśena yogena sthiratararatatvajñānaṃ kathaṃ syād iti pṛṣṭas tāṃ pratyāha athetyādi* // " 'Now' *(atha)* means: now, once, when Ādinātha had gathered together all the tantras for the amusement of his beloved and the good of the world, the goddess asked 'How does there arise the very permanent knowledge of reality by means of the yoga of those [tantras] which destroys old age and death?' He replied 'Now...' "
191 Originally, at all the occurrences of the word *vidyā* in the text it would have meant "mantra" and that is how I translate it everywhere except in this verse and at 3.55c and 3.69a, where it can be taken to mean "magical science" and refer to the name of the text. On the reasons for these different meanings of *vidyā*, see page 12 of the introduction.

192 "called Khecarī" *(khecarisaṃjñitām)* : *khecara°*, as the stem form of the adjective, is the more correct form and is attested by μMK_2 (cf. *NT* 7.32 *khecarākhyāṃ tu mudrām*); *khecari°*, however, preserves some of the ambiguity over whether the word is being used as an adjective or a substantive. In Śaivism Khecarī is a specific type of etheric Yoginī (e.g. *JRY* 4.2.644 f. 32r, 4.2.685 f. 33r; *KJN* 9.2, 20.10; *KMT paṭalas* 14–16 (where Khecarīs are distinguished from Yoginīs—*paṭala* 16 describes the circle of thirty-two Khecarīs in detail); see also page 25 of the introduction and Hanneder 1998:71 n.39), and a *mudrā* or mantra *(vidyā)* is named after the deity or deities with which it is associated. Thus the *khecarīmudrā* (written as a compound) of Śaivism can be both "the *mudrā* of Khecarī/the Khecarīs" (understood as a *tatpuruṣa* compound) and "the moving in the ether *mudrā*" (as a *karmadhāraya*). In the texts of *haṭhayoga* there are very few traces of the tantric Yoginī cult (one is at *SSP* 3.13 and 6.112 where Khecarī is mentioned in lists of female deities), *khecarī* has an adjectival rather than substantive force and *khecarī mudrā* (often written as two words—see e.g. *HP* 4.43) has only the latter meaning. Thus Ballāla (f. $2r^{2-3}$) understands *khecarīmudrā* to be so called because it causes the tongue to move in the hollow above the uvula: *khe vakṣyamāṇalakṣaṇarājadaṃtordhvamaṃḍale jihvāṃ cārayatīti*. The tantric and haṭhayogic *khecarīmudrās* are discussed in detail on pages 24 to 33 of the introduction.

193 I have adopted the reading *yayā vijñātayā ca syāl* of β_1 for two reasons: firstly, it is similar to μ's corrupt *yayā vijñāyate bhyāsāt*; secondly, it is more sophisticated and semantically apposite than the formulaic *°mātreṇa* constructions found in the rest of $\alpha\beta\gamma$.

194 "with one's whole heart" *(sarvabhāvena)* : Ballāla (f. $4r^2$) explains *sarvabhāvena* with *kāyena vācā manasā svasamarpaṇena vā*, "with body, word, mind, or by offering oneself".

195 "in letter and spirit" *(granthataś cārthataḥ)* : on this expression cf. *KhV* 1.9a, *MVUT* 19.54d, *KMT* 6.34c, 10.88d, 25.197d, *Bṛhatsaṃhitā* 2.13ab.

196 Ballāla analyses the compound *tadabhyāsaprayogataḥ* as a *dvandva* and explains it thus (f. $3v^7$): **pra*yogas tu maṃtravidyāyāḥ* / *evaṃ ca jihvordhvakramamaṃtrapuraścaraṇayor nityābhyāsād ity arthaḥ* / "The 'use' *(prayoga)* is of the mantra. Thus [the compound] means 'from regular practice of raising the tongue and reciting the mantra' ". The different layers of the text (see pages 12 to 13 of the introduction) use *vidyā* and *abhyāsa* in different ways. *Vidyā* as both "mantra" and "magical science" has been mentioned in note 191. *Abhyāsa*, which first occurs here, referred to the practice of repeating the mantra in the earliest layer of the text, but in later layers means the practice of drinking *amṛta* by lengthening the tongue and inserting it above the palate. Ballāla takes it to have the latter meaning throughout his commentary. I have tried to translate *abhyāsa* so that it can be interpreted either way. The two interpretations have resulted in confusion in the text, and corruption in its transmission. Thus, the translation of 1.5–7 is somewhat forced and I can only make sense of 1.42c–43b by taking *abhyāsa* to refer to the tongue practice alone.

197 Ballāla (f. $4v^1$) divides *abhyāsa*, "practice", into two types, internal *(āntara)* and external *(bāhya)*. He further divides the internal practice into two: entry into the

aperture above the palate *(tatpraveśa* cf. 2.102b) and *melaka* (see the next note). The external practice is the lengthening of the tongue described at 1.43–51.

198 All the witnesses except S have *melanaṃ* here. At the other occurrences of *melaka/melana* (1.5d, 6c, 7c, 8a, 9b, 12c, 16b, 41a; 3.56a, 59a) there is more complex disagreement between the witnesses over which form is used. In some witnesses the two do seem to be differentiated. This is particularly so in J_2PFCγ at 1.5–7, but this appears to be simply an attempt to make sense of a corrupt transmission in which there are two almost identical half-verses (5cd and 6cd). In *MaSaṃ* 17.1–31 *melana* means "meeting [with Khecarīs]" (see below) while at the one occurrence of *melaka* (17.31d) it is an adjective describing the guru who can effect *melana*. However, at *MaSaṃ* 17.52, 18.2 and 18.14 *melaka* is used as a substantive. Ballāla (f. $4v^5$) says that *melana* and *melaka* are synonyms: *melanaṃ melakaṃ vā paryāyaḥ*. To avoid confusion, I have decided to use only *melaka*, the form preferred in the texts of Śaivism from which the word originates. Only *U* and R_2 are similarly partisan, sticking to *melana*. (At 3.56a I have adopted *khecarīmelana* which is attested by all the witnesses.)

Melaka in tantric Śaiva texts implies *yoginīmelaka*, "a meeting with Yoginīs", in which the *sādhaka* causes a circle *(cakra)* of Yoginīs to surround him and grant him *siddhi*s. This reward of tantric *sādhana* is often mentioned in the texts and exegesis of the Bhairavāgama, e.g. *MVUT* 19.21; *JRY* 4.2.350 (f. 19v), 367 (f. 19v), 593 (f. 30r), 647 (f. 32v) etc.; *TĀ* 28:371–384; *KMT* 14.2. Cf. *Hevajratantra* I, *paṭala* 8. *KJN paṭala* 8 (particularly vv. 31–45) describes *yoginīmelaka* and its rewards in detail. Cf. *SYM paṭala* 8 which describes a meeting in the cremation-ground with various terrifying Yoginīs but does not use the word *melaka*. The *melāpasiddha*, "the master of effecting *melaka*", is described in Maheśvarānanda's *Parimala* commentary on 38ab of the *Mahārthamañjarī* (see also Silburn 1968:133–135). *Vātulanāthasūtravṛtti* 5 gives an esoteric interpretation of *siddhayoginīmelāpa* as the union of the perceiver *(grāhaka)* and the perceived *(grāhya)*. *Melaka* is never explicitly stated to be a meeting with Yoginīs in the *KhV*, but 3.56a suggests this by mentioning *khecarīmelana*. All the occurrences of *melaka* are found in the earliest layer of the text (in the context of the *vidyā*) and later tradition does not understand it as referring to a meeting with Yoginīs. Ballāla says that *melana* is a type of internal physical practice (f. $4v^1$), and defines it as the conjunction of the tip of the tongue and *amṛta*, i.e. the drinking of *amṛta* (f. $4v^{4-5}$): *jihvāgrasyādhomukhacandrasravadamṛtasya ca saṃyogas tatpānārtho melanaṃ*.

I have taken *melaka* to be the result of the practice *(abhyāsa)* and have translated accordingly. This interpretation, which I have found necessary in order to make sense of the corrupt transmission (see note 196), may be forced: see *MaSaṃ* 17.43 where even the *sādhaka* who does not practise *(anabhyāsī)* is said to gain everything as a result of *melana*. (The *MaSaṃ* passage is almost certainly derived from the *KhV*; it may thus be the composer's own attempt to resolve the difficulties found in the *KhV*.)

199 Only $\mu R_2 UT$ have 6c–7b. $S\alpha\beta\gamma$ (excluding $M\alpha_3 J_3 J_1$ which omit 6cd) repeat 5cd at 6cd and omit 7ab. The readings found in μ, which suggest *melana* with snakes, may preserve the original reading in some way but are obscure to me. Because it is

the only reading of which I can make sense, I have have had to adopt that of *U*, although it is likely to be the result of redaction by the compiler of the *upaniṣad*. It may be that originally there was one verse rather than two at 6–7. The common practice of scribes of tantric manuscripts writing a variant line immediately after that which has been adopted could be responsible for the confusing similarity of verses 6 and 7. I am grateful to Dominic GOODALL for making this suggestion.

200 The meaning of *siddhi* falls somewhere between "magical power", "perfection", "accomplishment" and "success".

201 "*Mahākāla*" could mean the *Mahākālasaṃhitā* attributed to Ādinātha. In *paṭala* 6 of its *Kāmakalākhaṇḍa* the *khecarīsiddhividhānam* is given. By means of a magical *guṭikā*, yantras, mantras and propitiation of deities, the yogin attains *khecarīsiddhi*. However, it is very likely that the *MKS* postdates the *KhV* (see page 12 of the introduction). The *Jayadrathayāmala* lists a *Mahākālīsaṃhitā* associated with the *Viṣṇuyāmala* and a *Mahākālyupasaṃhitā* associated with the *Yoginījālaśambara* at ff. 180r and 176r respectively (DYCZKOWSKI 1988:118 and 112). The *Mahāsiddhasāratantra* lists a *Mahākālatantra* among those of the northern Rathakrāntā (AVALON 1914:lxvi). WHITE (1996:472 n.73) mentions a *Mahākālatantrarāja* in the *Kanjur*, a manuscript of which from the NAK has been microfilmed by the NGMPP (reel E-1358/7). JHĀ (1976:9) describes in brief a Buddhist *Mahākālatantra* as found in a manuscript from the Kāśīprasād Jāyasavāl Śodh Saṃsthān.

202 *Vivekamārtaṇḍa* is the original name of the text now more commonly known as the *Gorakṣaśataka* or *Gorakṣasaṃhitā*, a treatise on *haṭhayoga* attributed to Gorakṣanātha. Several editions of the work exist, the best being that of Nowotny (1976), in which *khecarīmudrā* is described at 64–69 and 138–152. This mention of a known work provides us with a *terminus a quo* for the *Khecarīvidyā*. (It is possible that in the text from which the *Khecarīvidyā*'s framework was borrowed (see pages 12 to 13) the name of a work other than the *Vivekamārtaṇḍa* was originally found here and replaced by the redactor of the *Khecarīvidyā*.) See page 4 and note 9 in the introduction for further details.

203 Here $R_2S\alpha_1\beta\gamma$ have *śāmbhavam*, A has *śābharam*, J_6J_7 have *śāṃvaram* and α_3 has *śobhanam*. Apart from a mention in the *Jayadrathayāmala* (f. 179v—DYCZKOWSKI 1988:115) of a *Śāmbaramatatantra* associated with the *Brahmayāmala*, I have found no mention of tantras by these names and have made the conjecture that *śābaram* is the original reading. The *Śābaratantra* (or *Śābaratantras*; see GOUDRIAAN & GUPTA 1981:120–121) is associated with the Nātha order (DYCZKOWSKI 1988:28 and n. 144). The colophon of a manuscript entitled *Divyaśābaratantra* (No. 8355 in the Asiatic Society of Bengal Library) reads *iti śrīdivyaśābare gorakṣasiddhiharaṇe dattātreyasiddhisopāne nāma ekādaśapaṭalaḥ* (GHAROTE & BEDEKAR 1989:84–85) while MS No. 10542 in the same library, entitled *Śābaratantra*, ascribes the text to Gorakhanātha (ibid. 360). A *Śābaratantra* is quoted extensively in the *Mahākālasaṃhitā* and in the *Gorakṣasiddhāntasaṃgraha* (pp.14–15). *KJN* 9.6 and *HP* 1.5 include Śabara in lists of *siddhas*.

204 The *Nityāṣoḍaśikārṇava*, the root text of the cult of Tripurasundarī which was known (as the *Vāmakeśvarīmata*) to the thirteenth-century Kashmiri commentator Jayaratha, mentions a *Viśuddheśvaratantra* (1.21b). AVALON, citing the *Mahāsiddha-*

sāratantra includes a *Viśuddheśvaratantra* among the 64 tantras of the Viṣṇukrāntā in the east and the 64 of the Aśvakrāntā in the south (1914:lxv–lxvi). KAVIRĀJ (1972:597) mentions six relatively late East Indian texts which quote from a *Viśuddheśvaratantra*: Kṛṣṇānanda's *Tantrasāra* (1580 CE), the *Puraścaryārṇava*, the *Mantramahārṇava*, the *Tārābhaktisudhārṇava*, the *Tārārahasyavṛtti* and the *Āgamatattvavilāsa* of Raghunātha Vāgīśa (1687 CE). The *Tārābhaktisudhārṇava* consists mainly of quotations, including many from the *Mahākālasaṃhitā*. The *Viśuddheśvara* is quoted in two places (pp. 127 and 148). The Bombay University Library Catalogue of Manuscripts (s.v. *Mahākālayogaśāstra*) says that the *KhV* is also quoted in the *Tārābhaktisudhārṇava* but I have been unable to locate any such quotation (confusion between the *Mahākālasaṃhitā* and *Mahākālayogaśāstra* is probably responsible for this incorrect attribution).

205 Like the *Viśuddheśvara*, the *Jālaśaṃvara* is mentioned in the *Nityāṣoḍaśikārṇava* (1.14). A tantra called *Jālasaṃvara* is mentioned in a list of tantras given at *Kularatnoddyota* 1.13 (Chandra Sham Shere c. 348 f. $2r^3$). *JRY* f. 176a lists the twelve tantras and twenty Upasaṃhitās of the *Yoginījālaśambara* root tantra. The same work mentions *Śambarā* in a list of Mata tantras at f. 185r (DYCZKOWSKI 1988:121). *SYM* 29.16c mentions a *Savaratantra*. The *Mahāsiddhasāratantra* includes a *Samvaratantra* among the 64 tantras of the Rathakrāntā, the northern region of the subcontinent (AVALON 1914:lxvi). *KJN* 21.4 mentions *sambara* as the name of a Kaula school.

206 Ballāla (f. $6v^1$) lists more works in which *khecarīsiddhi* is described: the sixty-four Tantras, Lakṣmīdhara's commentary on the *Saundaryalaharī* and "the *Śivasaṃhitā* etc." *(śivasaṃhitādau)*.

207 "in the Khecarī doctrine" *(khecarīmate)* : a text called *Khecarīmata* is mentioned at *TĀ* 29.165b (and *Tantrālokaviveka ad loc.*) and in a list of sixteen *Mata*s in the *Manthānabhairavatantra* (NAK 5-4630, f. 209r) v. 28d. It seems unlikely however that a specific text is being referred to in this verse of the *KhV*. An inventory of religious teachings in the *Kularatnoddyota* (Bodleian Library Chandra Shum Shere Collection c.348 f. $2r^{1-2}$) also mentions *khecarīmata*. (I am grateful to Alexis SANDERSON for providing me with the above references.) A *Khecaratantra* is mentioned at *SYM* 29.16b.

208 See *SSP* 6.99–116 for a similar passage on keeping a text safe.

209 Cf. *JRY* 2.10.50d–51b (NAK 5–4650 f. $27r^1$): *nedaṃ gūḍhaṃ prakāśayet //50// prakāśayanti ye mohād yoginyo bhakṣayanti tān (tān] conj.* SANDERSON*); te codd.)* / "[The yogin] should not make this secret public. Yoginīs eat those who through ignorance make [it] public." Another passage describing Yoginīs eating negligent *sādhaka*s can be found in the Buddhist *Cakrasaṃvaratantra* (38.2–5: Baroda Oriental Institute Acc. No. 13290, f. 27v). I am grateful to Alexis SANDERSON for pointing out these parallel passages.

210 The *granthi* is the knot in the string that holds together the leaves of the book *(grantha)*.

211 i.e. a libation pertaining to Kaula tantric practice. *KJN* 11.20 says that alcohol should be used for *devatātarpaṇa*: *devatātarpaṇārthāya surā deyā yathocitā*. *KAT* 6.26–35 describes *kaulikatarpaṇa* in detail. Cf. *MaSaṃ* 17.26c–29b. On this verse,

Ballāla writes (f. 8v[7]) *kaulikatarpaṇaṃ nāma vāmamārgācaraṇaṃ*, "the *kaula* libation is a practice of the left[-hand] path". He goes on to say (f. 8v[9]–f. 9r[5]) that because the practices of the left-hand path conflict with Vedic practice *(vāmasya vedaviruddhatvena)*, *kaulikatarpaṇam* must have a different meaning. He quotes from *ŚS* 4.6: *pītvā kulāmṛtaṃ divyaṃ punar eva viśet kulam* and equates *kulāmṛtam* with the *amṛta* drunk by means of *khecarīmudrā* and *kulam* with the *nāga nāḍī*. Thus he explains the external tantric practice of *kaulikatarpaṇam* as an internal haṭhayogic technique of sprinkling the *nāga nāḍī* with *amṛta*. The variant readings in GTK_2K_5 are less subtle attempts at getting around the problem.

212 Ballāla (f. 9r[9]–f. 9v[1]) lists the following as suitable fragrances: *candana* (sandal), *tamāla* (laurel), *mustaka* (*Cyperus rotunda* Linn.—Dash & Kashyap 1980:25), *kuṅkuma* (saffron), *kuṣṭhaka* (*Sassurea lappa* C.B.Clarke—Dash & Kashyap 1980: 61), *rocanā* (? probably *gorocanā*, a bright yellow orpiment—Monier-Williams 1988: s.v.), *nakha* (*Unguis odoratus*—ibid.:s.v.), *tāmbūla* (betel) and *yakṣakardama*, which consists of *karpūra* (camphor), *aguru* (aloe), *kastūrī* (musk) and *kaṅkola* (cubeb).

213 Cf. *Yonitantra* 6.3: *etat tantram mahādevi yasya gehe virājate | nāgnicaurabhayaṃ tasya ante ca mokṣabhāg bhavet ||* "He who has this tantra in his house is in no danger of fire or theft and in the end he becomes liberated".

214 In 26d I have adopted the reading found only in W_1 (and with corruptions in N). The witnesses that usually preserve the oldest readings, μ and G (as well as α), have the verb *samīhate* rather than the *saṃvadet* of $S\beta\gamma$ and I have thus adopted *samīhate*. As the object of the verb, μ and G have *saṃsiddhīni* and *saṃsiddhāni* respectively; *saṃsiddhīni* is corrupt while *saṃsiddhāni* is semantically inappropriate—we want a word meaning "*siddhi*s" here. Perhaps the original reading was that of μ and *saṃsiddhīni* was an *aiśa* form meaning *siddhīḥ* but I have decided to adopt the more grammatically correct reading of W_1.

215 Ballāla (f. 11v[9–10]) understands *khecarīṃ yuñjan* to mean "practising *khecarīmudrā*", i.e. inserting the tongue into the cavity above the soft palate and looking between the eyebrows: *khecarīṃ yuṃjann iti | atra khecarīśabdena (°śabdena] conj.* Isaacson & Goodall; *°śabde* S) *taṃtreṇa kapālāṃtarjihvāpraveśo bhrūmadhyadṛṣṭiś ca nirdiśyate || yuṃjanpadasvārasyāt ||* He glosses *khecaryā* with *jihvayā*, "by means of the tongue" (f. 11v[8]), and *khecara* (in *khecarādhipatiḥ*) with *graha*, "planet", and *deva*, "deity" (f. 12r[6]). He then (f. 12r[7]–f. 12v[3]) cites *Yogasūtra* 3.50 and Vyāsa's commentary thereon in which it is said that upon reaching the second stage *(madhumatī bhūmi)* of yoga the gods will invite the yogin to their heavenly paradise. The conscientious yogin should decline this invitation to indulge in sensual pleasures and concentrate on *samādhi*.

216 The abode of the Khecaras or "ethereal beings" is the ether. The visualisation of the lord of ether at 2.57 describes a great circle containing the syllable *haṃ*, thus this phrase denotes the letter *ha*.

217 "Fire" is a common name for the letter *ra*. At *KhV* 2.51–52 the lord of fire is said to contain the syllable *raṃ*.

218 In the *Varṇanāmapaṭala* of the *Jayadrathayāmala* (f. 199r[3]–f. 201r[5]), at verse 6, *ī* is called Mahāmāyā (i.e. Ambā). I have adopted the reading *ambā°* rather than *ahnī°*

or *ambho*°, the readings of μ and G, in order to force the *mantroddhāra* to produce the seed-syllable *hrīṃ* which is attested by various witnesses (see note 225). I have found no instances of *ī* being called *ahnī* or *ambho* so have adopted *ambā* because of the (albeit not completely conclusive) identification in the *JRY*.

219 I take *maṇḍala* to refer to the dot representing *anusvāra*.

220 The Khecarī seed-syllable is thus *ha* + *ra* + *ī* + *ṃ* = *hrīṃ*.
1.32c–37d teaches three different types of Khecarī mantra: 32c–33b teaches the *bīja*, 33c–34b teaches the *vidyā*, and 34c–37d teaches the *kūṭa*.
In witness K_5 (f. $2v^{6}$) a later hand has interpreted the elements of the *khecarībīja*: above *khecarāvasathaṃ* is written *kha*, above *vahnim* an unclear *akṣara* which is probably *ra*, above *aṃvā* is *au*, and above *maṇḍala, candrabindu*. These combine to make the seed-syllable *khrauṃ* (their combination is not given in the manuscript). In the appendix of *MKSK* (p.134) the *khecarībīja* is also said to be *khrauṃ*. Just as in the case of *hrīṃ*, the extraction of *khrauṃ* from this *mantroddhāra* hinges on the identification of *ambā/ahnī/ambhas*. If *au* were anywhere clearly said to have one of these names then the balance would swing in favour of *khrauṃ* as the *khecarībīja*: *khecarāvasatha* could just as well stand for *kha* as *ha*. Gharote, in his introduction to the *Jogpradīpakā* (p. 22), says that the *khecarībīja* is "*Hskhfren*" but he does not report his source for this assertion. Whatever the source, it sounds more like an interpretation of the *kūṭa* mantra given in the *mantroddhāra* at 1.34c–37d; cf. the tantric Śaiva *piṇḍa-nātha* mantras given in note 225.

221 None of the witnesses of μ gives an interpretation of this *mantroddhāra* and I am unable to suggest one myself.

222 All the witnesses except μ_a have *tasyāḥ ṣaḍaṅgaṃ kurvīta* at 34c instead of *ṣaḍaṅga-vidyām vakṣyāmi*. Ballāla (f. $21v^{4-6}$) glosses *ṣaḍaṅgaṃ* with *ṣaḍaṅganyāsaṃ* which he explains at f. $21v^{9-10}$ thus: *sa ca nyāsaḥ aṃguṣṭhādiṣu hṛdādiṣu ca ṣaḍaṃgeṣu kartavyaḥ // yathā / oṃ hrāṃ gsnmphlāṃ aṃguṣṭhābhyāṃ namaḥ //6// oṃ hroṃ gsnmphlā* ṃ* hṛdayāya nama ityādi*. A marginal addition in a later hand cites the tantric maxim that the yogin who does not carry out *nyāsa* will be struck dumb (f. $21v^{mg}$): *nyāsahīno bhaven mūka iti taṃtrokteḥ*.

223 "correctly" *(yathānyāyam)* : Ballāla (f. $22r^{1}$) understands *yathānyāyam* to mean that the yogin should perform the mantra-repetition in exactly the way that he has heard it from his guru: *nyāyo 'tra guruvaktrāt tadgrahaṇaṃ / tad anatikramya yathā-nyāyaṃ /*.

224 33c–35b are found after 53d in all the witnesses. μ has the passage twice, with variants, both after 53d (μ_b) and here (μ_a). Its occurrence after 53d does not fit the context (the lengthening of the tongue) although attempts have been made to adapt it. Hence for *mastakākhyā mahācaṇḍā śikhivahnikavajrabhṛt* several witnesses have *śanaiḥ śanaiḥ mastakāc ca mahāvajrakapāṭabhit*, "[the tongue] gradually breaks the great diamond doorway out of the skull". It seems that the passage was originally where it is first found in μ, was then mistakenly transposed to its position after 53d, and, through conflation of sources, appears in both places in μ. Thus none of the manuscripts entitled *Khecarīvidyā* contains a description of the *khecarīvidyā*.

225 Seven witnesses give one or more interpretations of this *mantroddhāra* (for details see the descriptions of the individual sources): *U: bhaṃ saṃ maṃ paṃ saṃ kṣaṃ,* *bhaṃ saṃ saṃ ṭhaṃ saṃ kṣaṃ, haṃ saṃ maṃ yaṃ saṃ kṣaṃ, bhaṃ saṃ ṣaṃ phaṃ saṃ kṣaṃ, bhaṃ saṃ maṃ vaṃ saṃ kṣaṃ*; S: *gaṃ saṃ naṃ maṃ phaṃ laṃ*; W_1: *ga ma na sa pha laṃ, ga sa na sa pha laṃ, ga sa na ma pha laṃ, oṃ sa kha phroṃ, aṃ sa kha phroṃ*; K_1: *ga ma na sa pha laṃ*; J_4: *haṃ saṃ ṣaṃ phaṃ raṃ iṃ—hsphrīṃ [sic], haṃ saṃ khaṃ phaṃ raṃ īṃ—hskhphrīṃ*; V: *gaṃ saṃ naṃ maṃ phaṃ laṃ, aṃ saṃ khaṃ phreṃ*; O: **hs*phreṃ*. USW_1K_1V add that *hrīṃ* is the *khecarībīja*.

Upaniṣadbrahmayogin's interpretation of the *mantroddhāra* is straightforward: Someśa is *sa*; nine back from there (inclusively) is *bha*; 36ab describes *sa*; eight back from there is *ma*; five back from there is *pa*; the *bīja* of *indu* is *sa*; *kūṭa* is *kṣa*.

The variations on *gamanasaphalaṃ* seem to be attempts to give meaning to the mantra: *gamana[m]*, "going [into the ether]" is *saphalam*, "successful". Ballāla (f. 13v[4]–f. 13(2)v[2]) tries to extract *ga sa na ma pha la* from the *mantroddhāra* (presumably because *ga ma na sa pha la* would have required an impossible amount of verbal contortionism). He starts well: as many sources attest, Someśa is a name for *ṭa*. Nine syllables back from *ṭa* is *ga*. Thirty forward from *ga* is *sa*. He is then in trouble, however, and the remainder of his interpretation is forced.

The *Jogpradīpakā* (between vv. 655 and 656) gives *hāṃ hīṃ huṃ haiṃ hauṃ haḥ* as the *khecarīmantra* and *gaṃ, saṃ, naṃ, maṃ, huṃ* and *laṃ* as elements of a *khecarīnyāsa* which closely matches Ballāla's description given in note 227.

The interpretations found in J_4 and O, and as alternatives in W_1 and V, are more redolent of tantric Śaiva mantras than the others and appear to be variants of the *piṇḍanātha/mātṛsadbhāva* mantra (on which see PADOUX 1990a:422–426). Jayaratha, commenting on *TĀ* 16.160 says that *khecarīhṛdaya* is another name for the *piṇḍanātha*. In the *TĀ* the *piṇḍanātha* is given as *khphreṃ* at 4.189–191, 5.75–85, 30.45–46 and as *hshrphreṃ* at 30.47–49. *Ṣaṭsāhasrasaṃhitā* 1.1 gives it as *hskhphreṃ* (cf. J_4^{vl}'s *hskhphrīṃ*). Despite finding several identifications of Someśa, Candra and Indra in the *JRY*, *MVUT*, *KMT*, *MKS* and various *mantrakośa*s, I have been unable to edit the text in such a way that I can extract a variant of the *piṇḍanātha* (or indeed any recognised mantra) from the *mantroddhāra*.

At the end of its description of *khecarīmantrasādhana*, H_2 gives the mantra form of the *saptavarṇamayī devī khecarīṇām*: *aiṃ hrīṃ klśrīṃ klīṃ haṃ ūṃ sauṃ*.

226 "with many forms [and] residing in the faculties" *(virūpā karaṇāśrayā)* : Ballāla, together with all of the other witnesses except $\mu UT\alpha_3C$, has here the compound *virūpakaraṇāśrayā* which he interprets as meaning the process of ageing: *sā yoginaḥ pūrvarūpāt tāruṇyād viruddhaṃ rūpaṃ virūpaṃ vṛddhatvaṃ tasya karaṇaṃ kṛtis tadāśrayā jarety arthaḥ* (f. 14r[1–2]).

227 Here Ballāla quotes the following passage concerning the *japa* of the *khecarīmantra* which he ascribes to the *Kapilatantra* and other texts *(kapilatantrādau)*. This passage is also found at the end of N (see p.44).

japavidhiś coktaḥ kapilataṃtrādau yathā / ācamya deśakālau saṃkīrtya / asya śrīkhecarīmaṃtrasya / kapila ṛṣiḥ khecarī devatā / gasanamaphalaghaṭākṣaraṃ bījaṃ / hrīṃ śaktiḥ si(f. 14v)ddhir anāyāse⌈na⌉ khecarīmudrāprasādasidhyarthe jape viniyogaḥ / atha nyāsaḥ / gaṃ hṛdayāya namaḥ / saṃ śirase svāhā / naṃ śikhāyai vaṣaṭ / maṃ kavacāya huṃ / phaṃ netratrayāya vauṣaṭ / laṃ astrāya phaṭ / hrāṃ hrīṃ hrūṃ hraiṃ hrauṃ hraḥ // atha dhyānam // ādhārapadmavana khecarirājahaṃsam aṃtar mahā-

gaganavāsavibhāpralekhaṃ || ānaṃdabījakam anaṃgaripoḥ puraṃdhrīm ābrahmalokajananīm abhivādaye tvām iti || anyac ca | mūlālavālakuharād uditā bhavānīty ābhidya ṣaṭsarasijāni śirodalāṃte || bhūyo pi tatra vasasīva sumaṃḍaleṃduniṣpaṃdataḥ paramam amṛtapuṣṭirūpā || mānasopacārair laṃ haṃ yaṃ raṃ vaṃ saṃ bījapūrvair gaṃdhādibhiḥ saṃpūjya maṃtraṃ japed iti || (f. 14r[10]–f. 14v[4]).

228 As remarked in note 196 I can only make sense of this verse by taking *abhyāsa* to refer to the tongue practice. If the *vidyā* has not been obtained then *abhyāsa* cannot mean mantra-repetition. I have been unable to conjecture how the verse might have originally read from the many variants in the witnesses. μ's *yadi* has been adopted over the reading *yathā* of most of the other witnesses because *yathā* is unlikely to be paired with the correlative *tataḥ* found in the second line. The relative clause found in all the witnesses except those of α has been eliminated by adopting K_5's *na labheta* in 42d and, in 43a, the form *saṃmelakādau* found in μGUT rather than the reading *sa melakādau* found in most of the other witnesses. A similar form is found at 2.15d: *devaiḥ saṃmelanaṃ bhavet.*

229 Ballāla (f. 18r[7–9]) recommends using the tip of the right thumb *(dakṣiṇahastāṃguṣṭhāgreṇa).* He explains this practice as a necessary part of *malaśodhana*, "the cleansing of impurity", and as useful in loosening the palate (f. 18v[1–2]): *jihvālāghavasya chedanasādhyatvam iva samudgharṣaṇapūrvakamalaśodhanasya bilalāghavakārakatvāt.* Witnesses AJ7T have *samutkṛṣya* for *samudghṛṣya.* While this may simply be a mistake, it could also refer to a practice not taught in the text but described to me by several of my informants and by BERNARD (1982:67). In this practice the soft palate is loosened by being drawn forwards and upwards (hence *samutkṛṣya*), so as to facilitate the entry of the tongue into the cavity above. My informants said that the yogin should bend the thumb of the right hand and hook it behind the palate. BERNARD was taught to use a bent teaspoon. Cf. *KhV* 2.78c–79b, 2.80.

230 *Euphorbia nerifolia* Linn. (DASH & KASHYAP 1980:27). Ballāla (f. 18v[5]) explains *snuhī* with *snuhī kṣīrikaṃṭakivṛkṣaḥ yasya khaṃḍaṃ dākṣiṇātyāḥ ṣaṣṭhīpūjanadine dvāri sthāpayaṃti | deśīyāś ca thūhara iti vadaṃti* "Snuhī is the Milkthorn tree, part of which southerners place on their doors on the day of worship of the goddess Ṣaṣṭhī. Locally it is called *thūhara*". Nowadays most yogins recommend a razor blade. W_1 lists sixteen types of blade that can be used (see page 44). One of my informants said that a blade was not essential because by pulling the tongue forward and then moving it from side to side one can slowly scrape away the frenum with the lower teeth. The frenum or *fraenum linguae* is the tendon that binds the tongue to the floor of the mouth. See also 2.111 and note 233.

The practice of cutting the frenum can be dangerous and the majority of my informants said that it is unnecessary, including those who had done it themselves. WOODROFFE (1992:209) says that cutting is unnecessary, and results in "a physical injury which interferes with the *[sic]* putting out and withdrawing the tongue without manual help." Of the several texts that describe the haṭhayogic *khecarīmudrā* only the *Khecarīvidyā*, the *Mahākālasaṃhitā* (*MKSG* 11.174–5), the *Haṭhapradīpikā* (3.33-5), the *Haṭharatnāvalī* (2.130–7) and the *Gheraṇḍasaṃhitā* (3.21) deem it necessary that the frenum be cut (see also *KhV* 2.111 where the frenum is called *bandhamṛtyu*, "the fetter of death", and must be cut for freedom from death). The *Jogpradīpakā* (v. 12) says that there are two types of *khecarīmudrā*: with or without cutting. I have met two people (Dr. Thakur of Bombay and Mark Kidd of Cirencester) and heard of two others (Dr. Thakur's son and Mrs. J.Benson of Oxford) who are able to insert their tongues into the cavity above the palate without any preliminary physical exercise. Of course, to lengthen the tongue so much that externally it can reach the top of the head as described at 1.55d will require cutting. I have not met any yogins who have caused themselves serious problems through cutting the frenum, but two of my informants did have very pronounced lisps and I heard first-hand accounts of two yogins, an ascetic of the Caitanya Sampradāya called Svāmī Rāmānand (d. 1991) who lived at Kaivalya Dhām in Lonāvalā, Mahāraṣṭra, and a Rāmānandī Tyāgī from Jaipur, who both had difficulty in eating and talking as a result of their practice of *khecarīmudrā*. *Jogpradīpakā* v. 882 says that if done incorrectly, the cutting of the frenum can result in the loss of the ability to speak.

Ballāla (f. 18v^{9}–f. 19r^{1}) relates what gurus teach about the cutting process: *dakṣiṇahastasyāṃgulāṃgulanyūnasaṃyuktapūrvapūrvasthitatarjanīmadhyamānāmikābhir upary aṃguṣṭhena ca sruvavat dhṛtvā tataḥ ekāṃte dattakapāṭaḥ sāvadhānaḥ ekākī dhṛtādhobhājanaḥ tena dakṣiṇahastasthitaśastrasya madhyena saṃmukhaṃ pārśvena tiryak vā romamātraṃ keśapramāṇaṃ samu*(f. 19r)*chidet pratisomavāsaram iti guravaḥ / tasmin chinne raktam adhaḥ patati tat pūrvādhodhṛtabhājane saṃgṛhya tyajet / ⌈pṛthivyāṃ raktapatananiṣedhāt⌉* "Gurus say: [the yogin] should hold [the blade] like a sacrificial ladle with the thumb of the right hand above the index, middle and ring fingers, which should be joined together, each one below the next. Then in a solitary place, behind a locked door *(dattakapāṭaḥ?)*, carefully, alone, holding a vessel below [his face], with the middle of the blade held in the right hand, from the front, or the side, or obliquely, he should cut a hair's breadth every Monday. On cutting it blood flows. [The yogin] should gather it in a vessel held in front and below [the mouth] and get rid of it. ⌈Because of the prohibition against letting blood fall on the ground.⌉" The long *Haṭhapradīpikā* (witness H2, v. 5.139 f. 99v$^{5-6}$) and its derivative the *Jogpradīpakā* (v. 615) say that the cutting should be done by one's guru, one's pupil, one's friend, one's guru-brother or oneself. H2 adds (v. 5.143 f. 100r$^{2-3}$) *chedayed yo dayāhīno karaṃ tasya na kampate*, "If someone pitiless does the cutting, his hand will not tremble". Gervis (1970:201–2) gives a first-hand account of a guru cutting his disciple's frenum.

231 The cut is rubbed with this powder to prevent it from healing: *chinnabhāgayor asaṃyogārthaṃ* (*BKhP* f. 19r^{2}). About *saindhava*, "rock-salt", Ballāla (f. 19r$^{2-3}$) writes *saiṃdhavaṃ lavaṇam asiddhaṃ tac cāṃtaḥ raktavarṇaṃ paṃjābadeśodbhavaṃ grāhyaṃ*: "*Saindhava* is unrefined salt. [The yogin] should use that found in the Punjab, which has a red colour inside." Ballāla (f. 19r^{3}) glosses *pathyā* with *laghuharītakī* (*Terminalia chebula* Retz. (Meulenbeld 1974:610), an ingredient in *triphalā*: see note 473 in *paṭala* 4) and adds *(ibid.)* that the *pathyā* and *saindhava* are to be used in equal amounts: *samo bhāgo 'tra vivakṣitaḥ*. To rub the powder into the cut, the yogin should use the tips of his index finger and thumb or just the tip of his index finger: *tarjanyaṃguṣṭhāgrābhyāṃ tarjanyagreṇa vā* (f. 19r$^{3-4}$).

The *Jogpradīpakā* includes *sūṭh*, dried ginger, in the list of powdered substances to be rubbed into the cut, adding that a thin thread should be kept under the tongue at all times in order to prevent the cut from healing and that the yogin should eat nothing but small quantities of rice and milk (vv. 618–621).

232 Those of my informants who did cut the frenum told me that it was to be done daily in order to prevent the cut from healing. BERNARD (1982:67) cut his each morning. See also 1.54cd and note 243.

233 Ballāla (f. 19r$^{8-9}$): *rasanāmūlaśirābandhaḥ / rasanā jihvā tasyā mūle yaḥ śirārūpo nāḍīlakṣaṇo baṃdhaḥ / baṃdhanaṃ baṃdhaḥ jarāmṛtyusaṃsārarūpaḥ sa praṇaśyati / asya chedane punar api jananaṃ punar api maraṇam ityādi naśyati /* "The binding tendon at the base of the tongue: the bond at the base of the tongue which has the form of a tendon, which is like a vein, is bondage; that bond, which consists of the cycle of birth and death, is destroyed. When it is cut rebirth and redeath etc. are no more".

234 Ballāla (f. 20r$^{9-10}$) analyses *kālavelāvidhāna°* as a *dvandvasamāsa*. An addition in the margin at the top of f. 20v analyses it as a *tatpuruṣa*, as I have done. Ballāla interprets *kāla* as *prātaḥkālaḥ bhojanāt pūrvaḥ*, "in the morning, before eating" and glosses *velā* with *maryādā*, saying that the tongue should not be extended more than half a finger's breadth *('rdhāṃgulam eva)*.

235 "the tip of the tongue" *(vāgīśvarīdhāmaśiraḥ)* : Vāgīśvarī, "the goddess of speech", is Sarasvatī; her "abode" *(dhāman)* is the tongue (*BKhP* f. 19v^{2}).

236 None of my informants mentioned the use of a cloth but BERNARD (1982:67) writes "I started by 'milking' the tongue. This was accomplished by washing it and then catching hold of it with a linen towel. Any sort of cloth can be used, but I found this to be the most convenient. When the tongue has become sufficiently dry, it can be handled with the bare hands; but the slightest bit of saliva makes it impossible to handle it without the aid of a piece of cloth". Ballāla (f. 19v$^{3-9}$) quotes *Yogabīja* 91–98 for a description of the cloth (on which see note 366).

Ballāla then describes three techniques to be used on the tongue: *cālana*, "moving", *dohana*, "milking", and *tāḍana*, "striking". He says at f. 20r^{6} that although they are not mentioned in the *KhV* they need to be understood because they are a part of *utkarṣaṇa*, "drawing out [of the tongue]", *(utkarṣaṇāṃgatvāt)*. *Cālana* and *dohana* are mentioned at *HP* 3.32 which he quotes at f. 20r$^{7-8}$; cf. *SSP* 6.84. About *cālana*, in which the yogin uses his fingers to pull his tongue from side to side and round in circles in order to lengthen it, Ballāla writes (f. 19v^{10}–f. 20r^{2}): *tatra cālanaṃ nāma jihvādhobhāge kaṃṭhābhimukhadakṣahastāṃguṣṭhaṃ tathā tadupari tarjanīṃ dhṛtvā rasāṃ dṛḍhaṃ dhṛtvā krameṇa śanair vāraṃ vāraṃ sṛkviṇīdvayaṃ paryāyeṇa pīḍayet / evaṃ muhūrtadvayaparyaṃ⌈taṃ⌉ pratyahaṃ kāryaṃ / evam eva jihvāṃ dhṛtvā bhramaṇam api ⌈maṃḍalākāraṃ⌉ kāryaṃ tena sarvataḥ samā vivardhate iti /* Cf. *HPJ* 3.33: *cālanaṃ hastayor aṅguṣṭhatarjanībhyāṃ rasanāṃ gṛhītvā savyāpasavyataḥ parivartanam /* On *dohana*, another technique for lengthening the tongue in which the yogin rubs his tongue with *saindhava* and *pathyā* and milks it like a cow's teat, he quotes an author called Mohanadāsa (f. 20r$^{2-3}$): *jihvāṃ bahiḥ śvavan niṣkāśya tasyāṃ saiṃdhavapathyācūrṇaṃ saiṃdhavamaricacūrṇaṃ vā kṣiptvā dohayet gostanavat / tatprakāraś ca pūrvavat tarjanyaṃguṣṭhābhyāṃ tadūrdhvādhaḥ sthāpitābhyāṃ karābhyāṃ paryāyeṇa dohanam iti.* Ballāla adds that this is to be done *svastikasiddhordhvīkṛtajānvāsanādau sthitvā*, "sitting in postures such as *svastikāsana, siddhāsana,* or one in which the knees are held up", and mentions that the practitioner will dribble a lot *(bahulālāpātaḥ syāt). Dohana* by means of a cloth is described at H2 5.152–161 (f. 100v[5]– f. 101v[1]); the *dohana* described at *Jogpradīpakā* vv. 624–634 is a thorough cleansing of the pharynx. Ballāla then describes the third process, *tāḍana*, which he explains thus (f. 20r[4–6]): *tato ghaṃṭikāṃ tāḍayet | ghaṃṭāśabdas tanmadhyalolakaparaḥ ghaṃṭālolaka iva jihvā ghaṃṭikā ivārthe kan | ghaṃṭālolako yathobhayato lagnaḥ san śabdaṃ karoty evaṃ balenordhvādho daṃtapaṃktau lagnā jihvā ity etat tāḍanam |* The tongue is said to be like the clapper *(lolaka)* of a bell and vice versa (cf. CHAMBERS 1983:113, 231, 1360). It should be struck forcefully against the upper and lower rows of teeth. In 1996, at the Yoga Centre of Benares Hindu University, I met Dr. K.M.Tripāṭhī who demonstrated a technique in which the tip of the tongue is pressed against the front teeth and held there while the mouth is repeatedly opened wide and closed again. It is to be done at least a thousand times a day, he said, and the technique tugs on the *merudaṇḍa* causing Kuṇḍalinī to rise. Dr. Tripāṭhī told me that he had to give up this technique when he got married: householder practices that pull on the lower end of the *merudaṇḍa* are incompatible with the yogin's practice of tugging at the top. This is the only practice that I have come across in my fieldwork or other sources that resembles *tāḍana* in any way. Cf. *GBS* 219, 220 and *Jogpradīpakā* 867, 873–880, in which a single channel (identified with Suṣumṇā in the *Jogpradīpakā*) is said to join the tongue and the penis. The *Jogpradīpakā* passage associates the lengthening of the tongue with *laghutā*, "lightness" (="flaccidness"?), of the penis, the overcoming of sexual urges and the awakening of Kuṇḍalinī. On the connection between the tongue and Kuṇḍalinī, see also note 366.

237 "after regular drawing out" *(nityasaṃkarṣaṇāt)* : °*saṃkarṣaṇāt* seems the correct reading here, since it picks up the *utkarṣayed* of the previous line. μG*U*TSK6 have variants on *saṃgharṣaṇāt*, "rubbing", (S, at f. 20v[3], has *saṃkarṣaṇāt* as an alternative reading). This is explained by Ballāla as *tadadhaḥśirābhāgasyādhastanadaṃtapaṃktau saṃmardanaṃ*, "rubbing part of the tendon below [the tongue] on the lower row of teeth". This method of wearing away the frenum was described to me by one of my informants (see note 230) but its inclusion here in the text seems forced: we have already heard how to cut the frenum; now we want to hear how to lengthen the tongue.

238 *Metri causa*, the edition here has *cibukaṃ mūlaṃ* rather than the semantically preferable but unmetrical *cibukamūlaṃ* found in S and M.

239 "Adam's apple" *(kaṇṭhakūpa°)* : Ballāla (f. 21r[3]) glosses *kaṇṭhakūpa* with *urasa ūrdhvabhāgīyo 'vaṭaḥ*, "the cavity at the upper part of the chest". However, I have translated *kaṇṭhakūpa°* as "Adam's apple" because it must be somewhere between the *cibukaṃ mūlam* of 1.51a and the *kaṇṭhabila* of 1.53d. *VS* 3.70c–71b locates the *kaṇṭhakūpa* six finger-breadths up from the heart and four below the root of the tongue. At 1.53d all the witnesses except μ*U*F state that after six years the tongue reaches the *karṇabila*. This is clearly corrupt, for two reasons: firstly, we have already heard at 1.50d that after only six months it reaches the *karṇabila*;

secondly, 1.53c states that obliquely the tongue reaches the *cūlitala* so now we need a location below the mouth, not to the side. Thus at 1.53d I have adopted the reading *adhaḥ kaṇṭhabilāvadhi* of μ*UF*.

240 "the end of Suṣumṇā" *(brahmarandhrāntam)* : *brahmarandhra*, "opening of Brahmā", usually refers to either the region at the top of the Suṣumṇā *nāḍī* (*GŚ*$_N$ 16, *HP* 4.16, *ATU* 5, *VS* 3.39, *Śāktavijñāna* 16, *SSP* 1.66, 2.25, 2.26, 6.81, *ŚS* 5.134, *KAT* 5.107, *AM* 72.1; see also Silburn 1988:30–33) or the *nāḍī* itself (*HP* 3.4, *VU* 5.30, *VS* 2.17, 2.26, *ŚS* 2.18, *MaSaṃ* 17.13). I have translated it in the latter sense here and understand *brahmarandhrānta* to mean the region on the top of the skull corresponding to the *daśamadvāra*, "tenth door", mentioned in note 131. *SSP* 2.8, in a list of nine *cakras*, locates the *nirvāṇacakra* at the *brahmarandhra*, above the *tālu*° and *bhrū*° *cakras* (I have emended the edition's *bhū* to *bhrū*) and below the *ākāśacakra*. Rai (1982:194) says that according to the *Layayogasaṃhitā* the *brahmarandhra* is at the root of the palate (cf. *ŚS* 5.134–5 where it is said to be the opening of Suṣumṇā and is identified with the *sahasrārā cakra*). *ŚS* 4.22 and 5.159 (quoted by Ballāla at f. 24v^{5}) locate it at the lower end of Suṣumṇā. Thus it seems that often *brahmarandhra* does not refer to a specific place but simply describes somewhere from which the yogin can reach Brahmā.

The stem form *brahma* found here and in many other compounds in the *KhV* is ambiguous: it can denote the deity Brahmā or the ultimate reality *brahman*. In tantric texts and early works of *haṭhayoga* it usually refers to the deity (as in the system of the three *granthis*, *brahma*°, *viṣṇu*° and *rudra*°, at e.g. *HP* 4.70–76; cf. *KhV* 3.3b where *dhāma svāyaṃbhuvaṃ* is used as a synonym of *brahmadhāma*). The inherent ambiguity allows later authors to interpret such compounds in a Vedantic light: e.g. *HPJ* 3.106 where *brahmasthānam* is glossed by Brahmānanda with *brahmāvirbhāvajanakam sthānam*, "the place that reveals *brahman*". I have chosen to translate *brahma*° as Brahmā.

241 "the region above the nape of the neck" *(cūlitalam)* : as far as I am aware, *cūlitala* occurs only in the *MaSaṃ* (9.24a), the *KhV* and derivative texts. From the evidence of 2.49–59 it appears to mean the region above the nape of the neck, on the same level as the forehead and temples. This meaning fits well with the context here. Ballāla (f. 21r$^{6-7}$) agrees, taking *cūli* as a variant form of *cūḍā*, "the crown of the head", and *tala* as meaning "the area below": *tiryak cūlitalaṃ śikhādhobhāgaṃ yāti cūliḥ śikhā | śikhā cūḍā ity amaraḥ | ḍalayor abhedaḥ*. See also 2.18 and note 285.

242 See note 239.

243 "not all at once" *(yugapan na hi)* : Ballāla (f. 22r^{3}) glosses *yugapat* with *ekasamayāvachedena*, "cutting [the frenum] all at once". One of my informants, Govind Dās Jī Mahātyāgī, did cut his frenum all at once. He told me that the cut bled a great deal but that otherwise he had no problems. See also 1.46–48 and the notes thereon. Ballāla adds (f. 22r$^{2-3}$): *yady api abhyāsakāle kadā cid asvāsthyaṃ tadā taddine heyo 'bhyāso 'nyadine susthatāyāṃ kartavyo na jhaṭiti*, "if ill health should ever arise during the practice then it should be abandoned for that day and taken up on another day when good health has returned, not straight away".

244 *brahmabila* is synonymous with *brahmarandhra* in its first sense (see note 240).

245 "the bolt [of the doorway] of Brahmā" *(brahmārgalam)* : Ballāla (f. 22r^{9}) equates the

brahmārgala with the *brahmadvāra*: *brahmārgalaṃ brahmamārgapratibaṃdhakaṃ rājadaṃtordhvadvāraṃ*, "the *brahmārgala* is the door above the uvula which blocks the pathway of Brahmā" (on the *rājadanta* see note 258). In the text, however, the two seem to be distinguished. The *brahmārgala*, "the bolt", is to be rubbed away for three years, after which time the tongue enters the *brahmadvāra*, "the door". 2.1a and 3.44 mention the *brahmārgaladvāra*, "the bolted door of Brahmā". In descriptions of the goddess Kuṇḍalinī she is often said to be asleep blocking the *brahmadvāra* at the base of Suṣumṇā and this is its usual location (*HP* 3.5, $GŚ_N$ 47, *YCU* 37, *ṢCN* 3 and 50). In the *KhV* the *brahmadvāra* is at the other end of Suṣumṇā, at the opening at the base of the palate.

1.55c–57b is puzzling. After a total of seven years the yogin is instructed to start rubbing at the *brahmārgala* so that after a further three years the tongue might enter the *brahmadvāra*. This is the first time in the section on the physical practice that the yogin is told to try to turn his tongue back. As I have noted at 1.46a it is possible to insert the tongue into the cavity above the soft palate without any preparation. So what is the internal destination for a tongue that externally can reach the crown of the head? The cavity above the soft palate is surrounded by bone so it would seem that however much rubbing the yogin may do there is nowhere else for the tongue to go. And why should the yogin wait so long before turning back his tongue? Are the verses that describe the extreme extension of the tongue so much *arthavāda*, designed to put off prospective *khecarīsiddhas*? Or did some yogins actually lengthen their tongues this much in displays of ascetic self-mortification? None of my informants had particularly long tongues yet most claimed that they had perfected the practice. I have heard of one yogin, Sampat Nāth of Ajmer, Rajasthan, whose tongue could reach his *bhrūmadhya* (personal communication from Robin Brown, 1996). No other text (except the *MKS* whose description derives from that of the *Khecarīvidyā*) claims that such extreme lengthening of the tongue is necessary to practise *khecarīmudrā*. *HP* 3.32 states *chedanacālanadohaiḥ kalāṃ krameṇa vardhayet tāvat* / *sā yāvad bhrūmadhyaṃ spṛśati tadā khecarīsiddhiḥ* // "By means of cutting, manipulation and milking [the yogin] should gradually lengthen the tongue until it touches the centre of the eyebrows. Then [there is] *khecarīsiddhi*." Cf. *KhV* 1.73ab, where the *siddhi*s brought about by means of the practice are said to arise between the eyebrows. The two other texts that deem the cutting of the frenum necessary for the perfection of *khecarīmudrā*, the *Haṭharatnāvalī* (2.130–142) and the *Gheraṇḍasaṃhitā* (3.21–22), also state that the tongue need only be lengthened enough for it to reach the region between the eyebrows. There is one ancillary benefit of lengthening the tongue: it can be used internally to control which nostril the yogin is breathing through, thus eliminating the need to use the hands during *prāṇāyāma*. This was reported to me by several of the yogins I met during my fieldwork and is described by Bernard (1982:68).

246 It is hard for the gods to pierce "because they are intent on pleasure" *(bhogāsaktatvāt)* : Ballāla f. 22r[9].

247 "the door of Brahmā" *(brahmadvāra)* : in the *Khecarīvidyā*, *brahmarandhra*, *brahmabila* and *brahmadvāra* seem to be synonymous (see notes 240 and 244). Kavirāj (1987:51) reports that in the *Vairāṭapurāṇa* the *brahmadvāracakra* is above the forehead but below the *brahmarandhra* in the cranium.

248 "churning" *(mathana)* : where the word *mathana* occurs in the text (1.57–63, 2.101–104), witnesses μSM occasionally, but not consistently, read *maṃthana.* This reflects the two forms that the root can take: $\sqrt{math}$ and $\sqrt{manth}$ (WHITNEY 1988:117).

249 Ballāla (f. 23r[3–4]) explains that the thread is passed through a small hole in the probe, like that in a needle: *tena* ⌈*sūcyām iva*⌉ *śalākānuchidre protenety arthaḥ* /.

250 It is not clear to me how this practice is to be carried out. Ballāla adds little to what is found in the text, thereby indicating that he too is unfamiliar with the practice. In his commentary on 2.101 (f. 58r[4]) he explains the purpose of practising *mathana* as *sarvamalaśodhanārtham*, "to cleanse away all impurity". This is clearly not the main aim of the practice since 1.64 says that *mathana* brings about *saṃsiddhi* and identification of body and self with the universe. In the *Khecarīvidyā*, it appears that after the probe is inserted into the nasal cavity it is to be moved about by the tongue, which has entered the cavity via the palate. The word *mathana* usually refers either to the rubbing of wood to produce fire, particularly in a sacrificial context, or to the churning of milk to produce butter. It is used in this second sense in the archaic myth of the churning of the ocean of milk by the *deva*s and *asura*s (*MBh* 1.17–19; cf. *SYM* 21.7, 22.36; see also GONDA 1965:61). Both senses of the word seem applicable here. Firstly, at *KhV* 2.72–75 the yogin is instructed to churn the circle of fire *(mathitvā maṇḍalaṃ vahneḥ)* at the base of the tongue *(jihvāmūle)* and thereby melt the orb of the moon into *amṛta* (cf. *HP* 3.48). MONIER-WILLIAMS [1988:s.v.] reports that *śalākā* can mean "a match or thin piece of wood (used for ignition by friction)". Secondly, when the ocean of milk was churned, *amṛta* was among the fourteen items that were produced. No yogin that I have met practises *mathana* as described here but Dr. Ṭhākur of Mumbai did describe how during his practice of *prāṇāyāma* and *khecarīmudrā* his tongue would involuntarily start to "bang away like a drill going into a hole".

The *Jogpradīpakā* has the most coherent description of the haṭhayogic *mathana* and describes two varieties. In the first (v. 642) the yogin is to rub the *śivaliṅga*, which is also the *agnisthāna*, at the root of the palate with his thumb three times a day. In the second (vv. 643–653), the yogin is to use a metal peg *(kīla dhātamaya)* to churn, purify and produce *amī* (=*amṛta*) at four places: *ambikā*, the frenum, *lambikā*, the tongue, *tālu*, the palate and *ghaṇṭikā*, the uvula. These four places are said to be the teats of Kāmadhenu (v. 651). Cf. the *Vairāṭapurāṇa*, which locates an *amṛtacakra* in the upper part of the forehead from which "nectar is constantly flowing. This place is described as the abode of the Gāyatrī named Kāmadhenu (the 'wish-giving cow') figured like a milch-cow with four teats, viz. Ambikā, Lambikā, Ghaṇṭikā and Tālikā" (KAVIRĀJ 1987:50). The *Amaraughaśāsana*, describing practices akin to the haṭhayogic *khecarīmudrā*, mentions *kalāpamathana*, "tongue churning", (p.2 l.10, l.13). It says that the practice brings about *nāḍīmukhojjṛmbhaṇam*, "opening of the mouth of the *[śaṅkhinī] nāḍī*", but does not go into detail. *MaSaṃ* 27.7 describes massaging the body with a preparation which has among its ingredients *amṛta* that is *mathanaja*, "produced by churning", and *brahmarandhravinirgata*, "issued forth from the aperture of Brahmā" (see note 328). At *SSP* 2.8 the *nirvāṇacakra*, which is situated at the *brahmarandhra*, is described as *sūcikāgravedhya*, "to be pierced with the tip of a needle"; this, however, sounds more like cranial trepanning than the practice of *mathana* described in the *Khecarīvidyā*. The *SSP*'s reading °*vedhya* is uncertain. A variant °*lekhaṃ* is found in one witness. The passage also appears at *Saubhāgyalakṣmyupaniṣad* 3.8 where we find *sūcikāgṛhetaraṃ* and a paraphrase at *ŚP* 4359 reads *sūcikāgrābham*. Abhinavagupta (*TĀ* 5.22–24) describes an internal *mathana* in which *apāna* and *prāṇa* are churned to force the breath upwards into Suṣumṇā and ignite *udāna*. In one of the earliest textual references to Kuṇḍalinī, the c. eighth-century CE *Tantrasadbhāva* 1.214c–228d (NGMPP reel No. A188/22; the passage is quoted by Kṣemarāja *ad Śivasūtravimarśinī* 2.3 and Jayaratha *ad TĀ* 3.67) describes a technique whereby Kuṇḍalī is awakened through the churning of *bindu*. *KMT* 12.60–67 describes a *mathana* at the *maṇipūra* centre, in which the churning of a *liṅga* in a *yoni* results in *ajñānamalanāśana*, the kindling of *jñānāgni*, a bliss like that generated in sexual intercourse and, finally, *amṛta*, with which the yogin is to visualise his body being flooded. On the *Khecarīvidyā*'s corporealisation of these subtle practices, see page 27.

251 In the texts of *haṭhayoga*, the *jīva* is the vital principle, entering the fetus at the moment of conception (*SSP* 1.68) and leaving with the body's final exhalation (*YCU* 90). It moves about the body, propelled by the breath ($GŚ_N$ 38–39), unless restrained by means of *prāṇāyāma* ($GŚ_N$ 40–41). Ballāla (f. $23r^{10}$) glosses *jīva* with *prāṇa* which seems to be an oversimplification: $GŚ_N$ 37 describes the ten *vāyus* as flowing through the *nāḍīs* while "having the form of the *jīva*" (*jīvarūpinaḥ*). Cf. *ŚP* 4317. See also *KhV* 3.34-46, *VS* 5.4–7, *ŚS* 2.39–53, *ŚP* 4503–4504, *TŚBM* 60-62b, *KJN* 6.1–14 and *YBD* 3.253–293 for descriptions of the workings of the *jīva*.

252 Ballāla (f. $23v^{8}$) says that churning is not meant to be done constantly "because it is very difficult" (*kaṭhinataratvāt*).

253 BERNARD (1982:68) reports that he kept his tongue in the cavity above the soft palate at all times, removing it only "to speak, eat, or engage in some other activity that made its position inconvenient". Cf. *KJN* 6.25c–26d, *GhS* 3.7. Lāl Jī Bhāī told me that *khecarīmudrā* should be practised for two to three hours a day.
The "pathway" is the pathway mentioned at 1.65a.

254 Ballāla (f. $24r^{3-8}$) understands this to mean twelve years from the time of first cutting the frenum, thus equalling the time needed to achieve *siddhi* mentioned at 1.70. He reckons the various stages of the practice up to the perfection of *mathana* to total eight and a half years (in my edition they total ten and a half years), thus leaving three and a half to wait for *saṃsiddhi*. The *Jogpradīpakā* (v. 613) also teaches twelve years as the amount of time needed to master *khecarīmudrā*.

255 Cf. *AY* 1.95ab: *brahmāṇḍaṃ sakalaṃ paśyet karastham iva mauktikam*, "he sees the entire universe like a pearl in [his] hand"; see also *KJN* 14.62–65.

256 "the great pathway" (*mahāmārga*) : this refers to the top of Suṣumṇā (cf. *HP* 3.4 where *mahāpatha* is given as a synonym of Suṣumṇā).

257 "in the skull" (*brahmāṇḍe*) : in the *KhV* *brahmāṇḍa* means "skull" rather than the more usual "macrocosm"; see 2.36, 2.42, 2.67c–68b, 3.16–17d; cf. *ṢCN* 53d; *AM* 8.1, p.109; *ŚS* 1.51, 1.95, 1.97, 1.99, 2.5, 2.37, 3.9, 5.191 (in which the physical

body is called *brahmāṇḍa*); *GBS* 217; *Kathāsaritsāgara* 2.15; SHEA & TROYER (1843: 132) "the seventh region is that of the head, which is called by the Hindus *brahmāṇḍa*". Ballāla (f. 24r^{9}), however, takes it to mean "macrocosm". Later Sanskrit and haṭhayogic works have a system of 21 *brahmāṇḍa*s in (and above) the head. See *GBP* 19.0 and the *Vairāṭapurāṇa* (KAVIRĀJ 1987:52). At *TĀ* 4.133cd *brahmāṇḍa* (understood to mean the universe by Jayaratha *ad loc.*) is said to arise from the *sahasrāra cakra* at the top of the head.

258 "in the region above the uvula" *(rājadantordhvamaṇḍale)* : the Royal Tooth *(rājadanta)* is the uvula. *SSP* 2.6 locates it at the *tālucakra*, equating it with the *ghaṇṭikāliṅga*, the *mūlarandhra* and the "tenth door" *(daśamadvāra)*, which is the opening of the *śaṅkhinī nāḍī* (on which see note 131). Ballāla interprets *rājadanta* in two ways: firstly (f. 24v$^{1-3}$), it is the microcosmic equivalent of the macrocosmic Prayāgarāja; he thus seems to be putting it in the same place as *trikūṭa* (see note 259) when the text clearly states that it is below *trikūṭa*. Perhaps *trikūṭa* can be thought of as a peak above the confluence. Secondly, "some say" *(ke cit)*, in the body the *rājadanta* is the uvula (f. 24v^{11}–f. 25r^{1}): he describes it as a hanging piece of flesh *(māṃsalolakaḥ)* in the area above the root of the tongue *(jihvāmūlordhvabhāge)* like the clapper of a bell *(ghaṃṭālolakavat)*—cf. note 236. See also 2.29cd, 3.16c–17b and *AŚ* pp.10–11, *GŚ*$_{N}$ 147, *HP* 1.46, 3.21, *ŚS* 3.84, *KJN* 6.23, *KMT* 9.82, 23.167. *Taittirīyopaniṣad* 1.6.1 calls the uvula *indrayoni*, "the source of Indra".

259 "the Three-peaked Mountain" *(trikūṭam)* : this passage and 3.16–17 locate *trikūṭa* between the eyebrows; a variant reading at *SSP* 6.81 locates it at the *brahmarandhra*; see also *KhV* 2.81c, *SSP* 3.5, *YV* 20 (≃*BVU* 73), *AM* 85.2, *GBP* 11.2. *MBh Sabhaparvan* 2.39.11cd implies that *trikūṭa* is in the forehead: *lalāṭasthāṃ trikūṭasthāṃ gaṅgāṃ tripathagām iva*; *MBh Bhīṣmaparvan* supplement 6.3.88 locates it at the base of the palate: *tālumūle ca lampāyāṃ trikūṭaṃ tripathāntaram.* Ballāla (f. 24v$^{1-4}$) continues the theme of micro°/macrocosmic equivalence and takes *mahāmārga* to mean the rivers Gaṅgā, Yamunā and Sarasvatī. Thus *trikūṭa*, where the Iḍā, Piṅgalā and Sarasvatī *nāḍī*s meet, is the bodily equivalent of the confluence of the three rivers, the *triveṇīsaṅgama*, located at Prayāgarāja (the modern-day Allahabad). He explains *trikūṭa* as meaning *trayāṇāṃ mārgāṇāṃ kūṭaṃ*, "the peak of the three ways" (f. 25r$^{5-7}$). At f. 25r$^{3-4}$ he cites *ŚS* 5.132, where the conjunction of the three *nāḍī*s is equated with the confluence in Vārāṇasī of the Gaṅgā with the Varaṇa and Asi rivers.

At f. 25r$^{7-8}$ he cites a list of esoteric centres which he ascribes to the *Kapilagītā* of the *Pādmapurāṇa*: *trikūṭaṃ śrīhaṭhasthānaṃ golhāṭaṃ auṭapīṭhakaṃ // pūrṇādri* (corrected in the margin from *puṇyādri*) *bhrāmarīguṃphā brahmarandhram anukramād iti.* In the margin of f. 25r is a quote attributed to Gorakṣa in which *trikūṭa* is located at the mouth: *asyārtho gorakṣeṇa darśito yathā // mukhaṃ trikūṭam ākhyātaṃ pṛthvītatvam ācāraliṃgaṃ ṛgveda[ḥ] brahmadaivatam īśvaraṃ pītavarṇaṃ jāgrad-* (*em.* ISAACSON & GOODALL; jāgṛd S)*avasthā sthūladeha[ṃ] iti / śrīhaṭhasthānaṃ rasanā'pastatvaṃ guruliṃgaṃ yajurvedaḥ svapnāvasthā viṣṇur deva[ḥ] śvetavarṇaṃ tatvam iti / golhāṭaṃ tu nayanasthānaṃ tejastatvaṃ śivaliṃgaṃ sāmavedaṃ suṣuptāvasthā rudradevaṃ raktavarṇaṃ trimātrādehasaṃbhavam iti / pūrṇapīṭhaṃ ca nāsikauṭhapīṭhasaṃjñakaṃ / pādatatvaṃ ṛṣir vāyur jaṃgamaliṃgaṃ (em.* ISAACSON

& GOODALL; *jaṃgamaṃ liṃga°* S) *daivataṃ* / *atharvavedaṃ (em.; atharvedaṃ* S) *turīyā ca oṃkāraṃ nīlavarṇakam iti* / *puṇyādrir (em.; puṇyādir* S) *merur ity arthaḥ* / *bhrāmarīguṃphā śrotrasthānaṃ ākāśa ṛṣiḥ prāsādaliṃgaṃ sūkṣmavedakaṃ unmanī śivaliṃgaṃ kṛṣṇavarṇam iti* / *brahmaraṃdhre sahasrāre daśamadvāre sarvatatvaṃ tanmātrāśabdasparśādipaṃcakaṃ* // *caitanyaṃ sūkṣmadehaṃ ca parabrahmātmakaṃ mahad iti* /. I have been unable to find this passage in any other text. It is the most detailed description of these esoteric centres and their locations that I have come across. This system is usually found only in texts from the Marāṭhī-speaking region: a similar, but less detailed, passage is found at *AM* 42; see also *AM* 55.2, 63.2; *SSP* 2.27, 6.81–82; *YV* 20–21; *VD* 10. Some lists of *śāktapīṭha*s in SIRCAR (1998:s.v.) include Trikūṭa, Śrīhaṭha and Pūrṇagiri, while the goddess Bhrāmarī is associated with a *pīṭha* called Janasthāna whose microcosmic location is the chin. (As Alexis SANDERSON has suggested to me, Janasthāna may well be wrongly written for Jālasthāna (=Jālandhara).) The *brahmarandhra*'s macrocosmic location is Hiṅg Lāj in Baluchistan. Of the bodily centres listed in the *BKhP*'s citations quoted above, only *golhāṭa* and *auṭapīṭha* are not listed by SIRCAR (1998) as geographical locations. SANDERSON has suggested that they are variant spellings of *kollāṭa* (=Kolhāpur ?) and *auḍapīṭha* (=Oḍḍiyāna). A bodily centre called *gollāṭamaṇḍapa* is mentioned at *SSP* 2.27 with variants *kolhāṭa* and *kollāṭa*. The tentative identification of Kollāṭa with Kolhāpur is supported by a description of female Maharashtrian entertainers called Kolhāṭanīs by SONTHEIMER (1989:236).

A work entitled *Trikūṭārahasya* in the MS collection of the Bodleian Library (Chandra Shum Shere e.83(4)) describes tantric ritual of the Śrīvidyā tradition.

260 *Jogpradīpakā* 651 compares the uvula *(ghaṇṭikā)* to a chickpea sprout.

261 See *Kathāsaritsāgara* 34.69–73 and 56.212 for descriptions of *khanyāvādī* and *bilavādī* Pāśupata ascetics.

262 "the science of controlling the earth" *(mahīvāda)* : Alexis SANDERSON suggested this emendation. *Mahīvāda* is not found in lists of magical sciences, but a synonym *kṣetravāda* (whose meaning is never explicitly stated) is mentioned in Śaiva sources among the *mantravāda*s (see e.g. *Śivadharmottara*, Wellcome Institute for the History of Medicine, London, South Asian MS Collection, No. 16, f. 3r[7]–f. 3v[3], and *JRY* 1.45.150–151a (NAK 5-4650, f. 161v[3])). Most of the witnesses of S$\alpha\beta\gamma$ have °*mahāvāde* (interpreted as a vocative by Ballāla at f. 26r[1]) which seems corrupt. *Rasārṇava* 1.44 gives a hierarchy of *siddhi*s: *khanya°* (a variant found in witness M; the edition has *khaga°*), *bila°*, *mantra°* and *rasa°*. The emendation of *mahīvāda* to *mantravāda* would, however, be unmetrical. K_2's *svarṇādidhātuvādāni*, "the sciences of metals such as gold etc.", for the whole *pāda* is noteworthy but most probably a scribal emendation.

263 Many of my informants told me that the practice of *khecarīmudrā* enables the yogin to go without food and water, a skill necessary for extended periods of *yogābhyāsa*; this is also stated at *GŚ*$_N$ 65 (=*HP* 3.38), *AŚ* p.2 l.3, *GhS* 3.24, *ŚS* 3.93, 5.60 and by BERNARD (1982:68). An addition in the margin of S (f. 21r) quotes *Yogasūtra* 3.29 which suggests early origins for this idea: *kaṇṭhakūpe kṣutpipāsānivṛttiḥ* "[*saṃyama*] upon the hollow of the throat [brings about] the suppression of hunger and thirst". Cf. The passage from the *Suttanipāta* (p. 138, vv. 716–718) cited on pp. 18–19 of

the introduction and note 425 on extended *samādhi.*

Ballāla understands *vratasthaḥ* to mean "living as a *brahmacārin*", i.e. practising celibacy: *guptemdriyasyopasthasamyamaḥ* (f. 27r[2]).

264 This odd-sounding assertion probably means that the *siddhis* only arise as a result of the mental and physical practices which are focussed on the region between the eyebrows (cf. 1.66b). This emphasis on the importance of the region between the eyebrows contradicts 1.50a–55d, where the tongue is to be lengthened until externally it reaches the top of the skull (see note 245), suggesting that the two passages were not composed together.

At 2.22cd the *somamaṇḍala* is said to be between the eyebrows; this verse may be referring to that place.

265 "in the ether" *(ākāśe)* : here *ākāśa* means the cavity above the soft palate. See page 28 of the introduction. Cf. *JRY* 4.2.157a, *MVUT* 21.2, *TĀ* 3.137–140, *AM* 67.1, *GBS* 23; see also White 1996:240–242. The *Khecarīvidyā*'s subtle physiology does not include a system of bodily voids such as those found in some texts of Śaivism and *haṭhayoga* (on which see Vasudeva 2004:263–271).

266 There is disagreement both between the witnesses of the *KhV* and between other haṭhayogic texts over whether or not the teeth should be clenched during the practice. Witnesses A and K3, and *TŚBM* 92 and 146 say that they should not; all the other witnesses, *Mahopaniṣad* 5.75 and *ŚS* 3.87 say that they should. Clenching the teeth is the preference of the more ascetic tradition—it is mentioned in the passages from the Pali canon cited in the introduction (pp.17–19) and is consistent with the ideas of effort and force implicit in the name *haṭhayoga*. Not clenching the teeth is favoured by the tantric tradition: cf. *KMT* 23.161c (see page 23 of my introduction). In instructions for physical postures to be adopted during *sādhana* (but not specifically connected with *khecarīmudrā*) *Mṛgendratantra yogapāda* 19c, *Sarvajñānottaratantra yogapāda* 12a (see Vasudeva 2004:398 n.77) and *JRY* 4.2.683c instruct the *sādhaka* not to touch his teeth with his teeth.

267 "making the mouth [like] the hollow of a crow's beak" *(kākacañcupuṭaṃ vaktraṃ)* : during the practice fluid gathers in the mouth. By pushing out the lips into the shape of a bird's beak there is more room for fluid to collect. In the haṭhayogic practice of *jālandharabandha* (described at *GŚ*$_N$ 62–63, *HP* 3.70–72, etc.) the throat is constricted by letting the head hang forward. The fluid dripping from the moon is thus diverted into the mouth and prevented from falling into the solar region at the stomach (hence the suitability of the name of the practice, *jālandhara*, which can be interpreted as a *vṛddhi* derivative from *jalaṃdhara*, "holding water"). *Jogpradīpakā* 886–889 describes a *jālandharabandha* in which the tongue is placed in the middle of the *trighaṃṭī*, the three sets of orifices at the nostrils, eyes and ears. *Vivekadarpaṇ* 10 mentions the *kākīmukhī* attitude in connection with *jālandharabandha*. Instructions to make the mouth like a bird's beak when practising *khecarīmudrā* are also to be found at *JRY* 4.2.157, *KhV* 3.25, *GŚ*$_N$ 139, *ŚS* 3.85, *GhS* 3.66.

268 Ballāla (f. 27r[10]) glosses *khecaratvam* with *devatvam*: he does not equate *khecaratva* with the ability to fly. See note 113 in the introduction.

269 "all the magical powers" *(siddhi†samayam†)* : the meaning of *samayam* here is not clear. It is tempting to emend °*samayam* to °*santānam* (cf. *KhV* 2.70a). However, Ballāla (f. 28v^{7}) reads *siddhasamayaṃ* (he glosses it with *jhoṭiṃgādivīrādibhūtapretādi* and understands the verse to mean that the *sādhakottama* can quickly get control over all these beings), and I have found three instances of the compound *siddhisamaya* in Buddhist tantras—*Guhyasamājatantra*, prose section after 17.25: *kāyasiddhisamayavajram* (I am grateful to Harunaga Isaacson for providing me with this reference); *Saṃvarodayatantra* 18.30: *siddhisamayasaṃvaraḥ*; *Kṛṣṇayamāritantra* p. 100: *tathāgatasiddhisamayaḥ*.

A marginal note in S (f. 27v) adds that all these *siddhi*s are described in the *Dattātreyatantra* and other texts *(dattātreyataṃtrādau)*.

270 *Pādukāsiddhi* gives the yogin sandals that enable him to go wherever he wishes. Ballāla (f. 27v$^{1-2}$) says that this *siddhi* is explained in the *Nāgārjunatantra* and the *Tantrarāja*, and that the sandals can be used to cross water and travel long distances. *MaSaṃ paṭala* 30 (MS A f. 70v^{6}–f. 71r^{8}) describes *pādukāsiddhi* : the *sādhaka* is to make sandals out of various precious metals, go to a cremation-ground, drink alcohol and repeat a *saptakūṭamantra* one lakh times. The sandals will thus be empowered by the Yoginīs of the cremation-ground. Cf. *Kulacūḍāmaṇitantra* 6.25c–26b, Robinson 1979:258. *Tantrarājatantra paṭala* 17 describes the mantras and effects of sixteen *siddhi*s, including *pādukā*, *khaḍga*, *vetāla*, *añjana*, *ceṭaka* and *yakṣiṇī*.

271 *MKSK paṭala* 6 (pp.52–54) describes *khaḍgasiddhi* : by means of mantras, an offering of his own blood, and, if possible, a human sacrifice *(narabali)*, the *sādhaka* empowers a sword to guarantee him victory in any battle. Cf. *Kulacūḍāmaṇitantra* 6.26c–33d.

272 "power over zombies" *(vetālasiddhi)* : Ballāla (f. 27v^{3}) explains this *siddhi* as *piśācavaśitvam*, "control over ghouls". *MaSaṃ paṭala* 32 (MS A f. 74v^{8}–f. 75r^{11}) describes *vetālasiddhi* : the *sādhaka* should drink alcohol, repeat a *saptakūṭamantra* one lakh times and make a *tarpaṇa* offering of goat's blood. If performed correctly, a *vetāla* appears and becomes his lifelong servant. Cf. *Kulacūḍāmaṇitantra* 6.19a–25b.

273 Realgar *(manaḥśilā)* is red arsenic, an ingredient in elixirs: see e.g. *KhV* 4.9. *Picumata* 46.57 (NAK MS No. 3-370, f. 224v) includes *manaḥśilā* in a list of *siddhi*s, and a Buddhist Kriyātantra, the *Amoghapāśakalparāja*, describes how *manaḥśilā*, when applied to the eyes, can make the wearer invisible and able to move in the ether: *manaḥśilā añjanaṃ vā parijapya akṣiṇy añjayitvā tato 'ntarhito bhavati. ākāśena parikramati* (pp.2–3). Cf. *Kāmasūtra* 7.2.46, in which it is said that if one coats one's hand with the faeces of a peacock that has eaten *haritāla* and/or *manaḥśilā* and touches something, it becomes invisible. I am grateful to Alexis Sanderson for providing me with these references.

274 *MaSaṃ paṭala* 35 (MS A f. 78r^{11}–f. 81r^{9}) gives instructions for *añjanasiddhi* : after a mantra-repetition and visualisation, various recipes are given for the preparation of the ointment *(añjana)* whose ingredients include herbs, honey and, in one concoction, mercury. By applying this ointment to the eyes, the *sādhaka* "sees everything" *(sarvaṃ paśyati)*. Cf. *MKSK paṭala* 6 (p.55), *Kulacūḍāmaṇitantra* 6.34–39. Ballāla (f. 27v^{4}) says that this *siddhi* has been described in the *Nāgārjuna* and *Dattātreya* Tantras.

275 *Vivarasiddhi* is similar to the *bilasiddhi* mentioned at 1.68c. Ballāla (f. 27v[4–6]) glosses it with *bhuvas tatsādhanaṃ* and explains it as the ability to enter ponds, wells, tanks, caves and ditches, and retrieve treasure therefrom.

276 *Ceṭaka*s and *yakṣiṇī*s are genie-like male and female servants respectively. Ballāla (f. 27v[8]) describes *ceṭakasiddhi* as *parapreṣyakāritvam*, "the power to enslave others". He says that the best slave is the *gaṇeśaceṭaka* and gives his mantra. (μ's reading for *ceṭakam*, *kheṭakam*, "shield", may be original.) *Yakṣiṇī*s are usually associated with Kubera and can bestow wealth and sexual favours (see e.g. *KSS* 37.64–83, *BKhP* f. 28v[1]–f. 28v[5]). *MaSaṃ paṭala* 34 (MS A f. 76r[1]–f. 78r[10]) describes *yakṣiṇīsiddhi*: by means of a *trikūṭa* and other mantras, and a visualisation of the goddess, the *sādhaka* gets *yakṣiṇīmelaka*. Ballāla (f. 27v[10]–f. 27r[1]) gives a *yakṣiṇīsiddhimantra* and says that according to the *Nāgārjuna* and *Dattātreya* Tantras there are thirty-two *yakṣiṇī*s.

The syntax of this list of *siddhi*s is odd. 1.75cd is a plural *dvandva* compound while 1.76ab lists its *siddhi*s one by one. G omits 1.75cd, suggesting that the line may be a later addition to the text. Some of the witnesses seem to have attempted to split 1.75cd into separate elements, but it is metrically impossible to alter °*khadgavetāla*° to *khadgo vetālaḥ*.

277 The basic meaning of *kalā* is "a part", especially "a sixteenth part of the moon" (e.g. *Bṛhadāraṇyakopaniṣad* 1.5.14; see GONDA 1965:115–130). The moon waxes and wanes in periods of fifteen days; each day it gains or loses one *kalā*. The sixteenth *kalā* is the *amṛtakalā* (*SSP* 1.63; cf. *ṢCN* 46) which never dies, even at the dark of the moon. (Some tantric texts add a seventeenth *kalā*; see e.g. *TĀ* 3.137, Jayaratha *ad TĀ* 5.63–64, *Parātrīśikāvivaraṇa* 35.) Many texts also describe the *kalā*s of the sun and of fire (e.g. *KAT* 6.37–40, *SSP* 1.63–65, *GBS* 89). The moon's association with *soma* and *amṛta* has led to all of its *kalā*s being thought of as containing *amṛta*, and it is in the sense of a store of *amṛta* that the word *kalā* is used in the *Khecarīvidyā*. *Kalā* can also mean "tongue" (e.g. *HP* 3.33) and, in tantric descriptions of the phonematic emanation of reality, "vowel" (*TĀ* 5.63–64; PADOUX 1990a:89–91). See also note 311; WHITE 1996:36–44.

278 The four aims of man are *kāma*, *artha*, *dharma* and *mokṣa*. See 2.3–6. Cf. *KJN* 5.31, 8.41.

279 I have been unable to find parallels of this list of *kalā*s in other texts.

280 Thus *mokṣa* (see 2.1) is equated with *parameṣṭhīnām ādhipatyam*, "dominion over the highest gods" and subordinated to the end described in the next verse: becoming Śiva, liberated while living.

281 The witnesses here are unanimous in reading *dvādaśābdam*, "for twelve years", or corruptions thereof. One would, however, expect a word meaning "for twelve months" rather than "for twelve years" because of the passage at 2.10–17, in which are listed the rewards obtained each month from drinking the *parāmṛta* in the *brahmarandhra* over a period of a year, culminating in the attainment of Śivahood.

282 For *saha saṃvartate* G has *sadā saṃveṣṭito*: rather than merely associating with the beings listed, the yogin is forever surrounded by them.

283 Cf. *GBS* 138: *parcay jogī unman khelā ahanisi iṃchyā karai devatā syuṃ melā*, "the yogin in the *paricaya* state plays in *unmanī* day and night, and meets with deities

at will".

284 *Jogpradīpakā* 638–640, in a section on *praveśana* (see *Khecarīvidyā* 2.105), lists the rewards of placing the tongue at the *brahmavivara*: after one month the *nāḍī*s are purified, after two months the yogin hears the *anāhata nāda* (Hindī *anahad nād)*, after three months the body has a divine radiance, after four months the yogin has long-distance hearing, after five months the mind becomes like that of a child and after six months the yogin assumes the form of Śiva.

285 Kedāra is located between the eyebrows in *HP* 3.23 and *Darśanopaniṣad* 4.48, but *KhV* 2.49–56 clearly indicates that the *cūlitala* is at the back of the head, above the nape of the neck (see also note 241). The description at 2.22 of a further set of *kalā*s at the *somamaṇḍala* between the eyebrows confirms that the *KhV*'s Kedāra is not located there. White (1996:245–246) describes parallels between the site of the Himalayan shrine of Kedārnāth and the subtle body of haṭhayogic physiology.

286 On the connection between *amṛta* and Soma, see note 277, Dasgupta 1976:250–1 and Gonda 1965: ch. 2.

Instead of *vīravandite*, "o you who are worshipped by the extreme adepts", S$\beta\gamma$ have the *aiśa* sandhi form *'maravandite*, "o you who are worshipped by the gods". This is the only occurrence of an *aiśa* form in the *KhV* manuscripts being found in a correct form in μ. I suspect that this is because of an attempt to get rid of *vīra*°, a word that has strong connotations of left-hand tantrism. Cf. 2.110d, where almost all the witnesses read *saṃsthitā vīravandite*; only G has *saṃsthitāmaravandite* (in which the sandhi is correct).

287 The names of the next sixteen *kalā*s that are listed (eight at Kedāra, four at the *somamaṇḍala*, three at the *khecaramaṇḍala* and the first of the two at the *rājadanta*) match exactly the sixteen *saumyakalā*s listed at *Kulārṇavatantra* 6.37–38 and the lunar *kalā*s listed in a quotation from the *Merutantra* in the third *taraṅga* of the *Puraścaryārṇava* (p. 215; in this list Puṣṭi and Tuṣṭi are transposed). In Amṛtānandanātha's *Dīpikā* on *Yoginīhṛdaya pūjāsaṃketa* 104–105 he lists sixteen *saumyakalā*s: Amṛtā, Mānadā, Pūṣā, Puṣṭi, Prīti, Revatī, Hrīmatī, Śrī, Kānti, Sudhā, Jyotsnā, Haimavatī, Chāyā, Sampūritā, Rāmā and Śyāmā. Monier-Williams (1988:s.vv.), at the entries for each of the names of the eight *kalā*s here located at the *khecaramaṇḍala,* says that they are (in the same order) the names of the *kalā*s of the moon as described in the *Brahmapurāṇa*, but I have been unable to locate any such passage in that work.

288 In this and subsequent descriptions of groups of *kalā*s, it seems that the yogin should spend a month tasting the *amṛta* at each *kalā* because the rewards to be gained are obtained after the same number of months as *kalā*s at that particular *kalāsthāna*.

289 The Orb of Soma *(somamaṇḍala)* probably refers to the moon: the names of the *kalā*s here have particularly lunar connotations; furthermore, in the Kaivalyadhām edition of the *GŚ*$_N$ the moon is called *somamaṇḍala* in verse 56 (Kaivalyadhām 1991:314). *MKSG* 11.997 mentions a *mahācakra* called Soma above the forehead. *MVUT* 16.13 and *VS* 4.41 locate the *somamaṇḍala* at the heart.

290 *samāpibet*: the reading *samāviśet* found in almost all the witnesses seems odd, particularly after *samāveśya* earlier in the line. I have thus adopted Sanderson's

conjectural emendation *samāpibet*. One could understand *samāviśet* to mean "the yogin should enter [*samādhi*]" but there are no similar constructions elsewhere in the text. Ballāla (f. 32v[9]) understands *samāviśet* to mean that the yogin should remain with his tongue in place: *praviśyaiva sthito bhavet*.

291 I have conjectured *yogī* for the first word of 24c where G and the *KhV* manuscripts have *devi*. Nowhere else in the text does a vocative start a half-verse. The manuscripts of μ have *devabhāsacatuṣkoṇa (°keṇa J6)*, "a square of divine appearance", for 24c which does not fit the context and is probably a corruption of the reading found in the other witnesses.

292 Witnesses μG, which often preserve original readings, have *khecaramadhyagam*, "in the middle of Khecara", for *khecaramaṇḍalam*, but I have been unable to locate any other references to a place called Khecara in the body so have adopted the reading of the *KhV* manuscripts. *Khecaramaṇḍala* perhaps refers to the sun, in contrast to the lunar *somamaṇḍala* that has just been described.

293 "known as the Diamond Bulb" *(vajrakandākhyam)* : I have found no references to a *vajrakanda* in the body in other works on yoga. *RAK* 156 mentions a plant called *vajrakanda* in a description of a mercurial preparation. Several works describe an egg-shaped *kanda* or *kandayoni* at the navel as the source of the 72,000 *nāḍīs*, e.g. *GŚ*$_N$ 25 (=*YCU* 14c–15b), *VS* 2.11–12 (=*TŚBM* 58–59), *ŚP* 4307. On the analogy of this *kanda*, the *vajrakanda* may be a point of intersection or origin of *nāḍīs*. See also 2.49c–50b, 2.86 and note 448.

294 The reading found in various forms in the manuscripts of S$\beta\gamma$, *alakṣyaḥ sarvalekhakaiḥ*, is interpreted by Ballāla (f. 33r[10]) to mean "imperceptible by the gods", i.e. "invisible" *(adarśanīyaḥ)*.

295 *nāsikādho 'dharoṣṭhordhvam*: this is an emendation of the reading found in G and, in a corrupt form, in μ. The witnesses of S$\alpha\beta$ have *nāsikādhottaro°* or corrupt versions of it (γ has the nonsensical *nāsikādyotaroṣṭādhaḥ*). This form is the result of a double sandhi ("*ārṣa*" sandhi according to Ballāla at f. 33v[1]) of *nāsikādhaḥ+uttaro°*. I have taken *adharoṣṭha* to mean both the upper and lower lips (cf. MONIER-WILLIAMS 1988:19).

296 As we have seen in note 258 the *rājadanta* or "Royal Tooth" is the uvula, so its description as "below the nostrils and above the lips" is surprising and suggests that it means somewhere in the region of the front teeth. Presumably the description means that the *rājadanta* is on the same horizontal plane as the space below the nostrils and above the lips.

297 "the Base" *(ādhāram)* : this is the *ādhāra* or *mūlādhāra cakra* of tantric and yogic physiology. See e.g. *KJN* 14.15–24b, *KMT* 13.37–52, *ṢCN* 4, *GŚ*$_N$ 18, *YŚU* 1.168.

298 I have found no parallels for this or any of the subsequent lists of *kalās*.

299 i.e. by means of the haṭhayogic *mūlabandha*. Ballāla (f. 34v[1–2]) explains it to be the forcing of breath into the head by sitting in *padmāsana* or *siddhāsana*, contracting the Base and repeating *huṃ huṃ*: *ākuṃcanaṃ tu padmasiddhāsanasthatve sati huṃh* u* ṃkāreṇādhārakamalaṃ saṃkocya tatrasthavāyoḥ pṛṣṭhavaṃśe nayanāṃbhojavṛttau tu nābhimūlāt preritasya vāyoḥ śirasy abhihananam* /. Cf. *GŚ*$_N$ 58–59, *YKU* 1.64, *HP* 3.60–68 etc. In his commentary on *NT* 7.30, Kṣemarāja describes a forerunner of this practice in which the contraction and expansion of the anus cause Kuṇḍalinī to point upwards: *cittaprāṇaikāgryeṇa kandabhūmim avaṣṭabhya tanmūlam iti mattagandhasthānaṃ śanair iti saṃkocavikāsābhyāsena śaktyunmeṣam upalakṣya pīḍayet yathā śaktir ūrdhvamukhaiva bhavati* (see also *NTU* pp.157–158). This repeated contraction and expansion is a feature of the *Gheraṇḍasaṃhitā*'s *aśvinīmudrā* which is also said to awaken Kuṇḍalinī (*GhS* 3.64).

300 "up to his skull" *(brahmāṇḍakāvadhi)* : in the *KhV brahmāṇḍa* means skull. See note 257.

301 Ballāla (f. 35v[7–8]) explains *pañcabhūtalaya* as absorption into the subtle elements: *yady api sthūlānāṃ bhūtānāṃ layo ⟨'⟩saṃbhavas tathāpi tanmātrāṇāṃ lavarayahānāṃ bījabhūtānāṃ tatra tatra japeneṣṭadevatādhyānena ca laye tallayasyārthasiddhatvāt*. In haṭhayogic texts, *laya* is both an aim of yoga (see *KhV* 3.48–52; *AY* 1.21–98, *AŚ* p.5 ll.16–20, *HP* 4.3, 4.29–34 etc.) and a type of yoga itself (e.g. *DYŚ* 29–30 and 37–51, *HP* 4.103, *YB* 143, *ŚP* 4350–4363, *VU* 5.10). *μ*'s reading, *pañcabhūtajayaṃ labhet*, preserves an older idea of mastery over the elements found in the *Yogasūtra* (3.43) and many tantric works (see Vasudeva 2004:240–250). In his commentary on 3.65 (f. 97r[6–8]), Ballāla quotes a passage on *bhūtajaya* which he attributes to the *Mahābhārata*: *bhārate pauṣkare saptadaś⌈ā⌉dhyāye nīlakaṃṭh∗krameṇa pādādi jānuparyaṃtaṃ / jānvādi pāyvaṃtaṃ / pāyvādi hṛdayāṃtaṃ / tato bhrūmadhyāṃtaṃ / tato mūrdhāṃtaṃ / cakrapaṃcakaṃ (paṃcakaṃ] em.; paṃca* S) *paṃcaghaṭikāparyaṃtaṃ mano dhārayato bījāni japata uktadevān dhyāyataś ca tattadbhūtajayo 'vaśyaṃ bhavati /*. See also note 316.

302 "in the morning, in the evening and at midnight" *(trikālābhyāsayogataḥ)* : this is the conventional meaning of *trikāla* and it is understood thus by Ballāla (f. 36r[1–2]).

303 "the place of the penis" *(liṅgasthānam)* : the Svādhiṣṭhāna lotus is located in the region of the penis in $GŚ_N$ 22, *ŚS* 5.103, *ṢCN* 14 etc. Likewise Ballāla puts it *liṅgamūle*, "at the root of the penis" at f. 36r[7]. I have thus adopted G's reading over *μ*'s incorrect *nābhisthānam* and the vague *nābhisthānād adhaḥ* of the other witnesses.

304 As Ballāla notes (f. 37v[8–10]), this and the reward mentioned at 2.45b are presumably the reward described at 2.39.

305 "the Bamboo Staff" *(veṇudaṇḍam)* : I have not come across references to the *veṇudaṇḍa* in any other texts. Ballāla (f. 37r[1]) says that it is the lower part of the spine *(pṛṣṭhavaṃśākhyasya mūlaṃ)* and equates it with the *vajradaṇḍa* described in *YB* 131. G's reading of *vīṇā* may be original: *Tantrarājatantra* 27.35 says that the *vīṇādaṇḍa* is the spine—*suṣumnā pṛṣṭhavaṃśākhyavīṇādaṇḍasya madhyagā*; *YŚU* 6.8 describes the *vīṇādaṇḍa* as being in the region behind the anus and supporting the body *(dehabhṛt)*.

306 45c–48b appear to be a later addition to the text: 48c follows on directly from 45b.

307 Cf. $GŚ_N$ 32, *VS* 2.27–28 etc.

308 The edition's reading of *raviḥ proktaḥ* in 46a is attested only by B and is possibly a scribal emendation. It is tempting to adopt *μ*'s *raver bāhuḥ*, taking it to mean "a ray of the sun" but I have found no parallels for this usage of *bāhu*. The reading *raver vāhaḥ* found in a variety of forms in the other witnesses results in the unwanted repetition of *vāhaḥ*.

309 47a is puzzling and I suspect that the text is corrupt. I have found no parallel passages in other haṭhayogic texts. As Ballāla notes (f. 39r[10]), *dhāraṇā* can mean both fixing of the mind on a single object and fixing of the breath. (The two are linked: Vyāsa in his commentary to *YS* 2.52 states that mental *dhāraṇā* is brought about through breath-control; cf. *HP* 4.23.) I have interpreted this *pāda* with the former sense of *dhāraṇā*. It could also be interpreted with the latter sense, giving the meaning that the yogin is to inhale through the lunar channel but this would be somewhat redundant since the same is said in the next half-verse.

310 This lunar *prāṇāyāma* with its emphasis on inhalation through the Iḍā *nāḍī* has no parallel in the manuals of *haṭhayoga*, in which the yogin is usually instructed to use alternate nostrils for inhalation (e.g. *HP* 2.7–10, *ŚS* 3.24–25, *GhS* 5.38–53). There is one technique in which the yogin is to use only one nostril for inhalation: *sūryabhedana* (*HP* 2.48–50, *GhS* 5.58–63); however it is the Piṅgalā *nāḍī* which is to be used for inhalation and the Iḍā for exhalation.

311 The *kalā*s situated in the lower part of the body total twelve (five at the Base, three at the Svādhiṣṭhāna and four at the Bamboo Staff). This figure tallies with the descriptions of twelve *kalā*s of the sun (which is situated in the lower part of the body in yogic physiology: see e.g. *HP* 3.76–81) found in *SSP* 1.64 and *KAT* 6.39. This may be coincidence: here the *kalā*s are not said to have any connection with the sun while in the *SSP* and *KAT* passages the names of the *kalā*s are explicitly solar. Moreover, no such neat correspondence can be made for the twenty-two *kalā*s situated in the head. Indeed it is striking that the *kalā*s in the head do not total sixteen or seventeen (see note 277). (Ballāla (f. 38r[7]) omits the four *kalā*s at the *somamaṇḍala* and the single *kalā* above the *brahmārgaladvāra* to arrive at the scripturally prescribed total of seventeen *candrakalā*s.)

312 I usually translate *sudhā* as "nectar", *amṛta* as "*amṛta*", *parāmṛta* as "great *amṛta*", and *paramāmṛta* as "supreme *amṛta*". I have chosen to translate *parāmṛta* here as "ultimate *amṛta*" because Śiva is now teaching the location of the highest store of *amṛta* in the head.

313 The Diamond Bulb *(vajrakanda)* has been described at 2.25c-29b. See note 293.

314 For *yoginaḥ*, "yogins", μ has *yoginyaḥ*, "yoginīs". This may indicate a difference in doctrine between μ and the other witnesses, but could also be because of a scribal error.

315 On the *cūlitala* see note 241.

316 This description of five places in the head corresponds to descriptions of the qualities of the five elements to be meditated upon in the haṭhayogic *dhāraṇā* (e.g. *GŚ*$_N$ 155–159, *VS* 4.1–15, *DYŚ* 220–242, *ŚS* 3.72–74, *GhS* 3.59–63, *Śivasvarodaya* 209–213; cf. *MVUT* 13.21c–13.53d, *Mṛgendratantra Yogapāda* 39–44; Ballāla (f. 42(1)v) quotes similar passages from the *Kulaprakāśatantra* (see Kavirāj 1972:143), the *Śāradātilaka* and the *Mahākapilapañcarātra* (see ibid.:484)). These elemental qualities (appearance, colour, shape, *bīja* etc.) have been imposed (with some differences) upon different sets of five physical locations in different schemata of esoteric physiology. Thus they appear in the *ṢCN*'s description of the lower five *cakra*s at the perineum, the genital region, the navel, the heart and the throat (cf. *ŚS* 3.73–74); in the *GŚ*$_N$ they are found at the heart, the throat, the palate, between the eyebrows

and at the *brahmarandhra;* in the *DYŚ* they are in the regions between the anus and navel, at the navel, above the navel, between the navel and the eyebrows and above the eyebrows; here in the *KhV* the first four are at the cardinal directions in the head with the fifth above, in the centre. The order in which the elements are listed here is different from that found elsewhere. In the text from 49c to 58b and in its summary at 58c–59d the order is earth *(pṛthivī)*, fire *(sūrya)*, air *(anila)*, water *(jala)* and ether *(ākāśa)*, in contrast with the usual order of earth, water, fire, air, ether. They are, however, positioned in their usual order as one circumambulates the head (albeit anticlockwise): starting at the forehead with earth, there is water at the left temple, fire at the back of the head, air at the right temple and ether on top.

317 At f. 40v[10] Ballāla likens the four *liṅgas* with the fifth in the middle and a store of cooling *amṛta* above to the four columns of a temple with the *liṅga* in the middle and a *galantikā* or *kalaśa* dripping water onto the *liṅga* from above: *caturdikṣu galaṃtikāstambhās tadupari pragalajjalakalaśaḥ.*

318 "with the moon above it" *(ūrdhvacandram)* : the readings of μ and G (*ūrdhver ūrdhva°* and *ūrdhvaraṃdhra°* respectively), although corrupt, suggest that *ūrdhvacandram* may not be the original reading. The *Vairāṭapurāṇa* locates a *cakra* called both *ūrdhvarandhra* and *tālucakra* above the *sahasrāracakra* (Kavirāj 1987:51).

319 "perfect" *(heyopādeyarahitam)* : *heyopādeyarahita* literally means "free of those things which are to be rejected *(heya)* or cultivated *(upādeya)*", i.e. free of any hierarchised duality. Ballāla (f. 43r[10]) glosses *heya* with *saṃsāra* and *upādeya* with *mokṣa*. The *Mālinīvijayottaratantra* opens with a statement of what is *upādeya* and what is *heya* (1.14c–17b): "Śiva, Śakti and Sovereigns of Mantra-regents, Mantras, Mantra-regents, and individual souls" are to be cultivated. "Impurity, karma, Māyā, the entire universe deriving from Māyā" are to be rejected (Vasudeva's translation (2004:151)).

320 "to obtain the ultimate substance" *(paratattvopalabdhaye)* : here *paratattva* can be understood both physically and metaphysically. It is *amṛta*, the ultimate substance, beyond the five elements already mentioned, and it is the ultimate reality, the goal of many tantric and haṭhayogic practices (see e.g. *KT* 59.36, *HP* 4.37 and *KhV* 2.100c). That this practice is not entirely physical is indicated by phrases such as *manasā saha* at 64c and 65d, and *unmanyā tatra saṃyogam* at 67c. Most of the first *adhyāya* of the *Amanaskayoga* (vv. 21–98) is devoted to describing *laya*, by means of which the *paratattva* is obtained. (This first *adhyāya* is called *layayoga* when quoted from by later commentators; the second, which describes *amanaskayoga*, is called *rājayoga* (Bouy 1994:22, 69, 78)).

321 On Vāgīśā, "the goddess of speech", see 2.110cd.

322 "with her mouth upwards" *(ūrdhvavaktrām)* : i.e. with the tip of the tongue pointing upwards in order to lick at the *amṛta.* G's reading, *ūrdhvavaktre*, suggests the "upper mouth" at the opening of the *śaṅkhinī nāḍī* from which *amṛta* flows (cf. *AŚ* p.10).

323 The pot of *amṛta* is a recurrent theme in Indian mythology. When the ocean of milk was churned by the gods and demons Dhanvantri appeared carrying a white pot *(kamaṇḍalu)* of *amṛta* (*Mahābhārata* 1.18). Four drops of *amṛta* fell from this

pot at the sites of the triennial Kumbh Melā, "Pot Festival" (on this recent addition to the myth see LOCHTEFELD 2004). At *SYM* 21.7 Bhairava is to be visualised in the middle of the Umāmaheśvara *cakra* churning a pot *(kalaśa)* full of *amṛta*; at *SYM* 22.36 in a description of the fearsome Yoginīcakra, at the hub of the wheel the Yoginīs churn and drink from a white pot *(kalaśa)* full of *amṛta*. The inner shrine of the Nātha monastery at Caughera in Nepal contains a pot of *amṛta (amṛtapātra)* which is said to be the *svarūp* of Gorakhnāth (BOUILLIER 1997:31–32).

324 *Unmanī*, "the supramental state", is a common goal of tantric and haṭhayogic practices. At *HP* 4.3–4 it is included in a list of synonyms of *samādhi*. It is also frequently mentioned by Hindī poets of the *nirguṇa* tradition (CALLEWAERT & DE BEECK 1991:626).

325 "that consists of *nāda* and *bindu*" *(nādabindumayam)* : in tantric works, *nāda* and *bindu* (often combined with *kalā*—see note 277) have several different meanings. In particular, they refer to places in the body (e.g. *NT* 7.29, *KT* 58.56, *Vijñānabhairava* 36–37) and describe corresponding stages in the manifestation of the phonetic universe (e.g. *Śāradātilakatantra* 1.7–8, *TĀ* 4.175; see PADOUX 1990a:86–121). In some texts they are also listed among the six *lakṣyas*, "the six manifestations of Śiva as the 'goals', or 'targets', of yogic practice" (VASUDEVA 2004:253–292). In the texts of *haṭhayoga*, *nāda* is usually the internal, "unstruck" *(anāhata)* sound heard during yoga practice (see e.g. *HP* 4.66–106, *Nādabindūpaniṣad* 31–51). Meanwhile *bindu* is understood to be the *amṛta* secreted in the head, which the yogin must prevent from falling and being discharged as semen (*HP* 2.78, 3.42, *SSP* 2.13; but cf. *ŚS* 5.144 where *nāda* and *bindu*, together with *śakti*, are *pīṭhas* in the lotus of the forehead; cf. also *BKhP* f. 100v[3]: *pīṭhatrayaṃ bhāle biṃdunādaśaktirūpaṃ | tatphalaṃ janmāṃtarasmṛtiḥ | viparītajihvayā nādadhyānaṃ pāpanāśanaṃ | śaktau vāsanākṣayaḥ*, and *MaSaṃ* 17.14–16, in which the *viśuddhacakra* and an unnamed *cakra* somewhere above *viśuddha* are said to be *nādarūpaka* and *bindurūpaka* respectively). It is with the usual haṭhayogic meanings that Ballāla (f. 44v[3–4]) understands *nāda* and *bindu* (cf. *HPJ ad* 4.1). As such, the compound *nādabindu* joins two unconnected concepts and his interpretation seems forced. I suspect that in haṭhayogic works the compound is used more as a catchphrase, harking back to its use in tantric texts and thereby adding esoteric gravitas (see e.g. *HP* 4.1, *GBS* 163, 181, 184 etc., *YŚU* 6.70, *GhS* 6.12 and the *Nādabindūpaniṣad*, which, despite its title, concerns only the "unstruck" *nāda* and mentions *bindu* just once, at verse 50). On *nāda, bindu* and *kalā* see also KIEHNLE 1997:141.

At *HP* 3.46 in the description of *khecarīmudrā* the yogin is said to eat beef and drink wine (see page 28 of the introduction). The *jogī* is said to drink *vāruṇī* at *GBS* 137. Cf. *Rasārṇava* 1.26, *Rasendracūḍāmaṇi* 1.7–10. See also ROŞU 1997:413.

326 Ballāla (f. 45v[4–7]) takes this verse to be describing those entitled to teach and learn Khecarī yoga: the text is to be spoken by [a yogin] who has no desire for *siddhi (na kiṃ cit siddhim icchatā*—he interprets *siddhi* here as *śiṣyād dravya⌈sevā⌉diprāpti*, "obtaining goods, service etc. from a pupil"!) to one who has attained the means of *siddhi (siddhisopānam)* but does not know this yoga.

327 The *aiśa* anacoluthon in this verse has been emended in G, or one of its antecedents.

328 Practices involving massaging the body with various physical secretions are alluded to fleetingly in many haṭhayogic texts (see the references in the notes to 2.75a–77b). *Paṭala* 27 of the *Matsyendrasaṃhitā* (which is reproduced on page 154 of the appendices) describes several such techniques in detail, summarising them as "the ritual bath which is better than [bathing] at all the sacred bathing places" *(sarvatīrthādhikaṃ snānam* 27.1cd). (At *MaSaṃ* 27.2 faeces, urine, menstrual blood, phlegm (? *recaka*) and semen (? *sāraka*) are said to be the gods Lokeśa, Keśava, Rudra, Īśa and Sadeśvara.) These practices corporealise the techniques of *rasaśāstra*, alchemy. (On corporealisation see page 27.) The words used to describe the massaging of the body, *lepana* and *mardana*, are also used to describe *saṃskāras* in the process of fixing mercury (see e.g. *RAK* 80, 91, 150 etc. on *lepana* and 54, 89, 98 etc. on *mardana*). As with the substances to be rubbed into mercury in the alchemical *saṃskāras*, in *MaSaṃ paṭala* 27 minerals and herbs are added to the fluids to be massaged into the body. *MaSaṃ* 27.1 calls the knowledge of these practices *kṣetrajñāna*; at *Rasārṇava* 18.11, 18.15 and 18.19 the preparation of the human body for alchemical practice by the consumption of herbal preparations is called *kṣetrīkaraṇa* (see also WHITE 1996:265–273).

In verses 95 and 281c–282b of the *RAK* it is said that the urine and faeces of a man who eats certain herbal preparations (which do not include mercury) can transmute copper into gold (cf. *ŚS* 3.61 and *DYŚ* 197 quoted in note 336). At 146 it is said that by eating a preparation of calcined mercury, a man becomes *sparśavedhī* and his sweat can fix mercury.

The physical practices are attacked at *SSP* 6.90:

śaṃkhakṣālanam antaraṃ rasanayā tālvoṣṭhanāsārasam
vānter ucchadanam kavāṭam amarīpānaṃ tathā kharparīm /
vīryaṃ drāvitam ātmajaṃ punar aho grāsaṃ pralepaṃ ca vā
ye kurvaṃti jaḍās tu te na hi phalaṃ teṣāṃ tu siddhāntajam //

90b ucchadanaṃ] *em.*; ullaṭanaṃ Ed, uchuṭhanaṃ Ed^{vl} ◇ kharparīm] *em.*; kharparī Ed **90c** vīryaṃ] *em.*; vīrya Ed ◇ grāsaṃ pralepaṃ ca vā] grāsapradaṃ pañcadhā Ed^{vl}

"Those who practise emesis and enema [and] use the fluids from the palate, lips and nose with the tongue, who massage themselves with vomit, who practise *kavāṭa* (?), drink their own urine, use Kharparī (coryllium?), who use their semen after causing it to flow, and eat or massage [themselves with these fluids], are stupid and do not get the reward that is produced by the correct doctrine." (Several verses towards the end of *SSP paṭala* 6 appear to be later additions to the text since they contradict earlier verses: see e.g. 6.13 where the *avadhūta* who drinks his own urine is praised.) Cf. *AY* 2.33 (=*AP* 8): *ke cin mūtraṃ pibanti svamalam...*, "some drink urine, their own filth...", and *Rasārṇava* 1.11c–12b: *śukramūtrapurīṣāṇāṃ yadi muktir niṣevanāt* / *kiṃ na muktā mahādevi śvānaśūkarajātayaḥ* // "If liberation [comes] from using semen, urine and faeces, then why are dogs and pigs not liberated, o great goddess?"

329 Here Śiva teaches the physical locations of fire, the sun and the moon. As in the locations of the five elemental deities discussed in note 316, the system described

here is different from that found in other tantric and haṭhayogic texts. In the texts of *haṭhayoga*, the sun and fire are combined and said to dwell in the region of the navel, consuming the *amṛta* that drips from the moon which is situated at the palate (see e.g. *GŚ*$_N$ 133, *HP* 3.78, *GhS* 3.29).

In this verse, only μ has *bhālamadhye*, "in the middle of the forehead", (cf. *bhālajam* at 74b), which is almost certainly original in the light of both 2.75, where the *amṛta* that has dripped from the moon emerges from the nostrils, and 2.22, where the *somamaṇḍala*, i.e. the moon, is located between the eyebrows. Similarly, at *SSP* 2.21 the yogin is told to visualise a *candramaṇḍala* at the *bhrūmadhyādhāra* while *ŚS* 5.182 locates the moon at the Sahasrāra lotus at the top of the skull. The readings of the rest of the witnesses, which locate the moon at the palate, have probably originated through confusion with other texts, rather than through deliberate alteration.

330 On *mathana*, "churning", see 1.57c–64d.

331 Ballāla (f. 46v$^{1-3}$) describes how the orb of fire is to be awakened: *dakṣahastasya madhyamāṃguṣṭhābhyāṃ ḍamaruvan nāsikāpuṭe pūrayan recayaṃś (em.; pūraya*eca-yaṃś* S) *ca vādayitvā paścād gāḍhaṃ pūrayed recayed ity eṣātra bhastrā* (*em.*; *bhasrā* S) *tayā suṣumṇāvahane sati tadadhiṣṭhitavahner udbodhanaṃ bhavatīti*. This is a variation of the *bhastrā*/*bhastrikā prāṇāyāma* described at *YB* 108–112, *HP* 2.59–67 and *GhS* 5.70–72 (in the almost identical *YB* and *HP* passages the practice is said to be *kuṇḍalībodhakam* and bring about *śarīrāgnivivardhanam*, i.e. it awakens Kuṇḍalinī and increases the bodily fire).

332 *HP* 3.48 describes how *amṛta* flows from the moon after it has been liquefied by the heat produced when the tongue enters the opening above the palate: *jihvāpraveśa-sambhūtavahninotpāditaḥ khalu / candrāt sravati yaḥ sāraḥ sā syād amaravāruṇī //*. Cf. *TĀ* 4.131cd, 134ab.

333 "in a vessel" *(pātreṇa)*: *MaSaṃ* 40.8 (A f. 90v^2) says that the vessel used to hold the yogin's urine *(amarī)* should be made of gold or silver, or, if they are unavailable, copper or brass *(kāṃsya)*. *KJN* 12.11-16 describes the different materials that can be used to make the *pātra* that holds the *cāruka*, the Kaula *pañcāmṛta* libation, which consists of faeces, urine, semen, blood and marrow (*KJN* 11.11); cf. *TĀ* 11 (29) p. 130, ll. 5–8 where the five jewels are said to be urine, semen, menstrual blood, faeces and phlegm (Sanderson 1995:82)).

334 Cf. *MaSaṃ* 27.9. A corrupt passage at *HP* 3.93–94 describes the *amarolī* technique: *amarīṃ yaḥ piben nityaṃ nasyaṃ kurvan (nasyaṃ kurvan] tasya kuryād Ed*^{vl}*) dine dine / vajrolīm abhyaset samyag amarolīti kathyate // abhyāsān niḥsṛtāṃ cāndrīṃ vibhūtyā saha miśrayet / dhārayed uttamāṅgeṣu divyadṛṣṭiḥ prajāyate //* "He who always drinks urine, [also] using it as a nasally administered substance, every day [and who] correctly performs *vajrolī*, [his practice] is called *amarolī*. He should mix with ash the lunar [fluid] that has emerged after practice and put it on his head; he gets divine sight." (Translation by Goodall & Isaacson.) Brahmānanda (*HPJ ad loc.*) attributes this practice to Kāpālikas.

335 In haṭhayogic texts, *nāḍīśuddhi*, "purification of the channels of the body", is usually said to arise by means of *prāṇāyāma*. See e.g. *GŚ*$_N$ 95, *HP* 2.19, *GhS* 5.2, 5.35, *SSP* 6.79.

336 "the essence of immortality produced at the anus and penis" *(gudaliṅgodgatam amarīrasam)* : cf. *MaSaṃ* 27.6. *MaSaṃ paṭala* 40 describes *amarīsnāna* in detail and calls the process *kulācāra* (40.1). Ballāla (f. 47r$^{6-7}$) quotes a passage in this context which he attributes to "traditional teaching": *mūtrapurīṣayor alpatvaṃ ca / yallepāl lohasya svarṇatā gorakṣasyeva tadā vajrolyā sādhitaliṃganālo mūtrasyāgrimadhārāṃ viṣarūpāṃ tathāṃtimāṃ hīnaguṇāṃ saṃtyajya madhyamāṃ balapradāṃ gṛhītvaivam eva madhyamam alpaṃ malaṃ gṛhītvāṃgaṃ mardayed iti / paraṃparopadeśāt /*. For modern accounts of urine massage see Sarasvatī 1991 (especially pp. 74–76) and Armstrong 1994. At f. 47v$^{2-4}$ Ballāla describes the *amarī* and *ajarī kriyā*s in which the yogin is to consume faeces and urine respectively: *ke cit tu gudodgataṃ kakṣāmṛtena saṃloḍya *dharārasaiḥ saṃskṛtya yad bhakṣaṇaṃ sāmarī kriyā / tatphalaṃ nirāmayatvaṃ balavattvaṃ ceti / liṃgodgataṃ kakṣāmṛtena saṃloḍyādharārasaiḥ saṃskṛtya yat pānaṃ sājarī kriyā tatphalaṃ valītyāgādī(°tyāgādī°] em.; °tyādī° S)ty āhuḥ / amarī hy amarakāriṇī / ajarī ⌈a⌉jarākāriṇī /*. In contrast, Parry (1994:290) reports that present-day Aghorī ascetics call urine *amarī* and faeces *bajarī*. *GBS* 141 says that he who practises *bajarī* and *amarī* is Gorakhnāth's guru-brother. The *KhV*'s description of *amarīrasa* from the *guda* and *liṅga* and Ballāla's *amarī* and *ajarī kriyās* suggest that the Aghorī's coprophagy is more than just a combination of opposites in which "pollution becomes indistinguishable from purity" (Parry 1994:264).

ŚS 3.61 teaches how through perfection of *prāṇāyāma*, the yogin's urine and faeces can create gold or make it invisible: *viṅmūtralepane svarṇam adṛśyakaraṇaṃ tathā*. Cf. *DYŚ* 197: *malamūtrapralepena lohādīnāṃ suvarṇatā /*. See also *Rasārṇava* 18.28–29b.

HP 3.90 describes the *sahajolī* variant of *vajrolīmudrā*: *sahajoliś cāmarolir vajrolyā eva bhedataḥ / jale subhasma nikṣipya dagdhagomayasaṃbhavam // vajrolīmaithunād ūrdhvaṃ strīpuṃsoḥ svāṅgalepanam / āsīnayoḥ sukhenaiva muktavyāpārayoḥ kṣaṇāt //*. "*Sahajolī* and *amarolī* are types of *vajrolī*. [The yogin] should put good ash made from burnt cow-dung in water. Straight after sexual intercourse using *vajrolī*, it should be rubbed on the bodies of the man and woman, [when they are] sitting happily, free of activity". It seems likely that this passage has been redacted to conceal a practice in which the combined sexual fluids of the yogin and his consort are smeared on the body. *MaSaṃ* 40.48 describes a similar technique to be practised after intercourse although here it is only semen (mixed with gold, camphor, saffron and such like) that is to be smeared on the body: *tad vīryaṃ svarṇakarpūrakuṅkumādiviloḍitam / svadehaṃ mardayet kāntiś candravat saṃprajāyate*. *Jogpradīpakā* 677–683 describes the *varaṇaka mudrā* which it says is also known as *amarolī*. The yogin is to drink three handfuls of urine first thing in the morning before mixing his urine with *nirguṇḍī*, *bhaṃgaro* (=Skt. *bhṛṅgarāja* McGregor 1995:s.v.), *muṇḍī* and *giloī* (=Skt. *guḍūcī* ibid.:s.v.) and smearing the mixture on his body.

The *siddha* Karṇaripa added his "own water" to a potion and it became "as the essence of the alchemists" (Robinson 1979:88–9). The *siddha* Caparipa gave a child magical powers: "From his penis came the power to transform things into gold. From his anus came the elixir of immortality" (ibid.:206–7).

337 "the *amṛta* from the armpits" *(kakṣāmṛtam)* : the reading *kalāmṛtam* found in *μ*

may be original. Śiva has described *amṛtakalā*s at the anus and penis (2.32 and 2.40) but not at the armpits and *MaSaṃ paṭala* 27 does not mention *aṅgamardana* with sweat. However many haṭhayogic texts do teach that the sweat produced through yogic exertion should be rubbed into the body (e.g. $GŚ_N$ 53, *ŚS* 3.46, *HP* 2.13, *Dhyānabindūpaniṣad* 70–72, *DYŚ* 148) and it may be because of this idea that the reading *kakṣāmṛtam* supplanted *kalāmṛtam*. *ŚS* 3.46 adds the reason for the practice: *anyathā vigrahe dhātur naṣṭo bhavati yoginaḥ*, "otherwise the basic constituents in the body of the yogin are destroyed". Cf. Ballāla (f. 95r[8]): *evaṃ saniyamaprāṇāyāme jāyamānasya dehe svedasya mardanaṃ hastābhyāṃ kāryaṃ na tu vastreṇāpalāpaḥ | ⌈lāghava⌉ balanāśanāt |*. "The sweat produced when *prāṇāyāma* is practised in this way, [i.e.] according to the rules, should be rubbed into the body with the hands, not wiped away with a cloth. Otherwise suppleness and strength are lost." Like *lepana* and *mardana*, *svedana* is an alchemical *saṃskāra* (see *Rasārṇavakalpa* 98, 368–369 etc.).

338 "with fluid from the lower lip" *(cādharārasaiḥ)* : the feminine form *adharā* for *adhara* is probably *metri causa*. Monier-Williams (1988:19) does report that *adharā* can mean "Pudendum Muliebre" but such a meaning is unlikely here. Ballāla (f. 47r[10]) takes the plural *°rasaiḥ* to indicate that fluid from the lips, tongue and nostrils should be used.

AY 2.33 castigates those who rub saliva into their bodies: ... *atha tanau ke cid ujjhanti lālām... naiteṣāṃ dehasiddhir vigatanijamanorājayogād ṛte syāt ||* Cf. *SSP* 6.90 (quoted in note 328). See White 1996:311-2 for legends describing the initiatory and magical powers of yogins' saliva.

339 I have found no description of this practice in any other text. Ballāla (f. 47v[8–10]) identifies it as a supplementary practice to that described in 1.45a but he seems mistaken: at 1.45a it is the *tālumūla* which is to be rubbed and then all the impurity *(mala)* is to be cleansed. Here a potent "great fluid" (*mahādrava*; but n.b. μ's reading *madadrava*, "intoxicating fluid") is produced at the *jihvāmūla*.

340 "[the yogin] should push aside" *(sphoṭayet)* : Monier-Williams (1988:1270) gives "to push aside (a bolt)" as one of the meanings of the causative of the root *sphuṭ*. Ballāla (f. 48r[3–7]) takes this verse to refer to the practice of *tāḍana* (see note 236).

341 I have taken verses 80 and 81 to be summarising the practice of *khecarīmudrā* (unlike Ballāla who takes them with 78a–79d at f. 48r[1–9]). Verse 80 describes the process of inserting the tongue into the region above the palate. The tongue is to be pushed upwards (from its underside) while the uvula is to be brought forward thus making it easier for the tip of the tongue to reach the opening behind it (see note 229). The root *kṛṣ* normally has a sense of "pull" or "draw" but if one were to pull the tongue upwards with the fingers of the right hand, the uvula would be inaccessible to the fingers of the left hand. I have thus taken *utkṛṣya rasanām ūrdhvam* to mean that the tongue is to be pushed upwards (as was demonstrated to me by several of my informants).

342 I am here following Ballāla's interpretation of *ūrdhvavaktram* as meaning *laṃbikordhvakramam*, "going above the uvula" (f. 48r[8]). Alternatively it could mean "the upper mouth": see 3.23b and note 420.

343 "at the *kalā*s" *(candrāṃśe)* : a part of the moon *(candrāṃśa)* is a *kalā* (see note 277).

The *kalās* referred to here are the three at the Diamond Bulb *(vajrakanda*—see 2.25c–29b and note 293) which is said to be the place of Śiva at 2.49c–50b (cf. *HP* 1.48). For *candrāṃśe,* μ has *vajrāṃtyo* and G *vajrāṃte.* G's *vajrāṃte* may be the original reading, referring to the top of the *vajrakanda.*

344 In the *Khecarīvidyā, trikūṭa,* "the Three-peaked Mountain", is located between the eyebrows. See note 259.

345 For similar accounts of curing physical afflictions by means of haṭhayogic practices, see *HP upadeśa* 5, *YB* 102–112 and *DU* 6:25-30b; cf. *MKSG* 11.985. *ŚP* 4508–4513 describes *doṣopasargacikitsā* by means of visualisation.

346 I have found no parallels for this usage of *bhaṭa* and *naṭa.* The usual meaning of *bhaṭa* is "mercenary" or "warrior" and that of *naṭa* is "actor" or "dancer" (Monier-Williams 1988:s.vv.). The terms may thus refer to the different types of *sādhaka* that are afflicted by the problems listed. In Hindī, *bhaṭ* can mean "misfortune, curse" (McGregor 1995:757) while the Sanskrit root *naṭ* can mean "to hurt or injure" (Monier-Williams 1988:525). A Buddhist *vihāra* was established near Mathura by two brothers called Naṭa and Bhaṭa (*Paṃśupradānāvadāna, Divyāvadāna* No.26, p.349; see also *ibid.* pp.356 and 385, Edgerton s.v. *naṭabhaṭikā,* Böhtlingk and Roth s.v. *naṭa.* I am grateful to Peter Wyzlic for supplying me with these references.) G, S and most of α and β have *haṭa* or *haṭha* for *bhaṭa.* I have adopted *bhaṭa* over *haṭa/haṭha* for three reasons: firstly, *bhaṭa* is found in both μ and γ; secondly, the use of the word *haṭha* to describe a system of practices was only just beginning at the time of the *Khecarīvidyā*'s composition and is not attested elsewhere in the text; and, thirdly, the pairing of *haṭha* with *naṭa* seems unlikely. Witness K_5 lends weight to the idea that *haṭha* is a later emendation: at 84a and 99c it has *bhaṭa,* corrected to *haṭa* in the margin. Perhaps the first description of a systematised *haṭhayoga* named as such is to be found in the *Dattātreyayogaśāstra* (17–19 and 57–62) in which the term refers specifically to the practice of ten *mudrās.* The *DYŚ* is quoted extensively in the *Śārṅgadharapaddhati* (25 *ślokas* between *ŚP* 4376 and 4460) and was thus composed before 1363 CE.

In his commentary on *naṭa,* Ballāla devotes five folios (f. $48v^8$–f. $53r^7$) to quotations from various texts about *nāṭakādinibaddharasādi,* "the dramatic sentiments etc. involved in the various types of drama". The *Khecarīvidyā*'s *naṭabhedas* are physical manifestations of these sentiments. When they arise, actors are unfit for acting: *teṣu jāteṣu nartanayogyā naṭā na bhavaṃti* (f. $53r^8$). This is relevant to yogic practice because the sense organs are like the *naṭas*: *vastutas tu svasvavyāpāre nartanaśīlānāṃ naṭānām ivemdriyāṇāṃ netrādīnāṃ bhedā bhedakā naṭabhedā ity ucyaṃte* (f. $53r^7$). Concerning *haṭha* (S's reading for *bhaṭa*), Ballāla (f. $53r^9$–f. $53v^1$) writes that the four manifestations of *haṭha* given in 83cd are proof of success in *haṭhayoga* (!): *ete haṭhasya yogasya pratyayāḥ haṭhaḥ siddha iti pratītiṃ janayaṃti.*

347 "drying up of the body" *(aṅgaśoṣaḥ)*: at *Kubjikāmatatantra* 23.160 a practice similar to the haṭhayogic *khecarīmudrā* is said to get rid of *śoṣa, dāha* (cf. *KhV* 2.88d) and *vaivarṇa* (cf. *KhV* 2.87cd).

348 "sloth induced by hunger" *(kṣudhālasyam)* : in order for the varieties of *bhaṭa* to total four, *kṣudhālasya* must be taken as a single entity. I have chosen to take it as a *tatpuruṣa samāsa*; Ballāla (f. $53r^{9-10}$ and f. $53v^{8-9}$) understands it to be a *dvandva*

samāsa with the meaning "hunger and sloth".

349 "the essence of immortality" *(amarīrasam)* : see 2.76cd.

350 i.e. *aṅgaśoṣa*, "dryness of the body", (2.83c) is cured.

351 i.e. it should be done every four hours: *daśamadaśamaghaṭikāyām* (Ballāla f. 53v[6]). A *ghaṭikā* is 24 minutes.

352 See 2.25c–29b, 2.49c–50b and note 293 for descriptions of the Diamond Bulb *(vajrakanda)*.

353 "*amṛta* [from the anus and penis]" *(amarīm)* : see 2.76cd.

354 "trembling of the body" *(aṅgavepaḥ)* : I have adopted G's *aṅgavepaḥ* to avoid repetition of *aṅgaśoṣaḥ* from 2.83c.

355 "dizziness" *(bhrāntis)* : *bhrānti* usually means ignorance (see e.g. *KJN* 5.1). In the context here, however, it must refer to a more mundane physical affliction. Ballāla (f. 54v[2]) glosses it with *mānasī viparītadhīḥ*, "mental perversity".

356 "high fever" *(mahājvaraḥ)* : Ballāla says (f. 54v[7]) that *mahājvara* cannot be cured by doctors *(bhiṣagbhir acikitsyaḥ)* and adds that doctors' medicines are no use in curing any of the problems of *haṭha* and *naṭa*: *haṭhanaṭabhedeṣu bhiṣagauṣadhaṃ na calati*.

357 Ballāla (f. 54v[9]) takes the *tathaiva ca* that follows *netrāndhatvam*, "blindness", to imply *bādhiryam*, "deafness".

358 This is the practice described at 2.32c–39d. Only G has *mūlādhārāt suṣumnāyāṃ* at 2.92a; the other witnesses have variants of *svamūlāt śvāsasaṃbhinnām*, "from her base, together with the breath".

359 This technique involving internal sounds is similar to the haṭhayogic *nādānusandhāna* (see e.g. *SSP* 6.91, *HP* 4.66–106, *NBU* 31–51, *VS* 3.39–40, *GhS* 5.73–76), by means of which *samādhi* is realised (*HP* 4.81). Here, μ reads *jalanāda* for *mahānāda*. μ's reading may be original: in a passage which is found at both *HP* 4.83–89 and *NBU* 32–38 it is said that in the beginning of the practice one of the sounds that arises is that of *jaladhi*, "the ocean" (*HP* 4.85a). On the other hand, *HP* 4.84ab reads *śrūyate prathamābhyāse nādo nānāvidho mahān*, "in the first [stage of the] practice a great sound of many kinds is heard". *HR* 2.148 connects *khecarīmudrā* with the internal *nāda*. For a survey of descriptions of the technique of *nāda* and lists of the internal sounds found in tantric works see Vasudeva (2004:273–280).

360 "in his ears" *(karṇābhyām)* : *-ābhyām* is sometimes used for the locative and genitive dual *(-ayoḥ)* in Śaiva tantric works. See e.g. *Svacchandatantra* 2.231 and Kṣemarāja *ad loc.*, *JRY* 3.38.158c and *JRY* 3 *Yoginīsaṃcaraprakaraṇa* 1.63ab, 1.64. I am grateful to Alexis Sanderson for providing me with these references.

361 "the sound of the roar of a great elephant" *(mahāgajaravadhvanim)* : in the lists of the various sounds heard during *nādānusandhāna* given in haṭhayogic texts (see note 359 for references), no animal sounds are mentioned.

362 "the sound of Brahmā" *(brahmanādam)* : Ballāla (f. 56r[1–2]) offers two explanations of *brahmanāda*: firstly he takes *brahma*° to mean *bṛhat* and thus *brahmanāda* is the same as the *mahānāda* of 93b; secondly *brahmanāda* is the *anāhata*, "unstruck", *nāda* that is the focus of *nādānusandhāna* (see note 359). μ has *siṃhanādam*, "the sound of a lion", which may be original. The small whistle worn on a thread around

the neck by Nāthas is called *siṃhanāda*. Briggs (1938:11), however, reports that the Yogīs understand it to be called thus because ideally the whistle is made of *sīṃg*, "(deer-)horn". Cf. *SSP* 5.15a where it is called *śṛṅgī-nāda*, with a variant reading (from Mallik's edition) of *siṃhanāda*.

363 The sound of thunder, *meghanāda*, is given as one of the *anāhata* sounds at *GhS* 5.75 and *VS* 3.40. Aghora, "not terrific", is a name of Śiva and of one of his most important mantras (see e.g. *Pāśupatasūtra* 3.21–26, *KMT paṭala* 9 and the *Sisṭ* [sic] *Purāṇ* (Baḍathvāl 1960:236–237), a work ascribed to Gorakhnāth, in which Aghor is said to be the best mantra).

364 "knowing all the categories of reality" *(sarvatattvajñaḥ)* : Ballāla (f. $57v^{2-8}$) mentions four systems of *tattvas*: that described in the *Nārāyaṇayogasūtravṛtti* in which there are two types of *tattva*, *jaḍa* and *ajaḍa*, corresponding to the *prakṛti* and *puruṣa* of Sāṃkhya; a *śākta* system of twenty-five *tattvas*; a system said to be found in the *Śaivāgamas* comprising fifty *tattvas*, including the twenty-five just mentioned; and the (presumably twenty-five) *tattvas* described by Kapila in the *Bhāgavata[purāṇa]*. Ballāla adds that the system of fifty *tattvas* found in the *Śaivāgamas* has been described by him in the *Yogaratnākaragrantha*. Gharote & Bedekar (1989:208) list two manuscripts of works entitled *Yogaratnākara* but they are ascribed to Viśveśvarānanda and Rāmānandayogin.

365 "into this peaceful supreme reality" *(śānte pare tattve)* : cf. 2.63d. Ballāla (f. $57r^{10}$–f. $57v^{1}$) says that this *paraṃ tattvam* is the state reached by means of the four *mahāvākyas* of the Upaniṣads.

366 As Ballāla notes at f. $58r^{8-10}$, it is surprising to find *cālana*, "loosening", named as one of the four stages when in the first *paṭala*'s description of the practice *cālana* is only mentioned in passing (1.49) and not by name. The cutting of the frenum, however, is discussed in some detail (1.46–48) and one might expect *chedana* to be the first stage. In most of the other texts in which the practice is taught (e.g. *GhS* 1.28–31, 3.21, *Haṭhapradīpikā* (long recension) 5.147–151 (H2 f. $100r^{7}$–f. $100v^{5}$)), *cālana* is given much more emphasis than it is in the first *paṭala* of the *Khecarīvidyā*. In the *Siddhasiddhāntapaddhati* (2.19, 6.84) the tongue is to be lengthened by means of *cālana*; *chedana* is not mentioned. This suggests that *KhV* 1.44c–77b and 2.101c–105d were not composed together.

It seems likely that *cālana* here does not refer simply to the stretching of the tongue. Commenting on 1.49, Ballāla (f. $19v^{3-9}$) quotes *YB* 91–98 for a description of the cloth used to take hold of the tongue when practising *cālana*. He notes that the passage comes in the description of a *mudrā* for arousing Kuṇḍalinī, the *śakticālanamudrā*. Nowhere in the *YB* passage is it stated where the cloth is to be applied. The Hindī translation of the text supplies *nābhi*, "the navel" as the location. Similarly, in the description of *śakticālana* found in the *Gheraṇḍasaṃhitā*, a much later text, the cloth is to be wrapped around the *nābhi* (3.43). It is hard to imagine how such a practice could be performed. It is probably because Kuṇḍalinī is located in the lower part of the body that the practice is thought to be carried out there too. (Another description of *śakticālana* at *ŚS* 4.105–111 says that it is to be done by means of the *apānavāyu*; see also *ŚS* 5.11 and *YB* 124a; Satyānanda Sarasvatī (1993:385–6) says that *nauli*, churning of the stomach, should be used.) The description of the cloth at *YB* 91–92 is found in the *HP*'s description of *śakticālana* at 3.109 without any instructions as to what to do with it. Brahmānanda (*HPJ ad loc.*) takes the description to be of the internal *kanda* above which Kuṇḍalinī sleeps. Perhaps the earliest reference (pre-1450 CE; see Bouy 1994:40) to the haṭhayogic *śakticālana* is found in a text called the *Gorakṣaśataka* which is an unedited work, found in only four manuscripts, different from the more popular text of the same name (which is available in several editions; on the different *Gorakṣaśataka*s see note 9 in the introduction). Bouy (*loc. cit.*) has noted that the first eighty verses of the first chapter of the *Yogakuṇḍalyupaniṣad* (whose second chapter is taken from the *Khecarīvidyā*'s first *paṭala*) are taken from this unedited *Gorakṣasaṃhitā*. *YKU* 1.7–8 states that there are two methods of *śakticālana*: a technique called *sarasvatīcālana*, and *prāṇāyāma*. 1.9–18 describe *sarasvatīcālana*. Again the place where the cloth is to be applied is never explicitly stated. The wise yogin is to wrap it around *tannāḍīm* (1.11). The *sarasvatī nāḍī* ends at the tip of the tongue (*VS* 2.37, *DU* 4.21, *ŚP* 4311) and, as we have seen (*KhV* 1.49), *vāgīśvarī*, "the goddess of speech", i.e. Sarasvatī, has her abode at the tongue. This leads me to believe that *śakticālana* is performed by wrapping a cloth around the tongue, not the stomach. The *Haṭharatnāvalī* (c. 17th century) confirms this and seems to preserve an understanding of *śakticālana* that had already been lost before the composition of other, older texts such as the *Śivasaṃhitā*. *HR* 2.118–127 describes the practice in detail and states explicitly that the cloth is to be wrapped around the tongue. Ballāla connects the pulling of the tongue with the awakening of Kuṇḍalinī in his commentary to 2.40–42 (f. 36v^{4-5}): *vastraveṣṭitajihvācālanena ca śaktiṃ prabodhya...*, "awakening [Kuṇḍalinī-]śakti by moving the tongue wrapped in a cloth..." and also at f. 37v^{3-4} where he says that Kuṇḍalinī is to be awakened *āsanakuṃbhakarasanācālanamudrādinā*, "by *āsana*, breath-retention, moving the tongue, *mudrā* etc.". Touching the palate with the tongue is said to bring about immediate upward movement of the breath (which is the yogic forerunner of the awakening of Kuṇḍalinī) at *Kiraṇatantra* 59.35 (see page 20). Cf. the practice shown to me by Dr. Tripāṭhī described in note 236.

367 The witnesses here appear to be corrupt. They all have *cālana*, "loosening", as the first stage, *mathana*, "churning", second, *pāna*, "drinking", third and *praveśana/praveśaka*, "insertion", fourth (except G, which has *pramelanam* fourth). This presents two problems. Firstly, *praveśana/praveśaka* needs to precede *pāna*—the tongue must be inserted into the cavity above the palate before *amṛta* can be drunk. (Ballāla notes this at two places (f. 58r^{4-7} and f. 58v^{1-2}) and gives two conflicting explanations. At first he says that after *mathana* the upper *kalā*s start to produce *amṛta* and thus there is an intermediate *pāna* before that which follows *praveśana*. At the second instance he employs the Mīmāṃsakas' maxim that the order of words is sometimes subordinate to the order of their meaning: *śabdakramād arthakramasya kva cid balavattvāt.*) Secondly, in 102c–105d these stages are elaborated. No mention is made of *pāna* but a stage called *bhedana* is described between *cālana* and *mathana*. I have thus conjecturally emended 101d–102a from *dvitīyaṃ mathanaṃ bhavet // tṛtīyaṃ pānam uddiṣṭam* to *dvitīyaṃ bhedanaṃ bhavet // tṛtīyaṃ mathanaṃ śastam*.

5.125–6 in the long version of the *Haṭhapradīpikā* (witness H_2) describes the *khecarī* technique as having six ancillaries *(ṣaḍaṅga)* : *chedana, cālana, dohana, pāṇigharṣaṇa, praveśa* and *mantrasādhana.* The six ancillaries are described in detail over the next 93 verses. The *Jogpradīpakā* names six ancillaries of *khecarīmudrā* at verse 611, but has *mathana* for H_2's *pāṇigharṣaṇa.*

368 On "loosening" *(cālana),* see 1.45.

369 On "piercing" *(bhedanam),* see 1.56. Cf. *MKSG* 22.971 and 985. *NT* 7.29 locates the fourth of six *cakra*s at the palate and calls it *bhedana.*

370 On "churning" *(mathanam),* see 1.57c–64d. This passage (103c–104d) is corrupt. G omits 104cd while *μ* omits *bhedanam* and *mathanam* in 103cd and has *taṃ vadaṃti sma* ⊔⊔⊔⊔ *taṃtunā priye* at 104ab. I have been unable to conjecture a suitable emendation but the meaning of the passage is clear.

371 "into the ether" *(ākāśe)* : on this use of *ākāśa* to mean the hollow above the palate see note 265.

372 Detailed instructions on *praveśana* are given at *Jogpradīpakā* 635–640.

373 "By breaking the bolt of Brahmā" *(brahmārgalaprabhedena)* : for *prabhedena* all the witnesses except *μ* read °*praveśena* (N has *praveśe tālumūlena*). The idea of insertion is also present in *jihvāsaṃkramaṇena* (which I have translated with "inserting the tongue") so °*praveśena* is redundant. I have thus adopted *μ*'s °*prabhedena* and take the two *pāda*s to be referring to *bhedana* and *praveśana* respectively.

374 "a condition of bliss" *(ānandabhāvatvam)* : Ballāla (f. 59r^4) quotes (without attribution) the following to explain *ānanda*: *yathā ratau yathā ca miṣṭabhojane yathā suṣuptau iti* , "like [the feeling experienced] in love-making, eating sweets and deep sleep".

375 "a decrease in sleep" *(nidrāhāniḥ)* : *Khecarīmudrā* is said to remove the need for sleep at *HP* 3.38. In the *Haṭharatnāvalī* (f. 5v^5) the adept is described as *tyaktanidraḥ*, "not sleeping".

376 "social intercourse" *(saṃgamam)* : cf. *Yogasūtra* 2.40: *śaucāt svāṅgajugupsā parair asaṃsargaḥ*, "from purification [arises] disgust for one's own body [and] not mixing with others". Forsaking company *(janasaṅgavivarjana)* is said to lead to perfection of yoga at *HR* 1.78. Both *μ* and G read *saṃgamam* here while most of the other witnesses have *saṃgame.* Ballāla (f. 59r^8) understands *saṃgame* to mean *amṛtasthānajihvāgrasaṃyoge*, "on the conjunction of the tip of the tongue and the place of *amṛta*".

377 "food-consumption" *(bhojanam)* : in the texts of *haṭhayoga* and amongst today's *haṭhayogin*s there are two different attitudes towards food consumption. As a result of success in yoga, the yogin either eats very little (e.g. *HP* 4.75) or he can eat as little or as much as he likes without any effect (e.g. *DYŚ* 157). Before attaining *siddhi*, however, the aspirant must curb his appetite (e.g. *HP* 1.15, *ŚS* 3.20, *GhS* 5.16) but he should not fast (e.g. *GhS* 5.31, *ŚS* 3.36). Cf. *Bhagavadgītā* 6.16–17.

378 "With his seed turned upwards" *(ūrdhvaretāḥ)* : this is the only mention of semen-retention in the text. Other haṭhayogic texts put much more emphasis on *khecarīmudrā*'s usefulness in preventing the loss of semen (see e.g. *GŚ*$_N$ 69, which is reproduced at *HP* 3.41, and on page 29 of the introduction).

379 "endowed with the [eight] powers whose first is minuteness" *(aṇimādiguṇānvitaḥ)* :

the *locus classicus* for these eight *siddhis* is Vyāsa *ad Yogasūtra* 3.44: *aṇimā*, "minuteness", *laghimā*, "weightlessness", *mahimā*, "hugeness", *prāpti*, "the ability to reach anywhere at will", *prākāmya*, "the ability to do what one wants", *vaśitva*, "control over elements and animals", *īśitva*, "sovereignty" and *kāmāvasāyitva*, "effecting one's desires". Ballāla (f. 59v[3–4]) gives a list which has *garimā*, "heaviness", in place of Vyāsa's *kāmāvasāyitva*. *MaSaṃ* 18.36c–37b substitutes *garimā* for Vyāsa's *mahimā*. VASUDEVA (2004:364–365) translates Kṣemarāja's interpretation of the eight *siddhis* (or *guṇas*) as given in his *Svacchandatantroddyota ad* 10.1073 and adduces parallels from other tantric Śaiva works.

380 Śrī, "splendour", is a name of Lakṣmī, the consort of Viṣṇu. Ballāla calls her Yogīśā (f. 60r[3]).

381 Vāgīśā, "the goddess of speech", is a name of Sarasvatī, the consort of Brahmā. See 1.49 and note 366.

382 "the fetter of death" *(bandhamṛtyuḥ)* : this is the *fraenum linguae* or frenum, the binding tendon at the root of the tongue. It is called *bandhamṛtyu*, "the fetter of death" because it ties down the tongue, preventing it from reaching *amṛta*, "non-death". See 1.46 and note 230. One would expect this compound to be *mṛtyubandhaḥ*. Ballāla makes no comment on the odd order of its elements.

383 "o mistress of the host" *(gaṇāmbike)* : the host *(gaṇa)* is Śiva's troop of attendants.

384 This is the area in the middle of the skull described at 2.57.

385 "absorption in it" *(tallayam)* : Ballāla (f. 61r[1]) understands *tallayam* to mean either *tatra sthāne layam*, "absorption at the place of Śambhu", or *tasya manaso layam*, "absorption of the mind". I have taken *tat* to refer to *unmanī*.

386 "with [inner] vision" *(dṛśā)* : it is of course impossible to look at the tip of the tongue when it is in the cavity above the palate so we must assume some sort of internal "sight". Ballāla (f. 61r[4]) glosses *dṛśā* with *aṃtardṛṣṭyā*. After a passage on *laya* at *HP* 4.23–34, we hear of the *śāmbhavīmudrā* (which brings about the same result as *khecarīmudrā*—*HP* 4.37—and is called *khecarīmudrā* in one manuscript of the *HP* and in a quotation of the passage in the *BKhP* at f. 72r[2]) in which the yogin is to dissolve his mind and breath in the internal *lakṣya*: *antarlakṣyavilīnacittapavanaḥ* (4.37a). *SSP* 2.26–27 describes four *antarlakṣyas*. In the *HP* and *SSP*, however, there is no mention of "sight", as such; only forms from $\sqrt{}$*lakṣ* are used. Cf. *ŚS* 5.37; *MaSaṃ* 18.29 mentions a *lakṣa* at the forehead. It may be that G's *tadā* is the original reading. The reading *rasān* found in γ is perhaps inspired by the idea that the tongue tastes different flavours during the practice, an idea found in many other texts that describe the practice (see page 22 of the introduction), but not in the *Khecarīvidyā*.

387 "perfect" *(heyopādeyavarjitam)* : on this adjective see note 319.

388 In contrast with the rest of the *Khecarīvidyā*, 2.107–115 fits the first of the two yogic paradigms described at *ŚP* 4365a–4371b in which the yogin is to raise his mind and breath by way of the central channel and cause *bindu* to enter the void. Among other rewards, he becomes *ūrdhvaretāḥ*—his seed turns upwards. *Amṛta*, Kuṇḍalinī and *cakras* are not mentioned. On the two paradigms and their attempted synthesis in haṭhayogic works, see pages 28 to 30 of the introduction.

389 "The Ethereal Gaṅgā" *(ākāśagaṅgā)* : the homologue of the Gaṅgā in haṭhayogic

physiology is the Iḍā *nāḍī* (see *KhV* 3.10). However, Iḍā only goes as far as the left nostril (*TŚBM* 70, *VS* 2.39) and is never said to reach the cranial vault (*ākāśa*—see note 265). It is thus unlikely to be the referent of *ākāśagaṅgā*. On the macrocosmic level there is an ideal homologue of this *ākāśagaṅgā* in the high Himālaya: the Ākāśa Gaṅgā flows from Tapovan, above Gaumukh, the glacial source of the Gaṅgā.

390 "he instantly becomes a master poet" *(kavitvaṃ labhate kṣaṇāt)* : Sarasvatī (see note 235) bestows ***kavitva***. At $GŚ_N$ 147 (≃ *ŚS* 3.84) the yogin is said to become a ***kavi*** by pressing the tongue against the *rājadanta*, drinking *[amṛta]*, and meditating on the goddess that consists of *amṛta (amṛtamayīṃ devīm)*. Cf. *SYM paṭala* 12 in which the *sādhaka* attains ***kavitva*** by visualising the goddess Parā (who is associated with Sarasvatī: Sanderson 1990:43-51) as pouring nectar into his mouth.

391 Meditation on Lakṣmī bestows kingship. Cf. *MaSaṃ* 34.58 where the the *rājya-lakṣmī* mantra is said to make the Kaula practitioner a king.

392 "five innate constituents" *(sahajāḥ)* : I have not come across any parallels of this usage of *sahajā* nor a similar set of innate physical constituents in any other text.

393 "which embodies the supreme" *(paramātmake)* : this description of the body is odd. It is tempting to take ***paramātmake*** as a vocative addressed to the goddess (wrongly written for ***paramātmike***) but such a usage is not attested elsewhere.

394 "through the fall of the father" (***pitṛkṣayāt***) : witnesses μ and G have ***pitṛkṣaṇāt*** and ***parikṣaye*** respectively here, neither of which seems better than ***pitṛkṣayāt*** which is found in S$\alpha\beta$. This unusual compound is glossed by Ballāla (f. 62r[7]) with ***pitṛśarīrāt*** which has then been altered in the margin by a later hand to ***pitṛvīryāt***. ***Pitṛkṣayāt*** has a disparaging sense to it and Alexis Sanderson has suggested that it may be some sort of yogic slang, implying a condemnation of householders who do not retain their semen. In Āyurvedic works, ***kṣaya*** refers to the decline of a bodily element *(dhātu)*: see Meulenbeld 1974:458–9.

395 In the ninth month according to Ballāla (f. 62r[8]).

396 "he should insert" *(viśet)* : ***viśet*** is being used here with a causative sense; in 124b it may be taken as indicative or causative.

397 In 123a–124b, the gender of *sahajā/sahaja* is somewhat confused throughout the witnesses. In 121c–122d it takes the gender of its referent and I have kept these genders in 123a–124b. No other witness does the same but it is the only way I can see of being consistent.

398 "o Lady of the Kula" *(kuleśvari)* : Ballāla (f. 63r[1]) understands ***kuleśvari*** to mean the "Mistress of Kuṇḍalinī"—*kulā kuṇḍalinī tasyā īśvari niyaṃtre*. In Kaula tantric works, Kuleśvarī is the highest goddess, the consort of Kuleśvara. See also note 6.

399 "insert" *(praviśya)* : for similar instances of $\sqrt{viś}$ having an indicative form and causative sense see 2.123d and 3.3a. Ballāla (f. 63r[10]) also understands it thus, glossing *praviśya* with *praveśayitvā* and *praviśet* (3.3a) with *praveśayet* (f. 63v[1]). In this passage (3.1–4) the subjects of the verbs are not clear. This is indicated by the confusion among the witnesses over whether Kuṇḍalinī is the object or subject in verse 1. I have chosen to adopt the readings of μ and G in which she is the object of *praviśya* (the use of *praviśya* with a causative sense adds to the subject/object confusion). I thus take *yogī* to be the subject of all the verbs in this passage. It is tempting to take Kuṇḍalinī as the subject of *pītvā* and *viśrāmya* in 4a (cf. *ṢCN* 53a where Kuṇḍalinī

drinks the *amṛta* herself; at *KhV* 3.41c the tongue *(vāgīśī)* rests in the *amṛta*) but the yogin is clearly the subject of *vibhāvayet* and even in *aiśa* Sanskrit absolutives and main verbs usually share a subject.

400 Ballāla understands 3.1–31 to be an expansion of the description of the five *sahajās* given at 2.120–124. Thus Kuṇḍalinī is described at verse 1, Suṣumṇā at 8, the tongue at 16, the palate at 23 and the *brahmasthāna* at 28. This somewhat forced schema may be due to the corrupt reading *paṃcamam* found at 3.24a in all the witnesses except μ and G (which have the correct *pavanam*). At f. 71r[3] he takes *paṃcamam* to refer indirectly to the fifth *sahajā*, glossing it with *binduṃ sthāna-galitam*.

401 "the bolt of Śiva's door" *(śivadvārārgalam)* : the *śivadvārārgala* is the *brahmārgala*. See 2.11a and 2.12a where *brahmadhāma* and *śivadhāma* are identified with one another, and note 245.

402 "by holding the breath" *(kumbhakena)* : Ballāla (f. 63r[11]) takes *kumbhakena* with *bhittvā*. This seems unlikely since *kumbhaka* is not mentioned as necessary for piercing the *brahmārgala* in *paṭalas* 1 and 2 while breath-retention is often invoked as the means of forcing Kuṇḍalinī upwards (see e.g. 2.35, 2.41cd).

403 On *praviśet* being taken as having a causative meaning see note 399. I understand its object to be Kuṇḍalinī. It could perhaps be the tongue but I have decided against understanding it thus for two reasons: firstly, there is no need to use *kumbhaka* to insert the tongue into the passage above the palate; secondly, if Kuṇḍalinī were not meant here, there would have been little point in mentioning her in verse 1. Ballāla (f. 63v[1–2]) also takes Kuṇḍalinī as the object, explaining that she is to be cooled down after being heated up in the course of her awakening: *pūrvaṃ yā* ⌈*vā*⌉*yvagninā taptā* ⌈*sā*⌉*mṛtena śītā bhavatīti tātparyaṃ*.

404 "he becomes a Khecara" *(khecaratvaṃ prajāyate)* : as at 1.75, Ballāla (f. 63v[5]) glosses *khecaratvam* with *devatvam*.

405 "cheating death" *(vañcanaṃ kālamṛtyoḥ)* : see 3.43–47 for a description of *kālavañcana* by means of this technique. I have emended μ's *kālamṛtyuś ca* to *kālamṛtyoś ca* to avoid adopting the unlikely plural *kālamṛtyūnām* found in the other witnesses. Ballāla (f. 63v[9]) explains the plural as referring to the omens of death that he is about to describe (on which see note 430): *bahuvacanaṃ tu vakṣyamāṇāriṣṭanimittam*.

406 "wandering throughout the three worlds" *(trailokyabhramaṇam)* : Ballāla explains *trailokyabhramaṇam* with *aṃtarikṣamārgeṇa guṭikāvat* "by way of the atmosphere like [when] a pill *(guṭikā)* [is consumed]" (f. 63v[9–10]). A marginal note describes the pill: *sā ca siddhapāradāder vihitā* "it is made from fixed mercury etc.". Cf. the *khecarīsiddhi* described in *MKSK paṭala* 6 which is achieved by means of, among other techniques, a *guṭikā*.

407 On these eight powers see note 379.

408 "luminous" *(jyotirūpiṇī)* : this is an *aiśa* sandhi form, avoiding the correct *jyotīrūpiṇī* which would be unmetrical. Ballāla (f. 65r[8]) identifies Suṣumṇā with the Sarasvatī *nāḍī*: *suṣumṇākhyā sarasvatīti*. This is very unusual—they are normally differentiated: see e.g. *DU* 4.7 where Sarasvatī is said to be at the side of Suṣumṇā.

409 "free of the qualities of colour and shape" *(varṇarūpaguṇais tyaktam)* : Ballāla (f. 65r[9]) understands *varṇa*, *rūpa* and *guṇa* to refer to consonants, colours and the

three *guṇas*: *varṇāḥ kakārādayaḥ rūpaṃ śuklādi | guṇāḥ satvādayaḥ*. Surprisingly, for *tyaktam*, μ has *sākam* and G has *yuktam*, both meaning "with".

410 Cf. *HP* 3.106, *ŚS* 5.170. DASGUPTA (1976:97) quotes a passage from Ḍombīpāda (song No. 14) in which "the boat is steered through the middle of the Ganges and the Jumna". See note 259.

411 "an immortal body forever" *(sadāmṛtatanuḥ)* : the original reading here may well have been that of G and M, *parāmṛtatanuḥ*, altered in most of the *KhV* witnesses to suggest the idea of liberation in an eternal body. Cf. 3.31d.

412 "the place beyond the Supreme Lord" *(parameśāt paraṃ padam)* : i.e. the *liṅga* in the vessel of *amṛta* described at 2.60a–63b (which is above Parameśa, the Supreme Lord, whose location is taught at 2.57).

413 Only μ reads *sudhayā śiśirasnigdhaśītayā*; all the other witnesses have variants on *atha sā śaśiraśmisthā śītalā* "then, she, cool, sitting on a moonbeam". I might have adopted the picturesque latter reading were it not for *siñcantī* at 13a which requires a main verb before the sentence can be ended by a conjunction such as *atha* (the obvious emendation *siñcati* is unmetrical).
Ballāla (f. 65v[8]) interprets *siñcantī* with *dvisaptatisahasranāḍīgaṇam amṛtenāhlādayati*, "she refreshes the 72,000 *nāḍī*s with *amṛta*". Kuṇḍalinī's return to the *mūlādhāra* is described at *ṢCN* 53.

414 "into the Three-peaked Mountain" *(trikūṭe)* : on *trikūṭa*, "the Three-peaked Mountain", see note 259.

415 "free from the process of time" *(kālakramavinirmuktam)* : Alexis SANDERSON made the emendation *kālakrama°* which I have adopted here. I have adopted the same form at 3.20b and 20c where only J4 has *°krama°* and have emended 3.21a likewise. It is time that is under discussion here, not action, so *°krama°* is preferable to *°karma°*. Ballāla (f. 67r[3]) takes *kālakarma* to mean time and action, glossing *karma* with *kriyā calanādi*.

416 i.e. the yogin should hold his breath to stop it flowing in Iḍā and Piṅgalā. He thereby forces it into Suṣumṇā ("the place where day and night are suppressed"). Cf. *MaSaṃ* 44.23cd *nāḍīdvayaṃ divārātriḥ suṣumṇā kālavarjitā*, "the two channels are day and night; Suṣumṇā is timeless". See also Dādu *sākhī* 16.22 (CALLEWAERT & DE BEECK 1991:174). *KhV* 3.19 is found at *HP* 4.42. Brahmānanda, in his *Jyotsnā* commentary on the verse, understands *liṅga* to mean *ātman*. The next verse (*HP* 4.43) equates *khecarīmudrā* with the flow of the breath in the central channel: *savyadakṣiṇanāḍistho madhye carati mārutaḥ | tiṣṭhate khecarī mudrā tasmin sthāne na saṃśayaḥ ||*.

417 This is one of the few instances where I have adopted a reading of βγ *(cedam)* over that of μα (*devam/liṅgam*; J6 has *vedaṃ* while G's *(ahorātram avi)cchedam* is probably a scribal emendation). S does the same—*devam/liṅgam* makes no sense in the light of verse 17—and glosses *idam* with *pratyakṣaṃ viśvaṃ dehaṃ vā*, "the perceptible universe or the body" (f. 70v[2]).

418 "death is defeated" *(kālamṛtyujayo bhavet)* : Ballāla (f. 70v[7–8]) gives two possible ways of analysing the compound *kālamṛtyujayaḥ* : *kālasya mṛtyoś ca jayaḥ kālādhīno mṛtyur iti vā | tasya jayaḥ*, "defeat of time and death, or defeat of that death which is dependent on time". I have understood it to have the latter meaning.

419 "with the flower of thought" *(bhāvapuṣpena)* : *KJN* 3.24–27 lists eight *puṣpa*s with which the internal *liṅga* is to be worshipped. The *bhāvapuṣpa* is the fourth. The *Bṛhatkālottara* (NAK 1-89/NGMPP B 24/59) contains an *aṣṭapuṣpikāpaṭala* (f. 136v[1]–f. 137v[2]) which describes four varieties of this internal and abbreviated Śaiva worship. Only the first includes the *bhāvapuṣpa* which is last in the list of eight "flowers". See also *Harṣacarita* p.35 ll.5–8 and p.175. (I am grateful to Alexis SANDERSON for providing me with references from these last two sources.) See also *KT* 59.28–32.

420 "pointing towards the upper mouth" *(ūrdhvavaktragām)* : it may be that μ's *ūrdhvavaktrakām* was the original reading, with the sense of "having the mouth pointing upwards" where "mouth" refers to the tip of the tongue, with which *amṛta* is tasted. The reading *ūrdhvavaktragām* suggests a plan of the body found in many haṭhayogic texts (but not in the *KhV*) in which the *amṛta* tasted by the tongue flows through the *śaṅkhinī nāḍī* and emerges at the *daśamadvāra* which is situated at the *rājadanta* (the uvula). See e.g. *AŚ* p.11 l.1, where the aperture is called both *mukharandhra* and *śaṅkhinīmukha*, and *SSP* 2.6. Cf. *KhV* 2.81.

421 "with a whistling sound" *(śītkāreṇa)* : in the *sītkārī prāṇāyāma* described at *HP* 2.54–56 a whistling sound is made as the yogin inhales through his mouth.

422 "in the supportless space" *(nirālambe pade)* : i.e. practising *dhyāna* without an object. At *HP* 4.4, *nirālamba* is mentioned in a list of synonyms of *samādhi*.

423 "natural yoga" *(sahajaṃ yogam)* : like *nirālamba* and *unmanī* (on which, see note 324) *sahaja* is given as a synonym of *samādhi* at *HP* 4.4. In tantric texts *sahaja yoga* is a state that arises naturally, without being forced (personal communication from Alexis SANDERSON). DIMOCK, analysing the *Caryāpāda*s of the Vaiṣṇava Sahajīyas, writes "The state of sahaja is one of utter harmony, in which there is no motion, no passion, and no differentiation" (1991:42 n.3). Ballāla (f. 71r[4]) understands *sahajaṃ yogam* to mean *yoga* using the five *sahajā*s described at 2.120–124.

424 "on the circle of sixteen vowels" *(ṣoḍaśasvaramaṇḍale)* : this is the *viśuddhacakra* at the throat. See e.g. *KMT* 11.44a–99b, *ṢCN* 28, *ŚS* 5.121. Ballāla (f. 100r[5–6]) writes: *atha kaṃṭhe viśeṣeṇa śuddhir yebhyas te viśuddhayo 'kārādivisargāṃtāḥ ṣoḍaśārā(ṣoḍaśārā°*] *em.*; *ṣoḍaśā∗a°* S)*bhidhāḥ svarāḥ caṃdrakalās teṣāṃ tatra sthitākhyā yata iti tadākhyaṃ* /. Placing the chin on the throat is part of the *jālandharabandha* technique described in note 267.

425 During my fieldwork many people told me that *khecarīmudrā* was used by *haṭhayogins* to enable them to stay in a state of extended *samādhi*. Ballāla, commenting on this verse, writes (f. 72v[7]): *eṣa cirakālasamādhyupāyaḥ*, "this is the means to long-term *samādhi*". He goes on to say that it should be done in a mountain cave, in the ground or in a *maṭha* of certain specifications. There should be a *śiṣyasaṃrakṣaṇagrāmakam*, "a group of pupils to protect him" (or perhaps "a small village [nearby] to look after a pupil"), *yato dehasaṃrakṣaṇam āvaśyakam*, "because the body [of the yogin] must be looked after [by one of his pupils]" (f. 72v[8]).

Writing in 1342 CE, Ibn Battūta reported of the *joki*s (yogīs): "These people work wonders. For instance one of them remains for months without food and drink; many of them dig a pit under the earth which is closed over them leaving therein no opening except one through which the air might enter. There one remains for months and I have heard that some jogis hold out in this manner for a year" (HUSAIN 1953:164). HONIGBERGER (1852:127–131) recounts the celebrated story of the "faqueer" Hari Dās who in 1837 was buried for forty days in a locked chest in a garden in Lahore. He was exhumed in front of "a great number of the authorities of [Maharaja Ranjit Singh's] durbar, with General Ventura, and several Englishmen from the vicinity" and revived. Describing those who practise this technique, HONIGBERGER continues (ibid.:129): "those who do succeed must undergo a long and continual practice of preparatory measures. I was informed that such people have their *fraenulum linguae* cut and entirely loosened, and that they get their tongue prominent, drawing and lengthening it by means of rubbing it with butter mixed with some pellitory of Spain, in order that they may be able to lay back the tongue at the time they are about to stop respiration, so as to cover the orifice of the hinder part of the *fosses nasales*, and thus... keep the air shut up in the body and head". Sir Claude Wade witnessed the revival and reported that Haridas's servant "after great exertion opened his mouth by inserting the point of a knife between his teeth, and, while holding his jaws open with his left hand, drew the tongue forward with his right,—in the course of which the tongue flew back several times to its curved position upwards, in which it had originally been, so as to close the gullet" (BRAID 1850:13). BOILEAU (1837:41–44) describes a similar spectacle that took place at Jaisalmer adding that "the individual... is, moreover said to have acquired the power of shutting his mouth, and at the same time stopping the interior opening of the nostrils with his tongue" (ibid.:43). Cf. the seventeenth-century account given by TAVERNIER (1925:156). MONIER-WILLIAMS (1878:50–53) reports two such attempts at "Samādh", both duplicitous. In the first, the practitioner's "friends were detected by the villagers in pouring milk down a hollow bamboo which had been arranged to supply the buried man with air and food. The bamboo was removed, and the interred man was found dead when his friends opened the grave shortly afterwards" (ibid.:50). BRUNTON (1995:112–120) describes in detail a meeting with an Egyptian *fakīr* who used the *khecarīmudrā* technique to enter a state of catalepsy. The technique, says the *fakīr*, was originally developed by Indian yogins. At every Kumbh Melā since the 1992 Ujjain Siṃhasth, a yogin called Pilot Bābā, together with a Japanese disciple, have remained in an open pit for periods of up to a week, emerging with much ceremony in front of large crowds. See also SIEGEL 1991:168–170.

426 "at that place" *(tatpadam)* : Ballāla f. 72r$^{1-2}$ understands *tat* to be referring to *brahman*: *oṃ tat sad iti trividho brahmanirdeśaḥ*.

427 "lifeless" *(nirjīvavat)* : cf. *AY* 1.39, *KJN* 14.82–85, *MVUT* 17.22c–23b, *Svāyambhuvasūtrasaṃgraha* 20.33–35 (as edited by VASUDEVA, 2004:435). Ballāla (f. 71v^{10}) notes the objection that if the body seems lifeless then surely a bad smell and other signs of putrefaction *(daurgandhyādi)* that are found in a corpse will arise. But this is not the case, he says: it is contraindicated by the use of *bhāti* (his reading for *bhā vi°*).

428 Ballāla (f. 72v$^{6-9}$) describes the yogin's state here as *samādhi* and mentions in passing some bizarre techniques for both reaching and returning from *samādhi* practised by other schools: *anye bahvabhyāsena jñātābhyaṃtaranāḍīviśeṣamardanenāpi taṃ* *kurvaṃti kārayaṃti ca | eke tu śavāsanasthit* āḥ sv* obhayapādāṃguṣṭhāgrāṃtarmanasai[kā]gratāyāṃ ca taṃ kurvaṃti | ... tatra samādhyavatāropāyaḥ bāhyavāyusparśaḥ śirasi navanītaghṛtādimardanaṃ | tadavatāravelāyāṃ devamūrttyādi tannetrāgre dhārayen na śiṣyādis tiṣṭhed...* |. "Others, after lots of practice, use a special massage of an internal channel that they have discovered to enter *[samādhi]* (and cause others to enter it). Some enter it in the corpse pose, once they have focussed their minds on both their big toes... The touch of fresh air [or] massaging the head with butter, ghee etc. are the means of bringing [the yogin] round from *samādhi*. When bringing him round one should hold an image of a deity or such like in front of his eyes. Pupils etc. should not stand [in front of him]." At the 1998 Hardwar Kumbh Melā, Raghuvar Dās Jī Yogīrāj tried to induce *samādhi* in me by squeezing the sides of my neck. I backed away as I started to feel faint. The corpse pose practice is taught at *DYŚ* 46–48.

429 "which consists of an eternal body" *(nityadehamayam)* : S$\alpha\beta\gamma$ have *nitya°* here where μ and G have *tyaktvā*. This indicates a doctrinal difference between the earlier and later recensions of the text. In μ and G *śivatvam* happens after death; the later tradition wants *śivatvam* in an eternal body. The original idea behind 31ab was of Kuṇḍalinī breaking out of the top of the skull (resulting in physical death for the yogin) rather than just entering the abode of Brahmā (as has already been described at 28cd). The use of *vrajati* (in contrast to *vasati* at 28d) confirms that this was the meaning intended in μ and G.

The readings for 31d found in the later tradition are slightly awkward. That of α_2, *nityadehamayam*, is better than the *nityadeham imam* of the other witnesses and I have thus adopted it.

430 Cf. *DYŚ* 251–258 (=*YTU* 107-111), which describes how the yogin can leave and return to his body at will.

Ballāla here embarks on a long excursus about *ariṣṭāni*, ways of forecasting impending death, including, among several others, palmistry, pulse-reading, dream analysis and shadow-inspection (f. 73r^1–f. 75v^4). (*Ariṣṭajñāna* (or *kālajñāna*) is also taught at *MVUT* 16.48–52, *Dīkṣottara samudāyaprakaraṇa* 59 (Vasudeva 2004:361), *Mataṅgapārameśvara yogapāda* 4.98cd–100ab, *TĀ* 4.127–144, *KMT* 23.1–80, *Mārkaṇḍeyapurāṇa adhyāya* 43 (of which vv. 3–26 are cited at *ŚP* 4564–4590), *VS adhyāyas* 7–8, *YBD* 11.135–143, in the ninth *upadeśa* of the ten-chapter *HP* (*H3*) and in vv. 761–772 of the *Jogpradīpakā*. On *ariṣṭa* in medical literature see Meulenbeld 1974:442.) Then, at f. 75v$^{4-7}$, Ballāla gives three ways (corresponding to the techniques described in *KhV* 3.32c–43b, 43c–47d and 48a–55b) in which the yogin might deal with impending death: *itthaṃ kālamṛtyum upasthitaṃ vijñāya yadā yogino buddhir imaṃ dehaṃ tyaktuṃ bhavet sā ca trividhā | samādhāv aikyabhāvinī kālavaṃcanī atyaṃtamokṣagāminī ca | tatrāpi prathamā dvidhā | svadehe jīveśaikyabhāvinī | paradehe svātmabhāvinī | aichikā parakāyapraveśarūpā ceti || dvitīyāpi dvidhā | kevalasamādhyā kālātikramāṃtā | sarvadhāraṇayā tadaṃtā ceti | tṛtīyā tu svechotkrāṃtyā brahmaikyasaṃpādinī* |. "Having thus realised that death is at hand is 'when the resolve of the yogin is to abandon this body'. And it [i.e. the resolve] is of three kinds: bringing about unity in *samādhi*, cheating death and going to final liberation. Of these, the first can take two forms: bringing about in one's body the union of the vital principle with the Lord, and manifesting oneself in the body of another (this takes the form of willful entry into another's body). The second can also take two forms: by means of the highest *samādhi* until the time [of death] has passed, and by introspection of all [objects] until that [time] has passed. The third brings about union with Brahmā by means of voluntary yogic suicide."

431 I have taken *jīvānilam* as a *dvandva*; Ballāla (f. $76v^3$) takes it as a *karmadhāraya* (see also note 251).

432 Ballāla (f. $76v^{4-7}$) adds that the yogin is to inhale with the right nostril: *piṃgalā-mārgeṇa pūrakapūrvakaṃ kumbhakaṃ saṃprāpya.*

433 The Svādhiṣṭhāna centre is in the region of the genitals—see e.g. *GŚ*$_N$ 22. Here Śiva is describing Kuṇḍalinī's ascent through the six centres that are the basis of a system of subtle physiology found in some haṭhayogic texts (e.g. *GŚ*$_N$ 15–16, *ŚS* 5.77–155, *Yuktabhavadeva* 3.234–252—a seventh centre, the Sahasrāra, is added in these texts) and which has become today the most widely accepted model of the body. In the texts of *haṭhayoga* there are many different systems of *cakra*s (see e.g. *SSP* 2.1–9 which lists nine *cakra*s and Kavirāj 1987, who describes a list of 26 *cakra*s given in a manuscript of the *Vairāṭapurāṇa*) and this reflects the even greater variety of such systems found in earlier tantric works. The first systematic description of the six *cakra*s can be found in *paṭala*s 11–13 of the *Kubjikāmatatantra.* (An earlier, but vague, reference to six *cakra*s can be found at *Mālatīmādhava* 5.2; a description of raising the breath through six centres which are not called *cakra*s is given at *Bhāgavatapurāṇa* 2.2.19c–21d). White (1996:134) suggests that the earliest systematic description of the six *cakra*s is found at *KJN* 17.2b–4a. 17.2c–4b reads: *gūḍhaṃ guhyaṃ sanābhiñ ca hṛdi padmam adhomukham ||2|| samīrastobhakaṃ cakraṃ ghaṇṭikāgranthiśītalam | nāsāgraṃ dvādaśāntaṃ ca bhruvor madhye vyavasthitam ||3|| lalāṭaṃ brahmarandhraṃ ca śikharasthaṃ sutejasam |.* The text is obscure and possibly corrupt but there are clearly at least eight *cakra*s listed and probably as many as eleven. 17.4cd implies that they number eleven: *ekādaśavidhaṃ proktaṃ vijñānaṃ dehamadhyataḥ.* (In a later article (2003:147) White acknowledges that this passage describes eleven *cakras.*) As White also notes (ibid.:423 n.86), at *KJN* 5.25–28 there is another of the text's many lists of centres in the body, which, although again rather obscure, does describe seven centres, of which five have locations similar to those of the *cakra*s in the *KhV* and other haṭhayogic texts. At *KJN* 10.6–8 there is a list of eight *cakra*s of which six correspond to those described here in the *Khecarīvidyā.*

434 The Maṇipūra *cakra* is at the navel. See e.g. *GŚ*$_N$ 23. (But cf. *GŚ*$_N$ 25 where the *kanda,* which in verse 23 is situated at the *nābhimaṇḍala* and is the site of the *maṇipūrakacakra,* is said to be below the navel. This discrepancy (or, perhaps, textual corruption) is noted by Ballāla at f. $99v^7$.)

435 The Anāhata centre is located at the heart. See e.g. *ŚS* 5.113.

436 i.e. the Viśuddhi/Viśuddha *cakra* at the throat. See e.g. *KMT* 11.44a–99b, *ṢCN* 28–29. The mixing of metaphors in the description of this "lotus" as "sixteen-spoked" is curious. As a lotus, this centre is usually said to have sixteen petals (*GŚ*$_N$ 15c–16b); one would expect it to be called a wheel *(cakra)* when described as

sixteen-spoked. The emendation of *padme* to *cakre* is tempting but nowhere else in the *KhV* is *cakra* used in this sense.

437 The Ājñā centre is located between the eyebrows. See e.g. *ŚS* 5.128.

438 "rest" *(viśrāmam)* : see *JRY* 4.2.159 and *NT* 7.13 for similar descriptions of relaxation in the ocean of *amṛta*.

439 Here Ballāla has an excursus on *parakāyapraveśa*, "entering another's body" (f. 77v[8]–f. 79r[7]). *Jogpradīpakā* 797–804 describes this practice and Alexis SANDERSON has provided me with the following references to Śaiva passages on this topic: *Niśvāsamūla* (NAK 1-277/NGMPP A 41/14) 7.20; *Svacchandatantra* 7.328c–329b; *Picumata* (NAK 3-370) 3.228–232b, 5, 96.19–35; *MVUT* 21.9–19; *TĀ* 28.294–300; *JRY* f. 195v (vv. 197c–204b), 3.5.31–32b, 4.2.397c–400b; *Liṅgapurāṇa* 1.24.128–130; *Vāyupurāṇa* 1.23.209–211. RAMA (1978:437–463) tells of witnessing yogins abandoning their bodies and entering those of others.

440 *Kālavañcana*, "deceiving death", is a common motif of tantric and haṭhayogic texts. Indeed, mastery over death is the *sine qua non* of the perfected *haṭhayogin*: yoga is said to be *kālasya vañcanam* at $GŚ_N$ 5–6; the *mahāsiddhas* listed at *HP* 1.5–9 are said to have broken the rod of death (*khaṇḍayitvā kāladaṇḍam*); vernacular tales of Yama's rough treatment at the hands of the Nāths are common (see ELIADE 1969:313–317). Techniques of *kālavañcana* similar to that of the *KhV* but using visualisations of *amṛta* alone and not involving the tongue can be found at *SYM paṭala* 11, *MVUT* 16.53–54, *Svacchandatantra* 7.217d–226b, *NT* 7.37–53 and *VS* 4.41–46, 6.32–41. The methods taught at *KJN* 6.16–28, *ŚP* 4598–4612, *YBD* 11.144–161, in the last *upadeśa* of the ten-chapter *HP* (H_2) and at *Jogpradīpakā* 773–9 do employ the tongue. At *GBS* 219ab the tongue is associated with *kālavañcana: jibhyā indrī ekai nāl jo rākhai so baṃcai kāl*, "the tongue and the penis [are joined by] one channel; who knows this deceives death". On the corporealisation of subtle tantric practices see page 27 of the introduction.

441 "knowing the apportionment of [the locations of] death" *(kālavibhāgavit)* : i.e. knowing the division described at 3.44c–45b. Alternatively, the compound could be understood to mean "knowing the apportionment of the time of death", i.e. having *ariṣṭajñāna*—see note 430. As Ballāla says at f. 79v[1], *kāla* can of course mean both time and death: *kālo dvividhaḥ yamo 'tītādivyavahārahetuś ca* /.

442 "death" *(kālam)* : I am taking *kālam* to be an *aiśa* neuter and the subject of *vrajati*.

443 i.e. with Kuṇḍalinī in union with Śiva in the ocean of *amṛta* above the gateway of Brahmā.

444 "supremely content" *(paramasaṃtuṣṭaḥ)* : Ballāla (f. 81r[8]) glosses *paramasaṃtuṣṭaḥ* with *na tu kiṃcidicchayāsaṃtuṣṭaḥ / punarjanmaprasaṃgāt* / "not unsatisfied because of the slightest desire, because it would [then] undesirably follow that he would be reborn".

445 "the rock of Brahmā" *(brahmaśilām)* : this rock *(śilā)* is perhaps the same as that at the top of the forehead described at 2.25. Ballāla (f. 81r[10–11]) says that it is like a rock blocking the way to *brahman*: *brahmanirodhakām (em.; brahmaṇo rodhekām* S^{pc}, *brahmaṇaḥ rodhakāṃ* S^{ac}*) śilām iva*, and locates it at the crown of the head where the fontanelle is found in infants and where [dead] renouncers' skulls are to be smashed with a conch shell: *yatra bālaśirasi mṛdulaṃ tatraiva ca saṃnyā-*

sinām śaṃkhena mūrdhā bhettavyo 'ṃtarāla iti. Witness R2 has the variant reading *brahmasabhāṃ*, "Brahmā's assembly".

446 i.e. the yogin is to return the microcosmic elements, mind and sense-organs of his body to their macrocosmic origins. Cf. *ŚP* 4531–4541.

447 "untouched" *(aspṛṣṭaḥ)* : the conjectural emendation suggested by SANDERSON of *adṛṣṭaḥ* and its variants to *aspṛṣṭaḥ* is found in the *BKhP* as a marginal addition by a later hand (f. 82r[2]).

448 "the orb of the sun" *(sūryasya maṇḍalam)* : this is the only mention of the *sūryamaṇḍala* in the text. *Maṇḍalabrāhmaṇopaniṣad* 2.1.5 describes how the *agni°*, *sūrya°*, *sudhācandra°* and *akhaṇḍabrahmatejo° maṇḍalas* are seen in the process of *śāmbhavī mudrā* but these are unlikely to refer to places in the body. Ballāla (f. 82r[3]) associates the *sūryamaṇḍala* with the Piṅgalā *nāḍī*: *sūryamaṇḍalaṃ piṅgalā sūryanāḍī tanmārgeṇa tanmaṇḍalaṃ pūrakapūrvakakuṃbhakena bhitvā.* His interpretation seems forced: *sūryasya maṇḍalam* almost certainly refers to a region at the top of the head. *ŚP* 4591–4611 describes both *videhamukti* and *kālavañcanā*. To deceive death the yogin seals all ten apertures of the body (4602) and floods it with *amṛta.* To abandon the body he seals only nine doors (4594) and then, using his breath and his mind, he fires the arrow of his soul by way of the tenth door towards the supreme target (4595–6). This tenth door is in the region of the top of the head (see note 240). Cf. *Bhagavadgītā* 8.12–13; *VS* 3.54–56. Descriptions of methods of "yogic suicide" *(utkrānti)* are found in several tantric Śaiva works. See the testimonia to *MVUT* 17.25–34 in VASUDEVA 2004 and the editor's analysis on pp. 437–445; in the *KMT*, the yogin is instructed to perform *utkrānti* when the place of the uvula dries up (23.99a). Alexis SANDERSON has provided me with the following further references to Śaiva passages on *utkrānti*: *Skandapurāṇa* 182.973–977; *Niśvāsakārikā* (NAK 1-277/NGMPP A 41/14 f. 114v ff.) *paṭala* 33; *Sārdhatriśatikālottara* (NAK 5-4632/NGMPP B 118/7) 11.13–19b and Rāmakaṇṭha *ad loc.*; *Bṛhatkālottara Utkrāntyantyeṣṭipaṭala* vv. 1–7 (NAK 1-89/NGMPP B 25/49 f. 187v[3] ff.); *Mataṅgapārameśvarāgama Caryāpāda* 9; *Picumata* (NAK 3-370) *paṭalas* 5 and 100; *TĀ* 28.292–302; *Jñānasiddhānta* (Old-Javanese, ed. and tr. Haryati Soebadio, The Hague, 1971). *Yogayājñavalkya adhyāya* 10 teaches how to abandon the body by means of *samādhi.*

449 "absorbed in Śiva" *(śive līnaḥ)* : in the description of *utkrānti* at *Svāyaṃbhuvasūtrasaṃgraha* 22.2d (VASUDEVA 2004:441 n.214) the yogin is said to be *śivalīnamanāḥ*: his mind is absorbed in Śiva. At *ŚP* 4596 he becomes absorbed in *paramātman.*

450 Ballāla (f. 82r[6]–f. 82v[11]) here describes two types of liberation: gradual *(kramamukti)* and subitist *(kevalamukti)*, citing "Yājñavalkya", the *Tantrarājatantra*, the *Bhāgavatapurāṇa*, and the *Yogasūtra* with Vyāsa's *Bhāṣya*.

451 Cf. the description of *khecarīmudrā* in the *Haṭharatnāvalī* where it is said that the yogin abandons his body and enters the place of Brahmā at the end of the *kalpa*: *kāyaṃ tyaktvā tu kalpānte brahmasthānaṃ vrajaty asau* (f. 13v[1]).

452 From here to the end of *paṭala* three, witnesses μ and G vary considerably from each other and from the text as I have presented it. Analysis of their variant readings indicates that μ preserves the earliest version of the passage and that G represents an intermediate stage between μ and the other witnesses. μ's passage is in praise

of *madirā*, "alcohol", and this explicit Kaula ideology has been expunged from the other witnesses who have turned the passage into a eulogy of Khecarī and *śivabhakti*. See pp. 7–9 of the introduction for a detailed comparison of the different versions.

453 We return here to the oldest layer of the text (see pp. 12–13 of the introduction). Thus in this verse *vidyā* would originally have meant the mantra of Khecarī but can now be interpreted as meaning the teachings of the whole text.

454 On *melana/melaka* see note 198.

455 Here Ballāla has an excursus on the various methods of Śaiva worship (f. 85v–f. 86(3)v). Among more orthodox practices he includes at f. 86(1)r$^{2-3}$ a ten-fold physical worship from the *Rudrahṛdaya*: *kaṃṭhavikāragadgadākṣarajihvāspaṃdauṣṭhasphuraṇa śarīrakaṃpanaromāṃcasvedāvalaṃbanānirgamarodana pāravaśyatāḥ*. At f. 86(1)r^{10}–f. 86(1)v^{1} he gives a six-fold *mantranyāsa* from the *Śivārādhanadīpikā* to be performed when bathing in ashes: *om īśānāya namaḥ śirasi oṃ tatpuruṣāya namaḥ mukhe oṃ aghorāya namaḥ hṛdaye oṃ vāmadevāya namaḥ nābhau oṃ sadyojātāya namaḥ pādayoḥ oṃ namaḥ sarvāṃge evam uddhūlayed evaṃ snānaprakramaḥ*. At f. 86(1)v^{5} he mentions a *pāśupatavrata* from the *Atharvaśira[upaniṣad]*.

456 "to advance in all types of yoga" *(sarvayogābhivṛddhaye)* : the next nineteen folios of Ballāla's commentary (f. 87v–f. 106v) are devoted to a description of *sarvayoga*, all the various methods of yoga.

457 For descriptions of suitable places for the *haṭhayogin* to carry out his practice see e.g. *DYŚ* 107–114, *HP* 1.12–13. Vasudeva (2004:247–251) surveys similar descriptions in Śaiva tantric works. *Jogpradīpakā* vv. 671–5 says that while training to practise *khecarīmudrā*, the yogin should stay in a secluded hermitage or forest hut for six months, not speak to anyone, repeat his mantra day and night, eat rice and milk without salt, use the herbal preparations described in its verses 665–670 (which are based on those described in *Khecarīvidyā paṭala* 4), cut his frenum every Sunday, perform *dohana* every fortnight and *mathana* day and night. His tongue will grow by four fingers, he will attain both *bhukti* and *mukti* and have no fear of birth and death.

458 "furnished with all that is necessary for the practice" *(sarvasādhanasaṃyuktaḥ)* : Ballāla (f. 108r^{3}) understands *sarvasādhana* to refer to food and medicinal herbs: *svāhārasādhanāni taṃḍuladugdhādīni auṣadhāni śuṃṭhyādīni ca*, "the requisites for his food [such as] rice and milk etc. and medicinal herbs [such as] dried ginger etc.". At f. 108r$^{9-10}$ he says how the yogin is to obtain them: *dhanāḍhyarājāśrayeṇa... svīyadravyeṇa vā*, "by recourse to a rich king... or by means of his own wealth".

459 Ballāla (f. 109r^{11}) expands *uvāca* with *evaṃ karuṇārdrakaṭākṣeṇa tārakopadeṣṭrā śivena prollāsitā lakṣyabhinnā pārvatī taṃ pratyuvāca*, "thus gladdened by Śiva, the teacher of salvation, whose sideways glance was wet with [tears of] compassion, Pārvatī, whose purpose had been fulfilled, replied to him".

460 "whose diadem is the crescent moon" *(candrārdhaśekhara)* : by this epithet "Śambhu's altruism is proven—when he holds the moon that consists of *amṛta* at his heart, there is the destruction of [his] poison and fever, but he holds it at his diadem in order to appease the three-fold afflictions of others." (*amṛtātmanaś candrasya*

svahṛdaye dhāraṇenāpi viṣadāhopaśāṃtisaṃbhave sati śikhare dhāraṇaṃ tu pareṣāṃ trividhatāpaśāṃtaye eveti lokopakāraḥ siddhaḥ : *BKhP* f. 109v$^{6-7}$).

461 "who can be attained [only] by true devotion" *(sadbhaktisaṃlabhya)* : the reading *sadbhāva*°, "true essence", found in μW_1 and G (after 3.56d) may be original: see *KJN* 21.10 where, after giving an exposition of the different Kaula schools, Bhairava declares *"kathitaṃ kaulasadbhāvam"*; cf. ibid. 14.93–94 where *amṛta* is located in the *khecarīcakra* and identified with *kaulasadbhāva*.

462 This chapter is a later edition to the text. See page 12 for details.
The *Jogpradīpakā* (vv. 665–670) draws on this *paṭala* in its description of various herbal preparations useful in the practice of *khecarīmudrā*.
Four verses in this *paṭala* are not in *anuṣṭubh* metre: verse 2 is in *vasantatilakā*, 3 and 10 are in *upajāti*, and 4 is in *sragdharā*. These different metres have in places confused scribes and account for some of the variants and omissions in the witnesses.

463 "the highest limb of the mendicant" *(bhikṣūttamāṅgaparikalpitanāmadheyam)* : as explained by Ballāla (f. 110r$^{9-11}$), this compound is a riddle standing for the *muṇḍī* plant (which is mentioned by name in verses 9 and 12). The mendicant *(bhikṣu)* is the *saṃnyāsī* whose highest limb *(uttamāṅga)*, his head, is shaven *(muṇḍa)*. He is thus *muṇḍī*. *Muṇḍī* is *Sphaerantus indicus* Linn. (Dash & Kashyap 1980:54). (When reporting the botanical names of plants mentioned in this chapter I give only those primarily identified with the Sanskrit term; for alternatives the relevant references in Meulenbeld 1974 or Dash & Kashyap 1980 must be consulted.)
Ballāla (f. 110r^{9}) introduces his commentary on this verse with *atha muṇḍīkalpam āha*, indicating that he regards this practice as a form of *kāyakalpa*, a technique of physical rejuvenation still practised by *haṭhayogins* in which the yogin stays in darkness in a cave or specially built room for long periods (usually a month), restricting his diet to a single herbal preparation. Similarly, his commentary on verse 4 begins *atha vārāhīkalpam āha* (f. 111r^{1}). Tonics to be consumed in *kāyakalpa* are described in MS O (on which see p.54). The second *upadeśa* of the *Yuktabhavadeva* contains detailed descriptions of thirteen *kalpa*s, including *muṇḍī-kalpa*. See also the *Kākacaṇḍīśvarakalpatantra*. For a modern account of the technique, see Anantha Murthy 1986.

464 Ballāla (f. 110v$^{1-2}$) says that *takra* here is three parts buttermilk to one part water and cites *Amarakośa* 2.8.1280 for definitions of the different varieties of *takra*: *takraṃ hy udaśvin mathitaṃ pādāṃbv ardhāṃbu nirjalam ity amaraḥ* /.

465 On the use of *takra*, *āranāla*, *madhu* and *śarkarā* in Āyurveda see Meulenbeld 1974:465–7, 445, 486–7 and 507–8 respectively.

466 Verses 2 and 4 are written as instructions for a physician attending to the yogin—in this verse the verb is *dadyāt*, "he should give", while in verse 4 there is the causative *pāyayet*, "he should cause to drink". Anantha Murthy (1986:57–61, 235) explains the necessity of an attendant physician to oversee *kāyakalpa*.
According to Ballāla (f. 110v$^{4-5}$), the yogin should be fed the pills for either 49 or, ("some say"—*ke cit*), 40 days, in the morning and evening.

467 It seems likely that a half-line is missing at the end of this verse, in which the yogin would have been said to obtain the various benefits listed in *pāda*s 2e and 2f.

468 "vigour" *(vīrya)* : this may refer to semen—*MaSaṃ* 40.50 describes a herbal *rasāyana* useful for semen-retention.

469 Ballāla (f. 110v[8–9]) adds: *varāhaḥ sūkaraḥ sa ca viprakṛṣṭaṃ sūkṣmam api śabdam avadhārayati*, "*varāha* is a boar, and a boar can make out distant and subtle sounds".

470 *Vārāhī* is *Tacca aspera* Roxb. (Meulenbeld 1974:599–600). According to Ballāla (f. 111r[1]), *vārāhī* is known as *vilāī* in the vernacular *(bhāṣāyām)*. Under *bilāī-kaṃd*, McGregor (1995:735) writes "cat's root: a large climbing perennial, *Ipomoea digitata*, having tuberous roots which are eaten and used medicinally".

471 "he gets rid of blackness on the body" *(kṛṣṇabhedī śarīre)* : this epithet is odd. Most of the *KhV* manuscripts read *kṛṣṇabhedī śarīram*. *Śarīram* is clearly corrupt—none of the adjectives agree with it, nor can it be taken with a verb. The reading that I have adopted, *śarīre*, is not much better. The only way I can see to translate it is "on the body" which is quite redundant in the context. The three preceding adjectives must be referring to the yogin (μ's *valipalitaharo* for *hatavalipalitaḥ* could perhaps be referring to the therapy but this is very unlikely in the light of *kṛṣṇakeśī* which must refer to the yogin). For *kṛṣṇabhedī*, S and α_2 read *kārśyabhedī*, "destroying thinness", which is probably a scribal emendation of *kṛṣṇabhedī*. The reading *varṣabhedī* found in μ is perhaps due to a scribal error in which a copyist inadvertently looked back to °*varṣau kṛṣṇa*° earlier in the line, although *varṣa*° could perhaps be understood in its meaning of "seminal effusion" (Monier-Williams 1988:926). I have taken *kṛṣṇabhedī* to refer to the therapy's property of combating *kuṣṭha*, which, as Ballāla notes at f. 111r[3], can manifest itself in blackness: *kuṣṭhaṃ śvetaṃ kṛṣṇaṃ cety anekavidhaṃ* I.

472 *Guggulu* is bdellium, the gum of the *Commiphora* tree (*Commiphora mukul* Engl.—Meulenbeld 1974:570).

473 Ballāla (f. 111r[9–11]) describes the preparation of *triphalā* in detail: *laghveraṃḍaphalāny ānīyeṣat saṃbharjya kuṭṭayitvā tatra vipulaṃ jalaṃ nikṣipya pācayitvā vastrāṃtaritaṃ kṛtvā tata uparitanaṃ tailaṃ saṃgṛhṇīyāt tac chuddhaṃ tailaṃ tena saṃyuktaṃ gugguluṃ māhiṣākhyaṃ tathānyaṃ triphalāyutaṃ gaṃdhakaṃ ca triphalā tu*

> *ekā harītakī yojyā dvau yojyau ca vibhītakau* I
> *catvāry āmalakāni syus triphalaiṣā prakīrtitā*

"Get some young castor fruits, parch them a little, grind them, add a large amount of water, cook them, put them in a cloth and take the oil from the top. That is pure oil. The wise [yogin], who knows the qualities [of herbs], should eat the *guggulu* which is called Māhiṣa and the other [*guggulu*], mixed with that oil and *triphalā*, and sulphur. *Triphalā:* one *harītakī* [*Terminalia chebula* Retz.—Meulenbeld 1974: 610] should be used, two *vibhītaka* [*Terminalia bellerica* Roxb.—ibid. 1974:601] and four *āmalaka* [*Phyllanthus emblica* Linn.—ibid. 1974:527]. This is called *triphalā*."

Ballāla (f. 111r[11]) takes *jarādāridrya*° as a *karmadhāraya*: "the debility that is old age".

474 *Winathia somnifera* Dunal. (Dash & Kashyap 1980:46).

475 S is the only witness to read *viśvasarpikā* here but since I can make no sense of the other variants and Ballāla (f. 111r[12]) confidently asserts that *viśvasarpikā* is a synonym of *mothā* I have adopted his reading. (The Hindī word *mothā* means "a kind of grass, *Cyperus rotundus*, and its tuberous root"—McGregor 1995:836; Dash & Kashyap (1980:25) give *musta* as the Sanskrit name for *Cyperus Rotundus* Linn.)
The *MaSaṃ* manuscripts insert the following corrupt passage between 6c and 6d: *hastinā saha yudhyate // triphalā puṣkaro vrāhmī (vrāhmīḥ* J_6*)* †*niḥsākotilalaṃsanī*† / *punarnavā vṛddhatārā* †*na yayuḥ*† *snehamiśritā // ṣaṇmāsāhārayogena*. Thus the result of eating the preparation is the ability to fight with elephants, while to be free of disease and death the yogin must eat for six months a mixture of *triphalā*, *puṣkara* (*Iris germanica* Linn.—Meulenbeld 1974:570), *brāhmī* (*Bacopa monnieri* Pennell—Dash & Kashyap 1980:53), †*niḥsākotilalaṃsanī*†, *punarnavā* ("hog-weed," *Boerhavia repens* Linn.—Meulenbeld 1974:575) and *vṛddhatārā* (probably *vṛddhadāraka*, *Gmelina asiatica* Linn. or *Rourea santaloides* Wight et Arn.—ibid.:600) mixed with oil. The phrase *na yayuḥ* is likely to be a corruption of the name of an ingredient of the medicine.
476 *Sassurea lappa* C.B. Clarke (Dash & Kashyap 1980:61).
477 A marginal note in W_1 *(ghṛtamadhuśarkarā)* and two *pāda*s added after 14b in γ *(ājyaṃ guḍo mākṣikaṃ ca vijñeyaṃ madhuratrayam)* say that *madhuratraya* is ghee, honey and sugar, as does Ballāla at f. 110v[3], where he adds that they should be in equal proportions.
478 The identity of *kunaṣṭi* is uncertain. It is perhaps *kunāśaka* (*Alhagi maurorum*—Monier-Williams 1988:286).
479 *Muṇḍikā* is presumably a synonym of *muṇḍī* (see note 463).
480 *Eclipta prostrata* (Monier-Williams 1988:765).
481 *Vitex negundo* (Monier-Williams 1988:554).
482 *Amala* is a synonym of *āmalaka* : see note 473.
483 *Eleocarpus ganitrus* Roxb. (Meulenbeld 1974:596).
484 As White (1996:170) remarks in the context of this verse, Bernier reported in the seventeenth century that "certain *Fakires*... can prepare mercury in so admirable a manner that a grain or two swallowed every morning must restore a diseased body to vigorous health, and so strengthen the stomach that it may feed with avidity, and digest with ease" (1891:321).
485 "the silk-cotton tree" *(śālmali°)* : *Bombax ceiba* Linn. (Meulenbeld 1974:602).
486 See note 227.
487 See note 259.
488 The verse quoted is *abhakṣyaṃ bhakṣayen nityam apeyaṃ pīyate sadā // agamyāgamanaṃ nityaṃ sa yogī nātra saṃśaya iti gorakṣaḥ /*.
489 The passage cited is not found in the Lonavla edition of the *Haṭhapradīpikā*.
490 Ballāla wrote this text himself: *āsanāni tu asmābhir yogara⌈tna⌉kārikāsu svakṛtāsūktāni* (*em.*; *°ūkt*** S).
491 These citations are usually introduced with *sūtre* and *bhāṣye*.
492 The *Vāyupurāṇa* is quoted from regularly in Ballāla's lengthy excursus on *sarvayoga* at f. 87v–f. 116v, sometimes with *"upamanyuḥ"* to indicate the source of the citation

but often without attribution.

493 The verse cited is not in Avalon's edition.

494 This passage is about the different tastes of *amṛta.*

495 I have located some of the citations introduced with *"śivena"* in the *Śivasaṃhitā*. I have been unable to find those listed here.

496 *Śivapaṃjaramārkaṇḍeyastotra* is a correction of *śivapaṃcaratnamārkaṇḍeyastotra.*

497 The *Dattātreyayogaśāstra, Yogabīja* and *Śivasaṃhitā* are paraphrased at many places in the commentary (especially between f. 87v and f. 108v). These have not been reported.

498 This text has been published as the *Dattātreyayogaśāstra*. These citations are usually introduced with *"datta"* or *"dattātreya"*.

Bibliography

Where more than one edition of a work has been consulted, references given are from the first edition listed. The date of a text's first publication is given in square brackets.

Manuscripts of works other than the *Khecarīvidyā*

Kularatnoddyota. Bodleian Library, Oxford. MS Chandra Shum Shere c.348. Paper. Newari. 106 folios. Incomplete and missing its first folio.

"Khecarīvidyā". Rajasthan Oriental Research Institute, Jodhpur. MS No. 34946. A work different from the *Khecarīvidyā* but containing verses from it. Reported as '"Khecarīvidyā" (O)' in the testimonia apparatus. See pages 54–5 for more details.

Jayadrathayāmala. National Archives, Kathmandu. MS. No. 1-1468. NGMPP Reel No. B 122/4. Paper. Newari. Dated 1622/3 CE. I am grateful to Alexis SANDERSON for providing me with transcripts of passages from this manuscript.

Bṛhatkhecarīprakāśa. Scindia Oriental Research Institute Library, Ujjain. MS 14575. This is Ballāla's commentary on the *Khecarīvidyā*. See under "S" in description of sources (p. 40).

Matsyendrasaṃhitā. The Wellcome Institute for the History of Medicine, London. MS Sansk. β1115.*

——— MS No.1782, MMSL, Jodhpur.

——— MS No.1783, MMSL, Jodhpur.

——— MS No.1784, MMSL, Jodhpur.

——— MS No.1785, MMSL, Jodhpur.

Yogacintāmaṇi of Śivānandayati. Oriental Institute of Baroda Library. Acc. No. 13047. Paper. Devanāgarī.

Vivekamārtaṇḍa of Gorakṣadeva. Oriental Institute of Baroda Library. Acc. No. 4110. Paper. Devanāgarī. Dated Saṃvat 1534.

*For full details of the *Matsyendrasaṃhitā* manuscripts see the descriptions of witnesses A,J6 and J7 on pages 35 to 37 of the introduction.

Vivekamārtaṇḍa of Gorakṣanātha. Oriental Institute of Baroda Library. Acc. No. 2081. Paper. Devanāgarī.

Haṭhapradīpikā of Svātmārāma. Rajasthan Oriental Research Institute, Jodhpur. MS No. 6756. Paper. Devanāgarī. This is the long recension of the *Haṭhapradīpikā*. See under H2 in the description of sources (p. 55).

Haṭharatnāvalī of Śrīnivāsa. Oriental Institute of Baroda Library. Acc. No. 13,118. Paper. Devanāgarī.

Printed sources

Ajitāgama, ed. N.R. Bhatt, 2 vols. Publications de l'Institut français d'Indologie No. 24. Pondicherry. 1964, 1967.

Advayatārakopaniṣad, ed. A.M. Śāstrī in ŚĀSTRĪ 1920.

Abhaṅgamālā of Jñāndev, ed. and tr. C. Kiehnle in KIEHNLE 1997.

Amanaskayoga, of Gorakṣanātha, ed. Rām Lāl Śrīvāstav. Śrī Gorakhnāth Mandir, Gorakhpur. 1980.

Amarakośa, of Amarasiṃha, ed. Krishnaji Govind Oka. Poona City: Law Printing Press. 1913

Amaraughaprabodha, of Gorakṣanātha, ed. K. Mallik in MALLIK 1954.

Amaraughaśāsana, of Gorakṣanātha, ed. Pt. Mukund Rām Śāstrī. KSTS 20. Srinagar. 1918.

Amoghapāśakalparāja, as transcribed by the Taisho group: "Transcribed Sanskrit Text of the Amoghapāśakalparāja, Part I", *Annual of the Institute for Comprehensive Study of Buddhism, Taisho University, No. 20.* 1998.

Īśānaśivagurudevapaddhati, ed. T. Gaṇapati Śāstrī, part 4, Kriyāpāda *paṭala*s 3–64 & Yogapāda. Trivandrum Sanskrit Series 83. Trivandrum. 1925.

Kathāsaritsāgara of Somadevabhaṭṭa, ed. Pt. Durgaprasād and K.P. Parab. Bombay: T. Jāvajī. 1903.

Kākacaṇḍīśvarakalpatantra, ed. R. Sharma. Kashi Sanskrit Series 73. Benares. 1929.

Kāmasūtra, of Vatsyāyana with the *Jayamaṅgalā* commentary of Yaśodhara, ed. G.D. Shastri. Kashi Sanskrit Series 29. Benares. 1929.

Kiraṇatantra. Unpublished collation of *paṭala*s 58 and 59 by Dominic Goodall. 1998.

Kiraṇavṛtti of Bhaṭṭa Rāmakaṇṭha, chh. 1–6, ed. Dominic Goodall. IFP. 1998.

Kubjikāmatatantra, Kulālikāmnāya version, ed. T. Goudriaan and J.A. Schoterman. Leiden: E.J.Brill. 1988.

Kularatnoddyota, ed. Somdev Vasudeva. Unpublished edition. 2000.

Kulārṇavatantra, ed. Tārānātha Vidyāratna. Tantrik Texts 5 (ed. Arthur Avalon). Madras: Ganesh and Company, 1965. Reprinted Delhi: Motilal Banarsidass. 1975.

———, ed. R.K. Rai. Tantragranthamālā 5. Vārāṇāsi: Prācyaprakāśan. 1983.

Kṛṣṇayamāritantra, ed. S. Rinpoche and V. Dwivedi. Rare Buddhist Text Series 9. Varanasi: Central Institute of Higher Tibetan Studies, Sarnath. 1992.

Kaulajñānanirṇaya of Matsyendranātha, ed. Prabodh Candra Bagchi in *Kaulajñānanirṇaya and Some Minor Texts of the School of Matsyendranātha.* Calcutta Sanskrit Series, No. 3. Calcutta: Metropolitan. 1934.

Kṣurikopaniśad with commentary of Nārāyaṇa, in *Śrīnārāyaṇaśaṅkarānandaviracitadīpikāsametānām upaniṣadāṃ samuccayaḥ.* Ānandāśrama Sanskrit Series 29. Poona. 1895.

———, in *Ātharvvaṇopaniṣadaḥ Nārāyaṇakṛtadīpikāsahitāḥ*, ed. Rāmamaya Tarkaratna. Calcutta: Asiatic Society of Bengal (New Series No. 249). 1872.

———, ed. A.M. Śāstrī in Śāstrī 1920.

Guhyasamājatantra, ed. Y. Matsunaga. Osaka: Toho Shuppa Inc. 1978.

Gorakṣavijaya of Bhīmasena Rāy. Ed. Pañcānand Maṇḍal. Calcutta: Viśvabhārati Granthālaya. 1949.

Gorakṣaśataka$_{\mathrm{N}}$, attributed to Gorakṣanātha, ed. F. Nowotny: *Das Gorakṣaśataka*, Köln 1976 (Dokumente der Geistesgeschichte).[†]

Gorakṣaśatakam, ed. Svāmī Kuvalayānanda and S.A. Shukla, in *Yoga-Mīmāṃsā*, 7, 4. Lonavla: Kaivalyadhama S.M.Y.M. Samiti. 1958.

Gorakṣasiddhāntasaṃgraha, ed. Janārdhana Śāstrī Pāṇḍeya. Sarasvatībhavanagranthamālā Vol. 110. Vārāṇaseyasaṃskṛtaviśvavidyālaye. 1973.

Gorakhbāṇī, ed. P.D. Baḍathvāl. Prayāg: Hindī Sāhity Sammelan. 1960. Reproduced in Callewaert and de Beeck 1991 (q.v.). I have used the verse numbering of the latter.

Gheraṇḍasaṃhitā, ed. and tr. J. Mallinson. New York: YogaVidya.com. 2004.

———, ed. and tr. S.C. Vasu. London: Theosophical Publishing House. 1895.

———, ed. P. Thomi. Wichtrach: Insitut fur Indologie Reike Texte und Ubersetzungen 2. 1993.

Jogpradīpakā of Jayatarāma, ed. M.L. Gharote. Jodhpur: Rajasthan Oriental Research Institute. 1999

Tantrarājatantra, ed. Lakshmana Shastri. Delhi: Motilal Banarsidass. 1997 [1926].

[†] This work was originally called *Vivekamārtaṇḍa* but came to be known as *Gorakṣaśataka* (see note 9). To avoid confusion with the original *Gorakṣaśataka*, an unedited work, I have marked references to Nowotny's edition with a subscript N.

Tantrāloka of Abhinavagupta with commentary *(°viveka)* of Rājānaka Jayaratha, ed. Madhusūdan Kaul Śāstrī. KSTS 23, 28, 30, 35, 29, 41, 47, 59, 52, 57 and 58. Bombay and Srinagar, 1918–1938.

Tārābhaktisudhārṇava of Narasiṃha, ed. Pañcānana Bhaṭṭācārya. Calcutta: Sanskrit Book Depot. 1940.

Taittirīya Upaniṣad, ed. V.P. Limaye and R.D. Vadekar in *Eighteen Principal Upaniṣads*. Pune: Vaidika Saṃśodhana Maṇḍala. 1958.

Triśikhībrāhmaṇopaniṣad, ed. A.M. Śāstrī in Śāstrī 1920.

Dattātreyayogaśāstra, ed. Brahmamitra Avasthī. Delhi: Svāmī Keśavānand Yogasaṃsthān. 1982.

Darśanopaniṣad, ed. A.M. Śāstrī in Śāstrī 1920.

Divyāvadāna, ed. E.B. Cowell and R.A. Neil in *The Divyāvadāna: A Collection of Early Buddhist Legends*. Amsterdam: Oriental Press. 1970.

Nādabindūpaniṣad in *The Yoga Upaniṣads*, ed. Pt. A.M. Śāstrī. Madras: Adyar Library. 1920.

Nityāṣoḍaśikārṇava with Śivānanda's *Ṛjuvimarśinī* and Vidyānanda's *Artharatnāvalī*, ed. Vrajavallabha Dviveda. Varanasi: Vārāṇaseya Saṃskṛta Viśvavidyālaya. 1968.

Nityotsava of Umānandanātha, ed. A. Mahadeva Sastri. Gaekwad Oriental Series No. 23. Baroda. 1923.

Netratantra with commentary *(Uddyota)* by Kṣemarāja, ed. Madhusūdan Kaul Śāstrī. KSTS 46. Srinagar. 1926.

Paramatthajotikā of Buddhaghoṣa. Pali Text Society Translation Series No. 32. London: Luzac. 1960.

Parātrīśikāvivaraṇa of Abhinavagupta, tr. Jaideva Singh, Sanskrit text corrected and annotated by Swami Lakshmanjee, ed. B. Baumer. Delhi: Motilal Banarsidass. 1988.

Pāśupatasūtra with the commentary *(Pañcārthabhāṣya)* of Kauṇḍinya, ed. Ananthakrishna Sastri. Trivandrum Sanskrit Series No. 143. Trivandrum: The Oriental Manuscript Library of the University of Travancore. 1940.

Puraścaryārṇava, ed. Muralidhar Jha. Vrajajivan Prachyabharati Granthamala No. 10. Delhi: Chaukhamba Sanskrit Pratishthan. 1985.

Bṛhatsaṃhitā of Varāhamihira with the commentary *(vivṛti)* of Bhaṭṭotpala, ed. Sudhākara Dvivedī. 2 Parts. Vizianagaram Sanskrit Series No. 12, Vol. X. Benares: E.J. Lazarus and Co. 1895 and 1897.

Bṛhadāraṇyakopaniṣad, ed. P. Olivelle in *The Early Upaniṣads: Annotated Text and Translation*. New York: Oxford University Press. 1998.

Bṛhadyogiyājñavalkyasmṛti, ed. Swami Kuvalayananda and Pandit Raghunathashastri Kokaje. Lonavla: Kaivalyadhama S.M.Y.M Samiti. 1976.

Brahmapurāṇa, ed. Hari Nārāyaṇa Āpṭe. Ānandāśrama Sanskrit Series No. 28. Poona. 1895.

Brahmavidyopaniṣad, q.v. *Kṣurikopaniṣad*.

Bhagavadgītā, ed. J.A.B. van Buitenen in *The Bhagavadgītā in the Mahābhārata: Text and Translation*. Chicago: University of Chicago Press. 1981.

Bhāgavatapurāṇa, ed. E. Burnouf. Paris: Imprimerie Royale. 1860.

Majjhimanikāya, vol. 1, ed. V. Trenchner. Pali Text Society. London: Oxford University Press. 1948 [1888].

Mataṅgapārameśvarāgama (Kriyāpāda, Yogapāda et Caryāpāda), avec le commentaire *(vṛtti)* de Bhaṭṭa Rāmakaṇṭha, ed. N.R. Bhatt. Pondicherry: Publications de l'Institut français d'Indologie No. 65. 1982.

Matsyendrasaṃhitā, ed. Debabrata Sensharma. Bibliotheca Indica Series No. 318. Calcutta: The Asiatic Society. 1994.

Mahākālasaṃhitā of Ādinātha, *Kāmakalākhaṇḍa*, ed. Kiśoranāth Jhā. Allahabad: Gaṅgānāth Jhā Kendrīya Saṃskṛta Vidyāpīṭha. 1986.

Mahākālasaṃhitā of Ādinātha, *Guhyakālīkhaṇḍa*, ed. Kiśoranāth Jhā (3 Vols.). Allahabad: Gaṅgānāth Jhā Kendrīya Saṃskṛta Vidyāpīṭha. 1976, 1977, 1979.

Mahābhārata, ed. V. Sukthankar, with the cooperation of S.K. Belvalkar, A.B. Gajendragadkar, V. Kane, R.D. Karmarkar, P.L. Vaidya, S. Winternitz, R. Zimmerman and other scholars and illustrated by Shrimant Balasaheb Pant Pratinidhi. (Since 1943 ed. S.K. Belvalkar). 19 Vols. Poona: Bhandarkar Oriental Research Institute, 1927–1959.

Mahārthamañjarī with the *Parimala* commentary of Maheśvarānanda, ed. T.G. Śāstrī. Trivandrum Sanskrit Series No. 63. Trivandrum. 1919.

Mahopaniṣad, ed. Pt. Mahādeva Śāstrī in *The Sāmānya Vedānta Upaniṣads*. Madras: Adyar Library. 1921.

Mārkaṇḍeyapurāṇa, ed. K.M. Banerjea. Calcutta: Bishop's College Press. 1862.

Mālatīmādhava of Bhavabhūti with commentary of Jagaddhara, ed. M.R. Kale. Delhi: Motilal Banarsidass. 1967.

Mālinīvijayottaratantra, *adhikāra*s 1–4, 7, and 12–17, ed. Somdev Vasudeva in VASUDEVA 2004.

——————, ed. Madhusūdan Kaul Śāstrī. KSTS 37. Srinagar. 1922.

Mṛgendratantra, *vidyā* and *yoga pāda*s, with the commentary of Bhaṭṭa Nārāyaṇakaṇṭha, ed. Madhusūdan Kaul Śāstrī. KSTS 50. Srinagar. 1930.

Maitrāyaṇīyopaniṣad, ed. J.A.B. van Buitenen. The Hague: Mouton and Co. 1962.

Yājnavalkyasmṛti of Yogīśvara Yājnavalkya, with the commentary *Mitākṣarā* of Vijnāneśvara, ed. Narayan Ram Acharya. Bombay: Nirnayasagara Press. 1949.

Yuktabhavadeva of Bhavadeva Miśra, ed. M.L. Gharote and V.K. Jha. Lonavla: Lonavla Yoga Institute. 2002.

Yogakuṇḍalyupaniṣad, ed. A.M. Śāstrī in ŚĀSTRĪ 1920.

Yogacūḍāmaṇyupaniṣad, ed. A.M. Śāstrī in ŚĀSTRĪ 1920.

Yogatattvopaniṣad, ed. A.M. Śāstrī in ŚĀSTRĪ 1920.

Yogabīja, ed. Rām Lāl Śrīvāstav. Gorakhpur: Śrī Gorakhnāth Mandir. 1982.

Yogayājñavalkya, ed. K.S.Śāstrī. Trivandrum Sanskrit Series No. 134. Trivandrum. 1938.

Yogaviṣaya, ed. K. Mallik in MALLIK 1954.

Yogaśikhopaniṣad, q.v. *Kṣurikopaniṣad*.

Yogasūtra of Patañjali with the commentaries (*Bhāṣya*, *Tattvavaiśāradī*, and *Yogavārttikā*) of Vyāsa, Vācaspatimiśra, and Vijñānabhikṣu, ed. Nārāyaṇa Miśra. Benares: Bhāratīya Vidyā Prakāśan. 1971.

Yoginītantra, ed. Biswanarayan Shastri. Delhi: Bharatiya Vidya Prakashan. 1982.

Yoginīhṛdaya with the *Dīpikā* of Amṛtānandanātha and Bhāskararāya's *Setubandha*, ed. Gopināth Kavirāj. Varanasi: Sarasvatībhavana Granthamālā Vol. 7. 1979.

Yonitantra, ed. J.A. Schoterman. New Delhi: Manohar. 1980.

Rasārṇava, ed. P.C. Ray and H. Kaviratna. Calcutta: Asiatic Society of Bengal. 1910.

Rasārṇavakalpa, ed. and tr. M. Roy with B.V. Subbarayappa. Delhi: Indian National Science Academy. 1976.

Rasendracūḍāmaṇi of Somadeva, ed. Jādavjī Trikamjī Ācārya. Lahore: Motilal Banarsidass. 1932.

Rauravāgama, ed. N.R. Bhatt, 3 vols. Pondicherry: Publications de l'Institut français d'Indologie No. 18. 1961, 1972 and 1988.

Laghuyogavāsiṣṭha, ed. V.Sh. Panasikara. Delhi. 1985. (Reprint of 1937 Bombay edition).

Liṅgapurāṇa, ed. Vīrasiṃhaśāstrin and Dhīrānandakāvyanidhi. Calcutta: Vaṅgavāsī Steam Press. 1890.

Varāhopaniṣad, ed. A.M. Śāstrī in ŚĀSTRĪ 1920.

Vasiṣṭhasaṃhitā (Yogakāṇḍa), ed. Svāmī Digambar Jī, Dr. Pītāmbar Jhā, Śrī Jñānaśaṃkar Sahāy. Lonāvalā: Kaivalyadhām Śrīmanmādhav Yogamandir Samiti. 1984.

Vātulanāthasūtrāṇi with the *Vṛtti* of Anantaśaktipāda, ed. and tr. Madhusūdan Kaul Śāstrī. KSTS 39. Bombay. 1923.

Vāyupurāṇa, ed. Rājendralāla Mitra (2 volumes). Calcutta: Bibliotheca Indica. 1880 and 1888.

Vijñānabhairava, ed. and tr. J. Singh. See SINGH 1979.

Vivekadarpaṇ, attributed to Amarnāth, ed. V.D. Kuḷkarṇī in *Nāthparaṃparetīl gadya graṃtha: Viveka-darpaṇ*. Hyderabad: Marāṭhī Svādhyāya Saṃśodhan Pattrikā, Marāṭhī vibhāg, Usmāniyā Vidyāpīṭh, aṃk 6vā. 1971.[‡]

Vivekamārtāṇḍa of Viśvarūpadeva, ed. K. Sāmbaśiva Śāstrī. Trivandrum Sanskrit Series No. 119. Trivandrum. 1935.

Viṣṇusmṛti, ed. Julius Jolly. Varanasi: Chowkhamba Sanskrit Series No. 95. 1962.

Śatakatrayādisubhāṣitasaṃgraha of Bhartṛhari, ed. D.D. Kosaṃbī. Bombay: Bhāratīya Vidyā Bhavan. 1948.

Śāktavijñāna of Somānanda, ed. L. Silburn. See Silburn 1988:117–119.

Śāradātilakatantra, ed. Arthur Avalon. Delhi: Motilal Banarsidass. 1996.

Śārṅgadharapaddhati, ed. Peter Peterson. Bombay: Government Central Book Depot. 1888.

Śivasaṃhitā, ed. and tr. J. Mallinson. New York: YogaVidya.com. 2006.

——————, ed. Svāmī Maheśānandjī, Bābūrām Śarmā, Jñānśaṃkar Sahāy, Ravīndranāth Bodhe. Lonavla: Kaivalyadhām, Śrīmanmādhav Yog Mandir Samiti. 1999.

——————, ed. and tr. S.C. Basu. Allahabad: Panini Office. 1914.

Śivasvarodaya in *Svar Yog* by Svāmī Satyānand Sarasvatī. Muṅger: Bihār Yog Vidyālay. 1994.

Ṣaṭcakranirūpaṇa, ed. and tr. Sir John Woodroffe in Woodroffe 1992.

Ṣaṭsāhasrasaṃhitā Chapters 1–5, ed. J.A. Schoterman. Leiden: Orientalia Rhenotraiectina 27. 1982.

Saṃvarodayatantra, ed. S. Tsuda. Tokyo: Hokuseido Press. 1974.

Sarvadarśanasaṃgraha, ed. Mahāmahopādhyāya Vasudev Shastri Abhyankar. Poona: Bhandarkar Oriental Research Institute. 1978.

Siddhayogeśvarīmata, ed. Judit Törzsök. DPhil. thesis, Merton College, Oxford. 1999.

Siddhasiddhāntapaddhati of Gorakṣanātha, ed. M.L. Gharote and G.K. Pai. Lonavla: Lonavla Yoga Institute. 2005.

——————, ed. K. Mallik in Mallik 1954.

Suttanipāta, ed. D. Andersen and H. Smith. Pali Text Society. London: Oxford University Press. 1948.

Saubhāgyalakṣmyupaniṣad, ed. A.M. Sastri in *The Śākta Upaniṣad-s*. Madras: Adyar Library. 1916.

Skandapurāṇasya Ambikākhaṇḍa, ed. Kṛṣṇaprasāda Bhaṭṭarāī. Mahendraratnagranthamālā 2. Kathmandu: Mahendrasaṃskṛtaviśvavidyālayah. 1988.

[‡]I have not consulted this edition but have used quotations from it found in Kiehnle 1997.

Svacchandatantra with the commentary *(-uddyota)* of Rājānaka Kṣemarāja, ed. Madhusūdan Kaul, KSTS 31, 8, 44, 48, 51, 53, 56. Bombay. 1921–1935.

Haṃsopaniṣad, ed. A.M. Śāstrī in Śāstrī 1920.

Haṭhapradīpikā of Svātmārāma, ed. Svāmī Digambarjī and Dr. Pītambar Jhā. Lonavla: Kaivalyadhām S.M.Y.M. Samiti. 1970.

——— of Svātmārāma (10 chapters) with *Yogaprakāśikā* commentary of Bālakṛṣṇa, ed. M.L. Gharote and P. Devnath. Lonavla: Lonavla Yoga Institute. 2001.

Haṭhayogapradīpikājyotsnā of Brahmānanda in *The Haṭhayogapradīpikā of Svātmārāma*, ed. K. Kunjuni Raja. Madras: Adyar Library. 1972.

Haṭharatnāvalī of Śrīnivāsayogī, ed. M.L. Gharote, P. Devnath and V.K. Jha. Lonavla: Lonavla Yoga Institute. 2002.

Harṣacarita of Bāṇa. Vidyabhawan Sanskrit Granthamala 36. 1972.

Hevajratantra, ed. D.L. Snellgrove. London Oriental Series Vol. 6, Pt. 2. London: Oxford University Press. 1959.

Secondary material

Alper, Harvey. 1989. *Understanding Mantras.* Albany: State University of New York Press.

Alter, Joseph S. 2004. *Yoga in Modern India: the Body Between Science and Philosophy.* Princeton: Princeton University Press.

Anantha Murthy, T.S. 1986. *Maharaj.* San Rafael, California: The Dawn Horse Press.

Armstrong, John W. 1994 [1944]. *The Water of Life. A Treatise on Urine Therapy.* Delhi: Rupa & Co.

Avalon, Arthur. 1914. *Principles of Tantra, Part 1.* London: Luzac and Co.

Baḍathvāl, P.D. 1960. *Gorakhbāṇī.* Prayāg: Hindī Sāhity Sammelan.

Bernard, Theos. 1982 [1950]. *Hatha Yoga.* London: Rider.

Bernier, François. 1891. *Travels in the Mogul Empire A.D. 1656–1668.* A revised and improved edition based upon Irving Brock's translation by Archibald Constable. London: Archibald Constable and Co.

Bodewitz, H.W. 1973. *Jaiminīya Brāhmaṇa I, 1–65 Translation and Commentary with a study Agnihotra and Prāṇāgnihotra.* Leiden: E.J.Brill.

Böhtlingk, Otto and Roth, Rudolf. 1855-1875. *Sanskrit-Wörterbuch.* 7 Volumes. St. Petersburg.

Boileau, A.H.E. 1837. *Personal Narrative of a Tour through the Western States of Rajwara, in 1835; comprising Beekaner, Jesulmer, and Jodhpoor, with the Passage of the Great Desert, and a brief visit to the Indus and to Buhawulpoor; accompanied by various Tables and Memoranda Statistical, Philological, and Geographical.* Calcutta: N.Grant.

Bouillier, Véronique. 1997. *Ascètes et rois. Un monastère de Kanphata Yogis au Népal.* Paris: CNRS Éditions.

Bouy, Christian. 1994. *Les Nātha-Yogin et les Upaniśads.* Paris: Diffusion de Boccard.

Braid, James. 1850. *Observations on Trance or, Human Hybernation.* London: John Churchill.

Briggs, George Weston. 1938. *Gorakhnāth and the Kānphaṭa Yogīs.* Delhi: Motilal Banarsidass.

Brunner, Hélène. 1994. "The Place of Yoga in the Śaivāgamas", in *Pandit N.R. Bhatt Felicitation Volume*, ed. P.S. Filliozat, S.P. Narang and C.P. Bhatta. Delhi: Motilal Banarsidass.

Brunton, Paul. 1995 [1936]. *A Search in Secret Egypt.* Maine: Weiser.

———. n.d. *A Search in Secret India.* London: Rider.

Bühler, G. 1873. *A Catalogue of Sanskrit Manuscripts in the Private Libraries of Gujarat, Kathiawad, Kachchh, Sindh and Khandes.* Fascicle 4. Bombay.

Callewaert, Winand M., and de Beeck, Bart Op. 1991. *Devotional Hindī Literature. A Critical Edition of the Pañc-Vāṇī or Five Works of Dādū, Kabīr, Nāmdev, Rāidās, Hardās with the Hindī Songs of Gorakhnāth and Sundardās, and a Complete Word-index.* 2 volumes. New Delhi: Manohar.

Chambers. 1983. *Chambers 20th Century Dictionary.* Ed. E.M. Kirkpatrick. Edinburgh: W & R Chambers Ltd.

Clark, Matthew. 2004. *The Daśanāmī-Saṃnyāsīs: The Integration of Ascetic Lineages into an Order.* PhD thesis, School of Oriental and African Studies, London.

Dasgupta, Shashibhushan. 1976 [1946]. *Obscure Religious Cults.* 3rd edition. Calcutta: Firma KLM Private Ltd.

Dash, Bhagwan and Kashyap, L. 1980. *Materia Medica of Ayurveda.* (Based on the *Āyurvedasaukhyam* of Toḍarānanda). New Delhi: Concept Publishing.

De Michelis, Elizabeth. 2004. *A History of Modern Yoga.* London: Continuum.

Derrett, Duncan. 1973. *Dharmaśāstra and Juridical Literature.* History of Indian Literature 4. Wiesbaden: Harrassowitz.

Digby, Simon. 1970. *Encounters with Jogīs in Indian Ṣūfī hagiography.* Unpublished paper presented at a seminar on Aspects of Religion in South Asia at the School of Oriental and African Studies, University of London.

Dimock, Edward C. Jr. 1991 [1966]. *The Place of the Hidden Moon.* Delhi: Motilal Banarsidass.

DVIVEDĪ, Hazārīprasād. 1996 [1950]. *Nāth Sampradāy.* Ilāhābād: Lokbhāratī Prakāśan.

————. 1978. *Nāth Siddhoṃ kī Bāniyāṃ.* Vārāṇasī: Nāgarīpracāriṇī Sabhā.

DYCZKOWSKI, Mark. 1988. *The Canon of the Śaivāgama and the Kubjikā Tantras of the Western Kaula Tradition.* Albany: State University of New York Press.

EDGERTON, Franklin. 1953. *Buddhist Hybrid Sanskrit Grammar and Dictionary.* New Haven: Yale University Press.

ELIADE, Mircea. 1969. *Yoga: Immortality and Freedom.* Princeton: Princeton University Press.

FULLER, C.J. 1992. *The Camphor Flame.* Princeton: Princeton University Press.

GERVIS, Pearce. 1970. *Naked They Pray.* Delhi: Universal. (Reprint of Cassell's edition, n.d.).

GHAROTE, M.L. 1991. "A critical note on the Haṭhapradīpikā", *Journal of the Oriental Institute, Baroda* 40, 3–4, pp.243–8.

GHAROTE, M.L. and BEDEKAR, V.A. 1989. *Descriptive Catalogue of Yoga Manuscripts.* Lonavla: Kaivalyadhama S.M.Y.M. Samiti.

GODE, P.K. 1938. "Date of Nārāyaṇa, the commentator of the Upaniṣads," in *Journal of the University of Bombay,* 7, 2.

GOLD, Daniel. 1995. "The Instability of the King: Magical Insanity and the Yogi's Power in the Politics of Jodhpur, 1803–1843", in *Bhakti Religion in North India: Community Identity and Political Action,* ed. David N. Lorenzen. Albany: State University of New York Press.

GONDA, Jan. 1965. *Change and Continuity in Indian Religion* (particularly chapter 2, *Soma, Amṛta and the Moon,* and chapter 4, *The Number Sixteen*). The Hague: Mouton & Co.

GOODALL, Dominic. 1995. *An Edition and Translation of the First Chapters of Bhaṭṭa Rāmakaṇṭha's Commentary on the 'Vidyāpāda' of the Kiraṇāgama'.* DPhil. thesis. Wolfson College, Oxford University.

GOUDRIAAN, Teun and GUPTA, Sanjukta. 1981. *Hindu Tantric and Śākta Literature.* History of Indian Literature 2, 2. Wiesbaden: Harrassowitz.

GROSS, R.L. 1992. *The Sadhus of India. A Study of Hindu Asceticism.* Jaipur: Rawat Publications.

HANNEDER, Jürgen. 1998. "Śaiva Tantric Material in the *Yogavāsiṣṭha*", *Wiener Zeitschrift für die Kunde Südasiens* Band XLII, pp. 67–76.

HEESTERMAN, J.C. 1964. "Brahmin, ritual and renouncer", *Wiener Zeitschrift für die Kunde Süd-und Ostasiens* 8, pp.1–31.

HIRALAL, Rai Bahadur. 1926. *Catalogue of Sanskrit and Prakrit Manuscripts in the Central Provinces and Berar.* Nagpur.

Honigberger, John Martin. 1852. *Thirty-five years in the East. Adventures, Discoveries, Experiments, and Historical Sketches, relating to the Punjab and Cashmere; in connection with Medicine, Botany, Pharmacy, &c. together with an original Materia Medica; and a Medical Vocabulary, in four European and Five Eastern Languages.* London: H. Baillière.

Horner, I.B. 1954. *The Collection of the Middle Length Sayings.* Vol. 1. London: Pali Text Society Translation Series No. 29.

Husain, Mahdi. 1953. *The Reḥla of Ibn Battūta.* Baroda: Oriental Institute.

Iyengar, B.K.S. 1977. *Light on Yoga* (Revised edition). New York: Schocken Books.

Jhā, Kiśoranāth. 1976. Introduction *(prastāvanā)* to the *Mahākālasaṃhitā Guhyakālīkhaṇḍa* vol. 1. Gaṅgānāth Jhā Kendrīya Saṃskṛta Vidyāpīṭha. Allahabad.

Kaivalyadhama. 1991. *Yoga Kośa.* Lonavla: Kaivalyadhama S.M.Y.M. Samiti.

Kane, P.V. 1968–1975. *History of Dharmaśastra.* 5 vols. 2nd edition. Poona: Bhandarkar Oriental Research Institute.

Kavirāj, Gopīnāth. 1972. *Tāntrik Sāhity (Vivaraṇātmak Granthasūcī).* Lucknow: Rājārṣi Puruṣottam Dās Ṭaṇḍan Hindī Bhavan.

———. 1987 [1966]. "The system of cakras according to Gorakṣanātha", pp.47–55 in *Notes on Religion and Philosophy,* by G. Kaviraj, ed. Gaurinath Sastri. The Princess of Wales Sarasvati Bhavana Studies. (Reprint Series No. 3). Varanasi: Sampurnanand Sanskrit University.

Kiehnle, C. 1997. *Songs on Yoga. Texts and Teachings of the Mahārāṣṭrian Nāths.* Stuttgart: Franz Steiner Verlag.

Kielhorn, Franz. 1874. *A Catalogue of Sanskrit mss. existing in the Central Provinces.* Nagpur: Government Book Depot.

Kiss, C. *Matsyendrasaṃhitā,* a critical edition of selected *paṭala*s. Forthcoming DPhil. thesis, Balliol College, Oxford.

———. 2004. *Introduction to the Matsyendrasaṃhitā.* Unpublished DPhil. transfer paper, Balliol College, Oxford.

Kuvalayānanda, Swami & Shukla, S.A. 1958. *Gorakṣaśatakam* (Preface pp. iv–vi; Introduction, pp. 1–19) in *Yoga-Mīmāṃsā,* 7, 4. Lonavla: Kaivalyadhama S.M.Y.M. Samiti.

Lochtefeld, James G. 2004. "The Construction of the Kumbha Mela", *South Asian Popular Culture,* 2, 2, pp.103–126.

McGregor, R.S. 1995. *Hindi-English Dictionary.* Oxford: Oxford University Press.

Mallik, K. 1954. *The Siddha Siddhānta Paddhati and Other Works of Nath Yogis.* Poona: Poona Oriental Book House.

Mallinson, J. 2005. "Rāmānandī Tyāgīs and Haṭha Yoga", *Journal of Vaishnava Studies,* 14, 1, pp. 107–121.

Meulenbeld, G. Jan. 1974. *The Mādhavanidhāna and its Chief Commentary. Chapters 1–10.* Leiden: E.J.Brill.

———. 1989. "The search for clues to the chronology of Sanskrit medical texts, as illustrated by the history of *bhaṅgā* (Cannabis sativa Linn.)", *Studien zur Indologie Und Iranistik*, 15, pp. 59–70.

———. 1999(–2000). *A History of Indian Medical Literature.* Two vols. Groningen: Egbert Forsten.

Mitra, Rājendralāla. 1880. *A Catalogue of Sanskrit Manuscripts in the Library of His Highness the Mahārājā of Bikaner.* Calcutta.

———. 1886. *Notices of Sanskrit MSS., vol. VIII.* Calcutta.

Monier-Williams, M. 1878. *Modern India and the Indians.* London: Trübner and Co.

———. 1988 [1899]. *A Sanskrit-English Dictionary.* Delhi: Motilal Banarsidass.

Norman, K. 1992. *The Group of Discourses (Sutta-Nipāta)* vol. 2. Oxford: Pali Text Society Translation Series No. 45.

Padoux, A. (ed.). 1986. *Mantras et Diagrammes Rituelles dans l'Hindouisme.* Paris: Éditions du Centre National de la Recherche Scientifique.

———. 1990a. *Vāc.* Albany: State University of New York Press.

———. 1990b. "The Body in Tantric Ritual: the Case of the *Mudrās*", pp.66–75 in *The Sanskrit Tradition and Tantrism,* ed. T. Goudriaan (*Contributions of the panels of the VIIth World Sanskrit Conference,* Leiden 1987, vol. 1). Leiden: E.J.Brill.

Parry, Jonathan P. 1994. *Death in Banaras.* Cambridge: Cambridge University Press.

Peterson, Peter. 1883. "Prof. Peterson's Report on the Search for Sanskrit MSS. in the Bombay Circle 1882–3", *Journal of the Bombay Branch of the Royal Asiatic Society Extra Number.* (No. 41 Vol. 16). London: Trübner and Co.

Raghavan, V. 1966. *New Catalogus Catalogorum Vol. 2.* University of Madras.

———. 1969a. *New Catalogus Catalogorum Vol. 1.* University of Madras.

———. 1969b. *New Catalogus Catalogorum Vol. 5.* University of Madras.

Rama, Swami. 1978. *Living with the Himalayan Masters.* Honesdale, Pennsylvania: Himalayan Institute Press.

Ray, Ram Kumar. 1982. *Encyclopaedia of Yoga.* Varanasi: Prachya Prakashan.

Rieker, Hans-Ulrich. 1992. *Hatha Yoga Pradipika: Translation and Commentary.* London: Aquarian Press.

Robinson, James B. 1979. *Buddha's Lions: The Lives of the Eighty-four Siddhas.* Berkeley: Dharma Publishing.

Roşu, Arion. 1982. *Yoga et alchimie.* Zeitschrift der Deutschen Morgenländischen Gesellschaft 132, pp. 363–379.

————. 1997. "À propos de rapports entre Rasaśāstra et Tantra: étude sur un fragment du *Rasendracuḍāmaṇi*", pp. 408–423 in *India and Beyond*, ed. Dick van der Meij. London: Kegan Paul International.

Sanderson, Alexis. 1986. "Maṇḍala and Āgamic Identity in the Trika of Kashmir," pp.169–214 in Padoux 1986.

————. 1987. "Trika Śaivism" in Mircea Eliade (ed.), *The Encyclopedia of Religion.* London: Macmillan.

————. 1988. "Śaivism and the Tantric Traditions", pp. 660–704 in *The World's Religions*, ed. S .Sutherland, L. Houlden, P. Clarke and F. Hardy. London: Routledge.

————. 1990. "The Visualisation of the Deities of the Trika", pp. 31–88 in *L'Image Divine: Culte et Méditation dans l'Hindouisme*, ed. A. Padoux. Paris: Éditions du Centre National de la Recherche Scientifique.

————. 1993. "An Outline of Brahmanism (ca. 900 A.D.)." The text of seven lectures delivered at All Souls, Oxford.

————. 1995. "Meaning in Tantric Ritual", pp. 1–98 in *Essais sur le Rituel III: Colloque du Centenaire de la Section des Sciences religieuses de l'École Pratique des Hautes Études,* ed. Anne-Marie Blondeau and Kristofer Schipper. Bibliothèque de l'École des Hautes Études, Sciences Religieuses. Louvain-Paris: Peeters.

————. 2003. "The Śaiva Religion among the Khmers Part I", *Bulletin de l'École française d'Extrême-Orient,* 90–91 (2003–2004), pp. 349–462.

————. n.d. Unpublished translation of the thirty-second *āhnika* of the *Tantrāloka.*

Sarasvatī, Svāmī Praṇavānand. 1984. *Jñān Bherī.* Rishikesh: Vijñān Press.

Sarasvatī, Svāmī Satyānanda. 1991. *Amaroli.* Munger: Bihar School of Yoga.

————. 1993. *Hathayogapradipika.* Munger: Bihar School of Yoga.

Śāstrī, A.M. (ed.). 1920. *The Yoga Upaniṣads.* Madras: Adyar Library.

Schopen, Gregory. 1997. *Bones, Stones and Buddhist Monks.* Honolulu: University of Hawai'i Press.

Shastri, Haraprasada. 1905. *Report on the Search for Sanskrit Manuscripts (1901–1902 to 1905–1906).* Calcutta: Asiatic Society of Bengal.

————. 1939. *A Descriptive Catalogue of the Sanskrit Manuscripts in the Collections of the Royal Asiatic Society of Bengal.* Vol. 8, Pt. 1 Tantra Manuscripts. (Revised edition by Chintaharan Chakravarti.) Calcutta: Royal Asiatic Society of Bengal.

Shea, David and Troyer, Anthony. 1843. *The Dabistan: or School of Manners.* London: Oriental Translation Fund of Great Britain and Ireland.

SHUKLA, S.A. 1966. "The Five Haṭha Texts" in *Yoga-Mīmāṃsā* 9.2. Lonavla: Kaivalyadhama.

SIEGEL, Lee. 1991. *Net of Magic: Wonders and Deceptions in India.* Chicago: University of Chicago Press.

SILBURN, L. 1968. *Le Mahārthamañjarī de Maheśvarānanda.* Paris: de Boccard.

———. 1988. *Kuṇḍalinī: Energy of the Depths.* Tr. J. Gontier. Albany: State University of New York Press.

SINGH, Jaideva. 1979. *Vijñānabhairava.* Delhi: Motilal Banarsidass.

SIRCAR, D.C. 1998 [1973]. *The Śākta Pīṭhas.* Delhi: Motilal Banarsidass.

SONTHEIMER, Günther-Dietz. 1989. *Pastoral Deities in Western India.* (Tr. Anne Feldhaus.) New York: Oxford University Press.

STERNBACH, Ludwik. 1974. *Subhāṣita, Gnomic and Didactic Literature.* History of Indian Literature 4. Wiesbaden: Harrassowitz.

SVOBODA, Robert. 1986. *Aghora, at the Left Hand of God.* Albuquerque: Brotherhood of Life.

TAVERNIER, Jean-Baptiste. 1925 [1676]. *Travels in India.* Translated from the original French edition of 1676 by V. Ball. Second edition ed. William Crooke. London: Oxford University Press.

TRIMINGHAM, J. Spencer. 1973. *The Sufi Orders in Islam.* London: Oxford University Press.

TUCCI, Giuseppe. 1930. *"Animadversiones Indicae", Journal of the Asiatic Society of Bengal,* New Series XXVI, pp.125–160.

VAN DER VEER, Peter. 1989. *Gods on Earth. The Management of Religious Experience and Identity in a North Indian Pilgrimage Centre.* Delhi: Oxford University Press.

VASUDEVA, Somdev. 1997. "The Mudrās of the Mālinīvijayottaratantra." Paper given at All Souls, Oxford, in Professor Alexis SANDERSON's Tantric Studies Seminar series, May 5th 1997.

———. 2004. *The Yoga of the Mālinīvijayottaratantra.*. Pondicherry: Publications de l'Institut français d'Indologie No. 97.

VYAS, K. and KSHIRSAGAR, D.B. 1986. *A Catalogue of Manuscripts in Maharaja Man Singh Pustak Prakash, Jodhpur. Pt. 2.* Jodhpur: Maharaja Man Singh Pustak Prakash.

WEITZMANN, M.P. 1977. "Review of V.A. Dearing, 'Principles and practice of textual analysis' (Berkeley 1974)", *Vetus Testamentum* 27, pp.225–235.

WEST, M.L. 1973. *Textual Criticism and Editorial Technique.* Stuttgart: B.G. Teubner.

WESTERGAARD, N.L. 1846. *Codices Indici Bibliothecae Regiae Havniensis.* Copenhagen.

White, David Gordon. 1996. *The Alchemical Body.* Chicago: University of Chicago Press.

———. 2003. "Yoga in Early Hindu Tantra", pp. 143–161 in *Yoga: The Indian Tradition,* ed. Ian Whicher and David Carpenter. London: Routledge Curzon.

Whitney, William Dwight. 1988. *The Roots, Verb-forms and Primary Derivatives of the Sanskrit Language.* Delhi: Motilal Banarsidass.

Woodroffe, Sir John. 1992. *The Serpent Power.* Madras: Ganesh and Co.

Pāda index

कक्षामृतं च संलोड्य 2.77a
कण्डूर्देहविवर्णता 2.83d
कण्डूश्चापि प्रणश्यति 2.87d
कथिता मृत्युनाशिनी 2.82b
कपाटं कुम्भकान्वितम् 2.64b
कर्णे वराहो नयने गरुत्मान् 4.3a
कलाः पञ्च सुधाधाराः 2.34a
कलाचतुष्कं तत्रस्थं 2.1c
कलाचतुष्कं तत्रोक्तं 2.23a
कलाचतुष्कं तत्रोक्तं 2.43c
कलात्रयमुदीरितम् 2.40d
कलास्थानं चतुर्गुणम् 2.48d
कलेवरगदक्षयः 2.21d
कवित्वं लभते क्षणात् 2.118d
काकचञ्चुपुटं वक्त्रं 1.74a
कालं कालविभागवित् 3.43d
कालक्रमनिरोधेन 3.20c
कालक्रमविनिर्मुक्तं 3.17c
कालक्रमविनिर्मुक्तां 3.21a
कालक्रमस्वभावजम् 3.20b
कालघ्नी ज्ञानदायिनी 2.33d
कालमृत्युजयो भवेत् 3.20d
कालवेलाविधानवित् 1.49d
किं भूयः श्रोतुमिच्छसि 3.68d
कीर्तिताः सर्वसिद्धिदाः 2.34b
कुनष्टिकायष्टिरजो 4.9a
कुम्भकेन महेश्वरि 3.2d
कुम्भकेन सुरार्चिते 2.35b
कुर्यादादावतन्द्रितः 1.30b
कुर्यादेकैकमभ्यासं 3.67c
कुर्याद्देवि यथान्यायं 1.35a
कूटो ऽयं परिकीर्तितः 1.37d
कृत्वा कुम्भकमाश्रयेत् 2.92d
कृत्वा तदमृतं पिबेत् 1.74b
कृत्वा शीघ्रं फलं लभेत् 1.59b
कृत्वा सद्भावसाधितम् 1.7b
कृष्णांस्तिलांश्चा-
मलकं तदर्धम् 4.10b
केदारं प्राहुरीश्वरि 2.18b
केशान्तमूर्ध्वं क्रमति 1.52a
कोटिचन्द्रसमप्रभम् 2.60d
कोटिचन्द्रसमप्रभम् 2.62d
कोटिसूर्यप्रतीकाशां 3.33c
कोटिसूर्यसमप्रभाम् 3.41b
क्व चिच्छास्त्रान्तरे न हि 3.55d
क्व चित्तन्मेलकादिकम् 1.16b
क्व चित्स्पष्टं तथास्पष्टं 1.16a
क्षणात्सत्यं प्रजायते 2.106d
क्षीरधारामृतं शीतं 2.27a
क्षीरवर्णमफेनिलम् 2.10d
क्षुधालस्यं च नश्यति 2.86d

ख

खन्याबिलमहीवाद 1.68c
खेचरत्वं प्रजायते 2.22b
खेचरत्वं भवेत्सत्यं 3.5c
खेचरत्वमवाप्नोति 1.75a
खेचराधिपतित्वदा 3.54d
खेचराधिपतिर्भूत्वा 1.32a
खेचरावसथं वह्निम् 1.32c
खेचरीं तु समाश्रयेत् 1.2d
खेचरीं वेत्ति भूतले 1.3b
खेचरीबीजपूर्वया 1.31d
खेचरीमन्त्रसिद्धस्य 1.58c
खेचरीसिद्धिभाग् भवेत् 1.31b
खेचरेषु सदा वसेत् 1.32b
खेचर्या खेचरीं युञ्जन् 1.31c
खेचर्यानन्दितो योगी 3.65c
खेचरी नाम या देवि 3.57a
खेचरीमेलकाद्येषु 3.59a
खेचरीमेलनं देवि 3.56a

ग

गङ्गा च यमुना चैव 3.10a

प

Index